RADIOPHARMACEUTICALS FOR
POSITRON EMISSION TOMOGRAPHY

Developments in Nuclear Medicine

VOLUME 24

Series Editor: Peter H. Cox

The titles published in this series are listed at the end of this volume.

Radiopharmaceuticals for Positron Emission Tomography

Methodological Aspects

edited by

G. STÖCKLIN
Institut für Nuklearchemie,
Forschungszentrum Jülich GmbH,
Jülich, Germany

and

V.W. PIKE
MRC Cyclotron Unit,
Hammersmith Hospital,
London, U.K.

KLUWER ACADEMIC PUBLISHERS
DORDRECHT / BOSTON / LONDON

Library of Congress Cataloging-in-Publication Data

Radiopharmaceuticals for positron emission tomography--methodological aspects / edited by G. Stöcklin and V.W. Pike.
p. cm. -- (Developments in nuclear medicine ; 24)

1. Tomography, Emission--Methodology. 2. Radiopharmaceuticals.
I. Stöcklin, Gerhard. II. Pike, V. W. III. Series.
[DNLM: 1. Tomography, Emission-Computed--methods.
2. Radioisotopes. W1 DE998KF v.24 1993 / WN 420 R1287 1993]
RC78.7.T62R33 1993
616.07'572--dc20
DNLM/DLC
for Library of Congress 93-1703

ISBN 978-90-481-4285-9

Published by Kluwer Academic Publishers,
P.O. Box 17, 3300 AA Dordrecht, The Netherlands.

Kluwer Academic Publishers incorporates
the publishing programmes of
D. Reidel, Martinus Nijhoff, Dr W. Junk and MTP Press.

Sold and distributed in the U.S.A. and Canada
by Kluwer Academic Publishers,
101 Philip Drive, Norwell, MA 02061, U.S.A.

In all other countries, sold and distributed
by Kluwer Academic Publishers Group,
P.O. Box 322, 3300 AH Dordrecht, The Netherlands.

Printed on acid-free paper

MEDICAL AND HEALTH RESEARCH PROGRAMME OF THE EC

BIOMEDICAL ENGINEERING IN THE EUROPEAN COMMUNITY

The involvement of the European Community (EC) in the field of Medical and Health Research started in 1978 with the first Programme which contained three projects. Since then, it has steadily expanded and it will include around 120 projects by the end of the fourth Programme (1987–1991).

The *general goal* of the programme is clearly to contribute to a better quality of life by improving health, and its *distinctive feature* is to strengthen European collaboration in order to achieve this goal.

The main objectives of this collaboration are:

- increase the *scientific efficiency* of the relevant research and development efforts in the Member States through their gradual coordination at Community level following the mobilization of the available research potential of national programmes, and also their *economic efficiency* through sharing of tasks and strengthening the joint use of available health research resources,
- *improve scientific and technological knowledge* in the research and development areas selected for their importance to all Member States, and promote its *efficient transfer into practical applications*, taking particular account of potential industrial and economic developments in the areas concerned,
- *optimize the capacity and economic efficiency of health care efforts* throughout the countries and regions of the Community.

The current programme consists of *six research targets*. Four are related to major health problems: CANCER, AIDS, AGE-RELATED PROBLEMS, and PERSONAL ENVIRONMENT AND LIFE-STYLE RELATED PROBLEMS; two are related to health resources: *MEDICAL TECHNOLOGY DEVELOPMENT* and HEALTH SERVICES RESEARCH.

Funds are provided by the Community for relevant "concerted action" activities which consist of research *COLLABORATION and COORDINATION* in EC Member States and/or in other European participant countries. *NETWORKS* of research institutes can be set up and supported by means of meetings, workshops, short-term staff exchanges/visits to other countries, information dissemination and so on; centralized facilities such as data banks, computing, and preparation and distribution of reference materials can also be funded. The funds are *not* direct research grants; the institutes concerned must fund the research activities carried out within their own countries – it is the international coordination activities which are eligible for Community support. Each such research network is placed under the responsibility of a *PROJECT LEADER* chosen from among the leading scientists in the network, with the assistance of a *PROJECT MANAGEMENT GROUP* representing the teams participating in the network.

The Commission of the European Communities is assisted in the execution of this programme by a Management and Coordination Advisory Committee (CGC – Medical and Health Research), and by Concerted Action Committees (COMACs) and Working Parties, composed of representatives and of scientific experts respectively, designated by the competent authorities of the Member States.

Other European countries, not belonging to the EC but participating in COST (Cooperation on Science and Technology) may take part in the Programme.

The present work was conducted according to the advice of *COMAC-BME* which supervises the coordination of research in *biomedical engineering* (BME) within the Medical Technology Development target.

More information may be obtained from: Commission of the European Communities
Directorate General XII-F-6
200 Rue de la Loi
B - 1049 Brussels

CONTENTS

LIST OF CONTRIBUTORS

Dr Claude Brihaye
Centre de Recherches du Cyclotron,
Bât. 30 - Sart Tilman,
Université de Liège,
B-4000 LIÈGE
Belgium

Dr Robert Cantineau
Centre de Recherches du Cyclotron,
Bât. 30 - Sart Tilman,
Université de Liège,
B-4000 LIÈGE
Belgium

Mr John C. Clark
MRC Cyclotron Unit,
Hammersmith Hospital,
Ducane Road,
LONDON W12 OHS
U.K.

Professor Heinz H. Coenen
Nuklearchemie und Radiopharmazie,
Klinik für Nuklearmedizin,
Universitätsklinikum-GHS-Essen,
Hufelandstrasse 55 (IG1),
D-4300 ESSEN 1
Germany

Dr Christian Crouzel
Service Hospitalier Frédéric Joliot,
CEA/DRIPP,
4 Place du Général Leclerc,
F-91401 ORSAY Cedex
France

Dr Marcel Guillaume
Centre de Recherches du Cyclotron,
Bât. 30 - Sart Tilman,
Université de Liège,
B-4000 LIÈGE
Belgium

Dr Christer Halldin
Department of Psychiatry and Psychology,
Karolinska Hospital,
S104 01 STOCKHOLM
Sweden

Dr Hans J. Helmeke
Medizinische Hochschule Hannover,
D-3000 HANNOVER 61
Germany

Professor Bengt Långström
Department of Chemistry,
University of Uppsala,
Box 531,
S-751 21 UPPSALA
Sweden

Dr Christian Lemaire,
Centre de Recherches du Cyclotron,
Bât. 30 - Sart Tilman,
Université de Liège,
B-4000 LIÈGE
Belgium

Dr Christian Loc'h
Service Hospitalier Frédéric Joliot,
CEA/DRIPP,
4 Place du Général Leclerc,
F-91401 ORSAY Cedex
France

Dr Sajinder K. Luthra
MRC Cyclotron Unit,
Hammersmith Hospital,
Ducane Road,
LONDON W12 OHS
U.K.

Dr André Luxen
Cyclotron,
Hôpital Erasme,
Université Libré de Bruxelles,
808 Route de Lennik,
B1070 BRUXELLES
Belgium

Dr Bernard Mazière
Service Hospitalier Frédéric Joliot,
CEA/DRIPP,
4 Place du Général Leclerc,
F-91401 ORSAY Cedex
France

Professor Geerd-J. Meyer
Medizinische Hochschule Hannover,
D-3000 HANNOVER 61
Germany

Dr Bruno Nebeling
Institut für Nuklearchemie,
Forschungszentrum Jülich GmbH,
Postfach 1913,
D-5170 JÜLICH
Germany

Dr Victor W. Pike
MRC Cyclotron Unit,
Hammersmith Hospital,
Ducane Road,
LONDON W12 OHS
U.K.

Dr Syed M. Qaim,
Institut für Nuklearchemie,
Forschungszentrum Jülich GmbH,
Postfach 1913,
D-5170 JÜLICH
Germany

Professor Gerhard Stöcklin
Institut für Nuklearchemie,
Forschungszentrum Jülich GmbH,
Postfach 1913,
D-5170 JÜLICH
Germany

Professor Sharon Stone-Elander
Karolinska Pharmacy,
Box 60024,
STOCKHOLM
Sweden

Dr Karel Strijckmans
Institute for Nuclear Sciences,
Universiteit Gent,
GENT
Belgium

Professor Willem Vaalburg
Department of Nuclear Medicine,
University Hospital and Department of Organic Chemistry,
University of Groningen,
GRONINGEN
The Netherlands

Dr Stephen L. Waters
MRC Cyclotron Unit,
Hammersmith Hospital,
Ducane Road,
LONDON W12 OHS
U.K.

PREFACE

Positron Emission Tomography (PET) is becoming an increasingly important tool for studying physiological, biochemical and pharmacological functions at a molecular level in living man, whether in health or in disease. More than a hundred PET groups have been established worldwide, about thirty of which are in Western Europe (Figure 1).

A Concerted Action was held on 'PET Investigations of Cellular Regeneration and Degeneration' (coordinator Professor D. Comar) from 1989 to 1992 within the Medical Health Programme of the European Community (EC). It consisted of working groups in the fields of cardiology, neurology, psychiatry, oncology, radiochemistry, instrumentation and modelling.

This book has emerged from the Concerted Action and especially from the work of several task groups on PET radiochemistry. While some reports from such task groups have been published previously in scientific journals (Clark *et al.*, 1987; Coenen *et al.*, 1987; Crouzel *et al.*, 1987, 1992; Luxen *et al.*, 1992; Mazière *et al.*, 1992; Vaalburg *et al.*, 1992; Pike *et al.*, 1993) and in other books within this series (Baron *et al.*, 1991; Comar *et al.*, 1993), it seemed worthwhile to publish reports on the methodological aspects of radiopharmaceutical production and analysis as a collection. The time for a state-of-the-art review seemed right since this field has advanced over the past fifteen years to reach a level where guidelines can now be suggested for the main methodological aspects.

Radiochemical methodology constitutes the most important base for the successful functioning of a PET group in the routine production and development of radiopharmaceuticals. The development of a new radiopharmaceutical is long and problematic, and involves several stages (Figure 2).

Once an objective has been established with regard to radiopharmaceutical development, the radionuclide for labelling and its production parameters must be chosen. This process starts from nuclear data. Their use is mandatory for achieving optimal production yield and radionuclidic purity. Many details of the targetry have to be specified in order to obtain the desired chemical form of the radionuclide in a high total radioactivity and in a high specific radioactivity; in-target chemistry during irradiation plays a major role.

The next step is the production of the radioactive labelling agent. This is already connected to the choice of the target. Some irradiation products can be used to label some compounds directly. Generally, however, rapid off-target conversion, or rather on-line procedures, are needed to convert the main irradiation product into a more useful labelling agent.

The labelling process itself should not only be simple, fast and efficient but should also allow for easy automation. Development of a labelling procedure generally starts with the scaling down of classical syntheses to non-stoichiometric micro-syntheses and then to radiochemistry at the no-carrier-added (n.c.a.) state, which has its own special problems and solutions. It includes 'high-tech' radioanalytical work to separate nanomolar amounts of the radiopharmaceutical from micro- to milli-molar amounts of the cold educt or by-products. After this has been achieved on an analytical scale at low radioactivity levels in the kBq–MBq range,

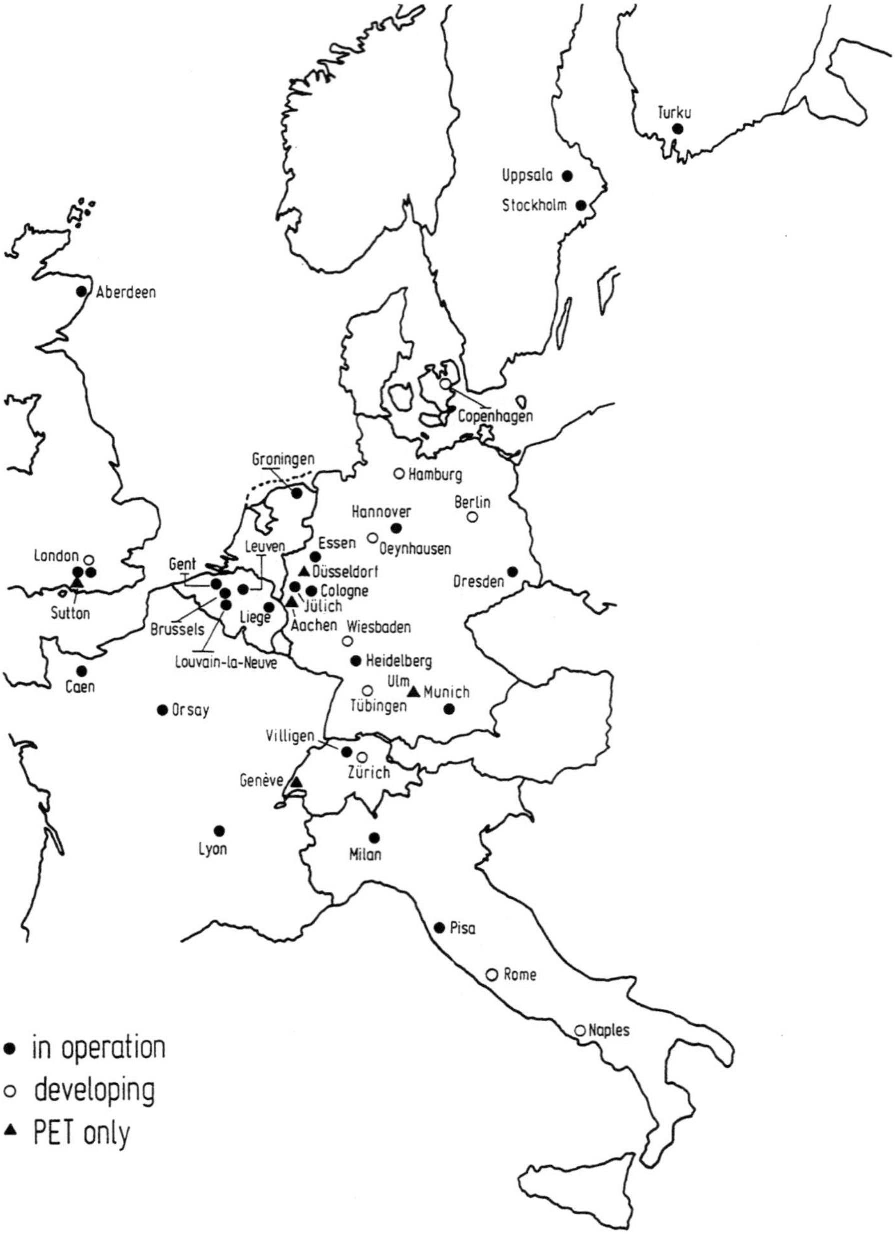

Figure 1. The distribution of West European PET centres (1993).

- **CONCEPT**

- **RADIONUCLIDE PRODUCTION**
  - Nuclear data
  - Targetry
  - Total radioactivity
  - Radionuclidic purity
  - Specific radioactivity

- **LABELLING AGENT**
  - In-target chemistry
  - On-line/off-line conversion
  - Total radioactivity
  - Specific radioactivity

- **LABELLING**
  - Position of label
  - Radiochemical yield
  - Time
  - Specific radioactivity
  - Purity

- **AUTOMATION**
  - Activity scale up
  - Reliability

- **QUALITY ASSURANCE/QUALITY CONTROL**
  - Efficacy
  - Safety

- **BIODISTRIBUTION/METABOLISM (rodents)**
  - Stability *in vivo*
  - Fate of the label
  - Pharmacokinetics
  - Target to non-target ratio
  - Metabolite analysis

- **PET PHARMACOKINETICS *IN VIVO* (primates)**
  - Dosimetry
  - Routine plasma analysis
  - Modelling

- **CLINICAL EVALUATION**

Figure 2. Development of a PET radiopharmaceutical. Key considerations at each stage are shown under the appropriate heading.

Table 1. PET Radiopharmaceuticals covered with respect to chemical methodology by chapters in this volume (√) or in published reports from EC task groups (a-f). See key below.

Radiopharmaceutical	**Formula**	**Automation**	**QA**	**Metabolite Analysis**
[1-^{11}C]Acetate		√	√	
S-[*carbonyl*-^{11}C]CGP 12177	I		√	√
L-[*N-methyl*-^{11}C]Deprenyl	II	√	√	
[*N-methyl*-^{11}C]Flumazenil	III	√	√ a	√ a
[*S-methyl*-^{11}C]Methionine	IV	√	√	√
L-[1-^{11}C]Methionine	V		√	
3-*N*-[^{11}C]Methylspiperone	VI		√ b	√
m-[*N-methyl*-^{11}C]Hydroxyephedrine	VII			√
[*N-methyl*-^{11}C]MQNB	VIII	√		√
S-[*N-methyl*-^{11}C]Nomifensine	IX	√	b	
[*N-methyl*-^{11}C]PK 11195	X	√	a	
[*O-methyl*-^{11}C]Raclopride	XI	√	√ b	√ b
[*N-methyl*-^{11}C]Scopolamine	XII			√
[*N-methyl*-^{11}C]SCH 23390	XIII	√	b	√ b
L-[1-^{11}C]Tyrosine	XIV			√
[^{13}N]Ammonia		*	√	√
n-[^{15}O]Butanol		√	√	
[^{15}O]Carbon dioxide		*	√ c	
[^{15}O]Carbon monoxide		*	√ c	
[^{15}O]Oxygen		*	√ c	
[^{15}O]Water		√	√ c	
[^{18}F]Altanserin	XV	√	d	√
2-[^{18}F]Fluoro-2-deoxy-D-glucose	XVI	√	√ e	
[^{18}F]Fluoride		*	√	
L-6-[^{18}F]Fluoro-DOPA	XVII	√	√ f	√f
[^{18}F]Fluorometaraminol	XVIII			√
L-4-[^{18}F]Fluoro-*m*-tyrosine	XIX	√		√
3-*N*-(ω-[^{18}F]Fluoroethyl)spiperone	XX	√	√	√
L-2-[^{18}F]Fluorotyrosine	XXI	√		√
3-*N*-[^{18}F]Methylspiperone	XXII	√	√	√
[^{18}F]Setoperone	XXIII		d	√
[^{76}Br]Bromolisuride	XXIV		b	√

Key: √ - see chapter in this book. a - Pike *et al.* (1993). b - Mazière *et al.* (1992). c - Clark *et al.* (1987). d. - Crouzel *et al.* (1992). e - Coenen *et al.* (1987). f - Luxen *et al.* (1992). Numbered formulae are shown in Figure 3. * - Production discussed in chapter on PET Radionuclide Production.

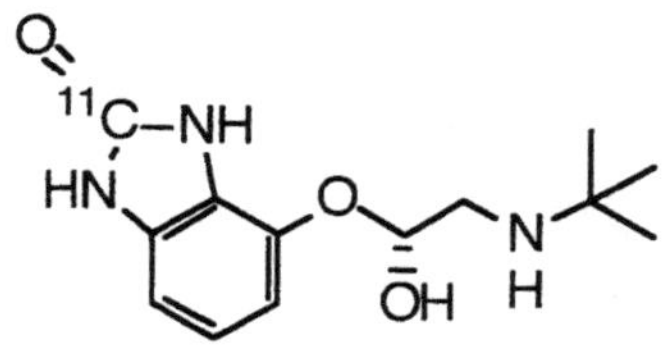

(I) *S*-[*carbonyl*-^{11}C]CGP 12177

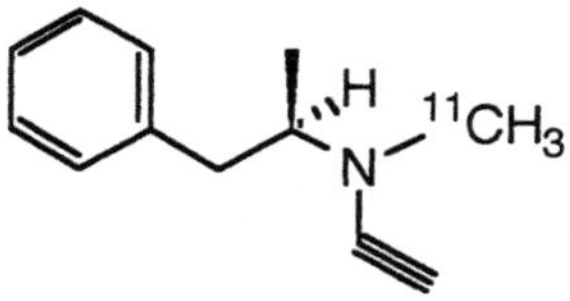

(II) L-[*N-methyl*-^{11}C]Deprenyl

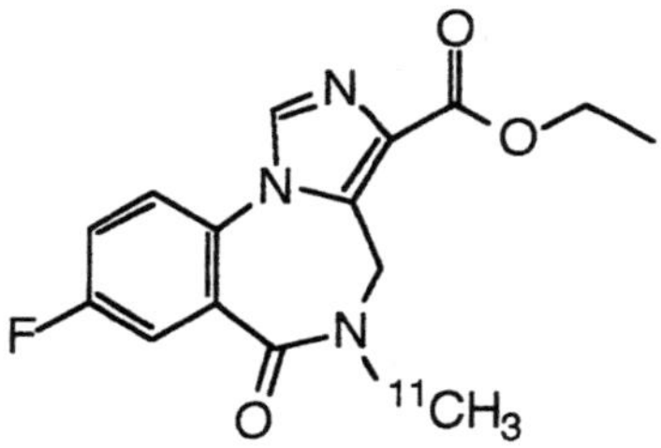

(III) [*N-methyl*-^{11}C]Flumazenil

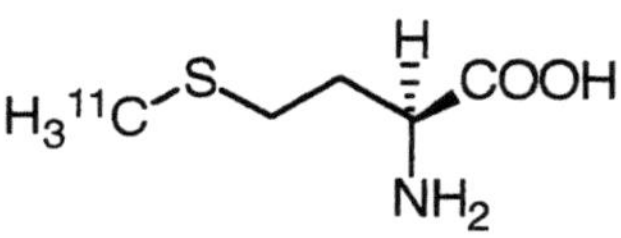

(IV) [*S-methyl*-^{11}C]Methionine

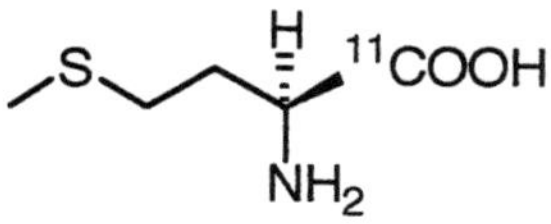

(V) L-[1-^{11}C]Methionine

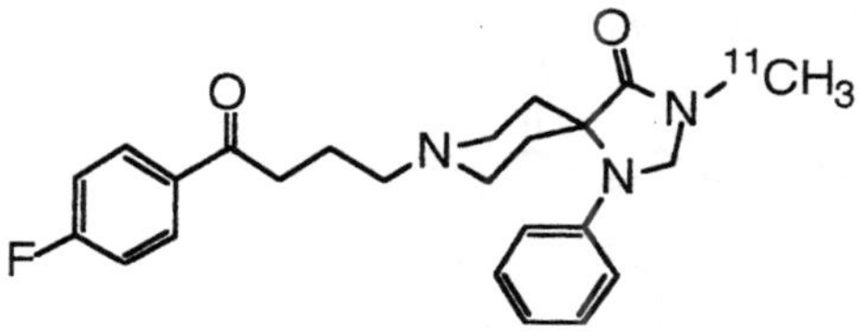

(VI) 3-*N*-[^{11}C]Methylspiperone

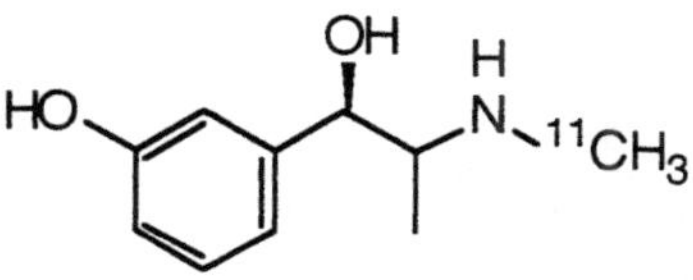

(VII) *m*-[*N-methyl*-^{11}C]Hydroxyephedrine

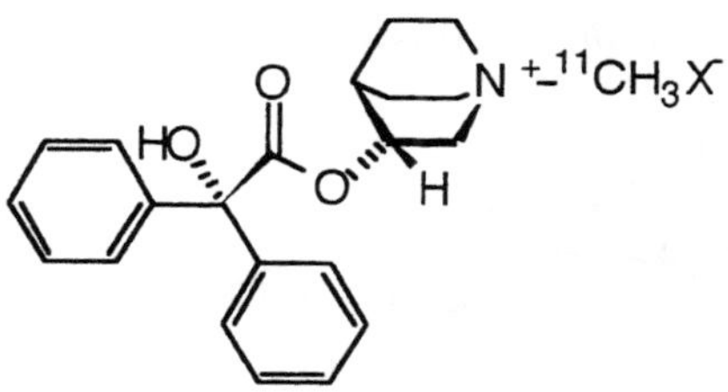

(VIII) [*N-methyl*-^{11}C]MQNB

Figure 3. Structures of radiopharmaceuticals numbered in Table 1.

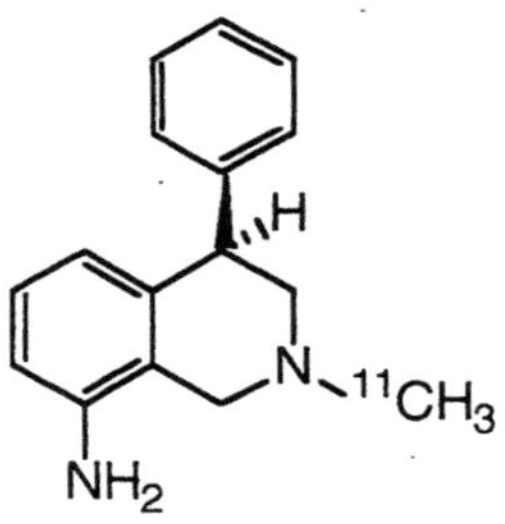

(IX) *S*-[*N-methyl*-^{11}C]Nomifensine

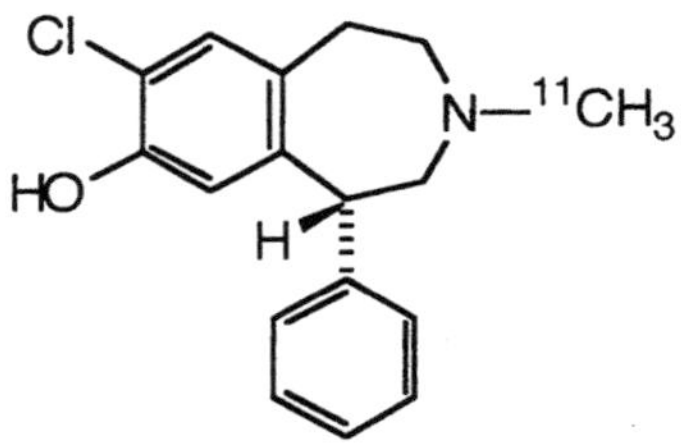

(XIII) [*N-methyl*-^{11}C]SCH 23390

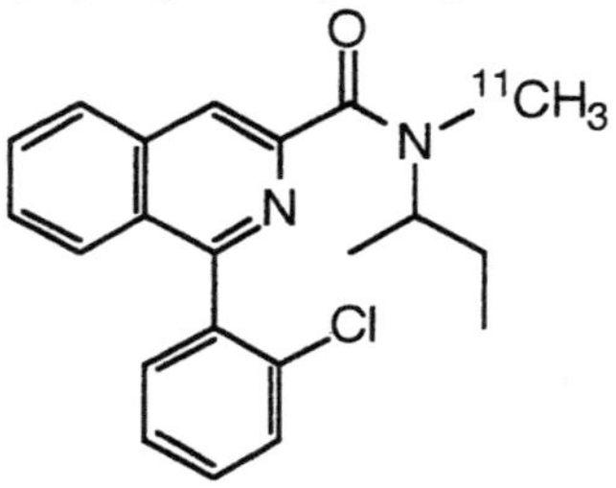

(X) [*N-methyl*-^{11}C]PK 11195

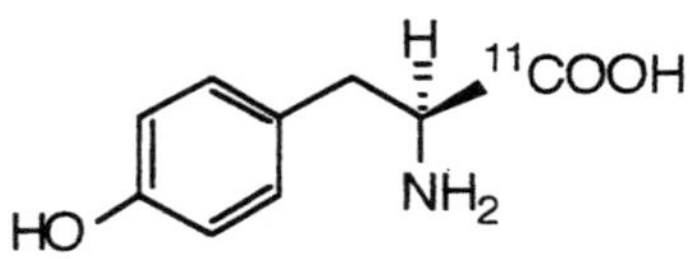

(XIV) L-[1-^{11}C]Tyrosine

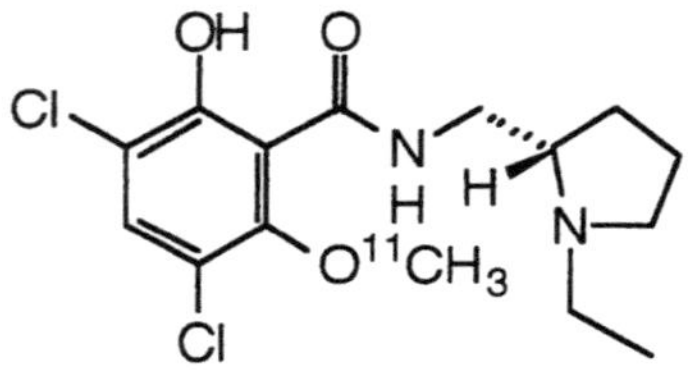

(XI) [*O-methyl*-^{11}C]Raclopride

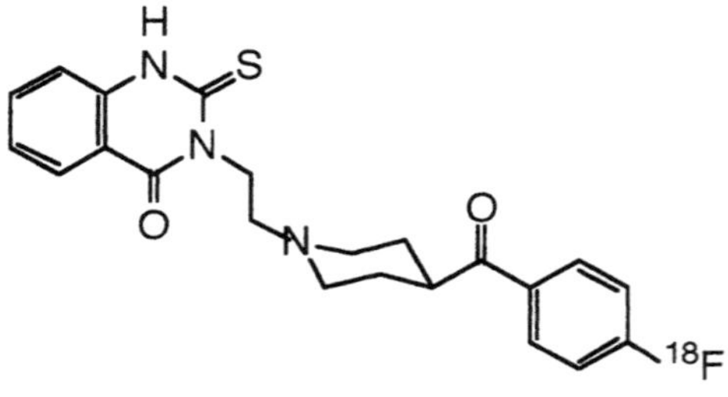

(XV) [^{18}F]Altanserin

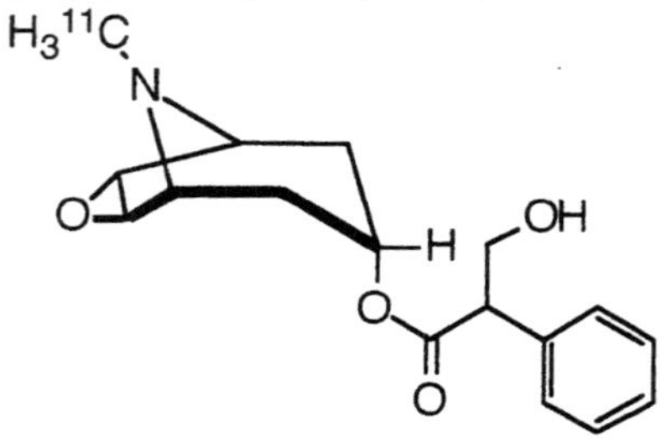

(XII) [*N-methyl*-^{11}C]Scopolamine

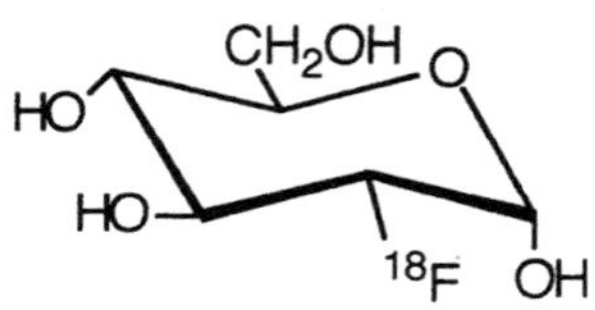

(XVI) 2-[^{18}F]Fluoro-2-deoxy-D-glucose

Figure 3 (Cont'd). Structures of radiopharmaceuticals numbered in Table 1.

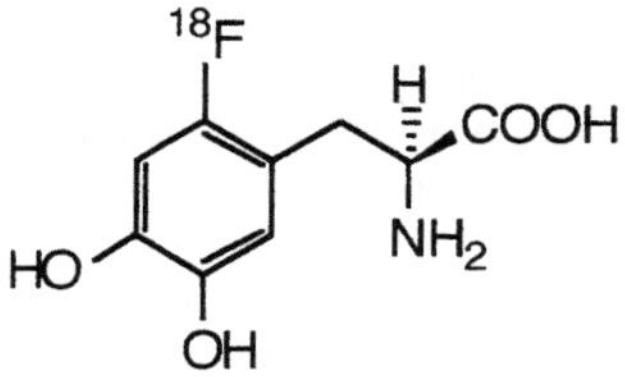

(XVII) L-6-[^{18}F]Fluoro-DOPA

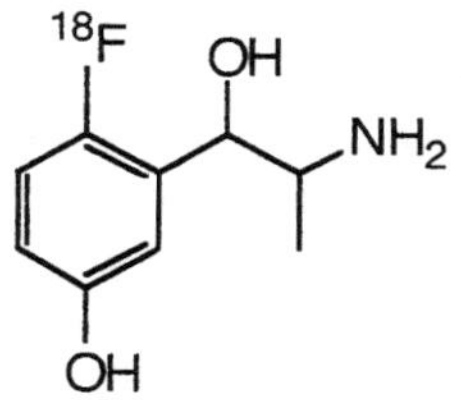

(XVIII) [^{18}F]Fluorometaraminol

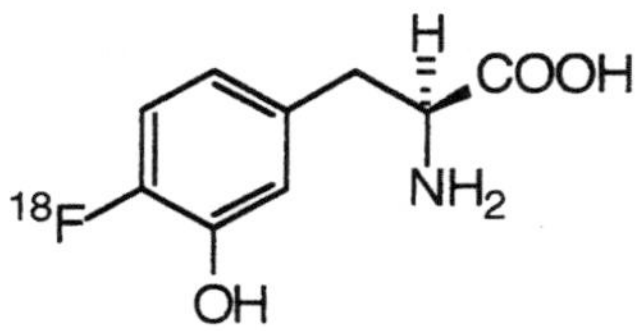

(XIX) L-4-[^{18}F]Fluoro-*m*-tyrosine

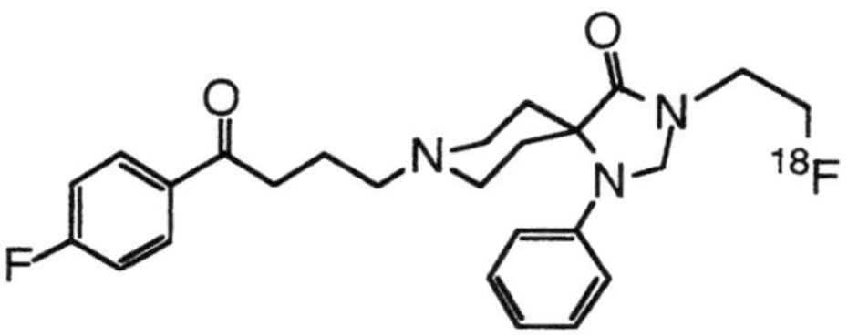

(XX) 3-*N*-(ω-[^{18}F]Fluoroethyl)spiperone

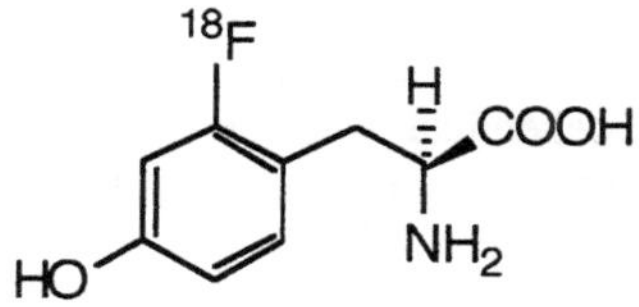

(XXI) L-2-[^{18}F]Fluorotyrosine

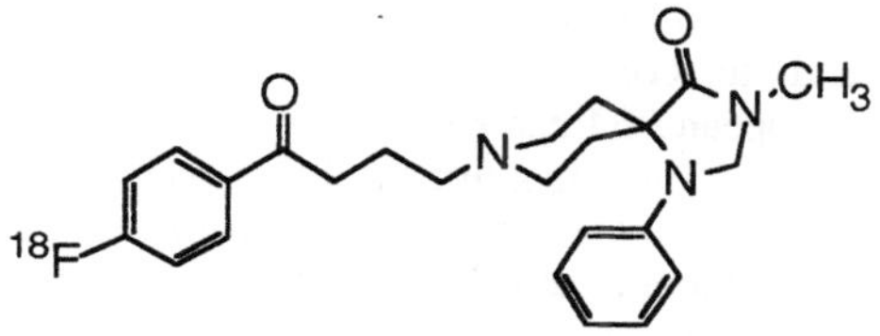

(XXII) 3-*N*-[^{18}F]Methylspiperone

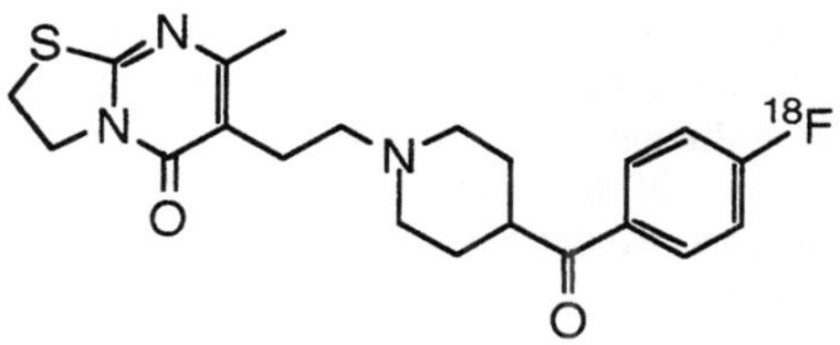

(XXIII) [^{18}F]Setoperone

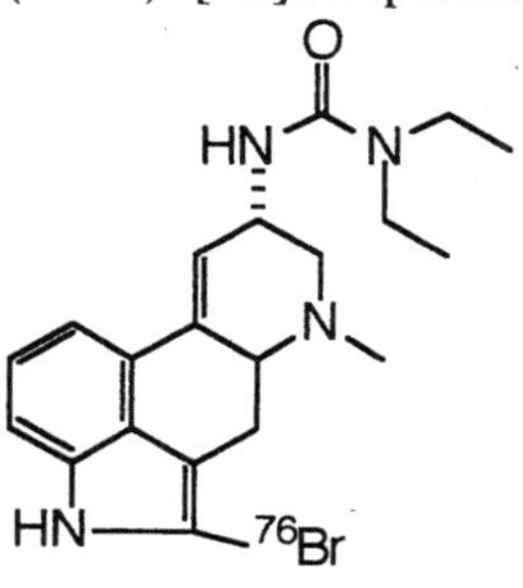

(XXIV) [^{76}Br]Bromolisuride

Figure 3 (Cont'd). Structures of radiopharmaceuticals numbered in Table 1.

scale up to a practical radioactivity level of several tens of GBq is required. This often leads to surprises due to the increased amounts of target material and/or solvents and impurities, which in turn affect radiochemical yields and HPLC purification. Once a radiopharmaceutical is routinely produced, automation becomes mandatory both for safety to personnel and for achieving reproducibility and reliability.

Prior to final automation and clinical evaluation of the radiopharmaceutical, many chemical questions have to be solved in relation to the measurement of biodistribution and pharmacokinetics in rodents. These preclinical studies include assessment of stability *in vivo*, the fate of the label, target-to-non target uptake ratios, and metabolite analysis in tissue and plasma. Efficient, fast and sensitive radioanalytical methods are needed for metabolite analysis.

Chapters of this book deal with each of the main methodological aspects of the chemistry needed to develop an effective radiopharmaceutical, namely radionuclide production, automation and metabolite analysis. The individual chapters were written by leading chemists from major European PET centres.

There is a further obligation to ensure that the radiopharmaceutical is not only effective but also safe for administration to humans. If the biochemical evaluation of the radiopharmaceutical in rodents turns out to be promising, routine Quality Assurance (QA) and Quality Control (QC) become mandatory. It includes an assurance of radionuclidic purity, appropriate specific radioactivity, radiochemical purity, chemical purity and pharmaceutical quality. The chapter on QA/QC is written by a broadly based expert group. It is meant to provide a guideline and a base for future monographs and regulations on major PET radiopharmaceuticals of today. The style of this chapter is therefore different from that of the others. At the expense of some repetition, the material for each individual radiopharmaceutical is presented as a virtually self-contained unit, including its own bibliography, for ease of consultation.

Of the several hundred products which have been labelled with positron-emitters during the past two decades about 35 are presently considered to be of major interest in Europe and are reviewed with respect to methodology, either in this book or in reports emanating from the Concerted Action or preceding EC task groups (see Table 1). The structures of the more complex radiopharmaceuticals are collected together in Figure 3, for easy reference.

The Editors hope that this book will help the increasing numbers of scientists who are now entering the field of PET to appreciate the methodological aspects that are normally addressed by chemists in relation to PET radiopharmaceuticals; we especially hope that it provides many useful practical guidelines and will promote early success in their own endeavours, since these will often necessarily begin by establishing chemical methodology of the kind discussed here.

G. Stöcklin and V.W. Pike (Editors).

References

Baron J.V., Comar D., Farde L., Martinot J.L. and Mazoyer B. (Eds) (1991) *Brain Dopaminergic Systems. Imaging with Positron Emission Tomography.* Kluwer Academic Publishers, Dordrecht, Boston, London.

Clark J.C., Crouzel C., Meyer G-J. and Strijckmans K. (1987) Current methodology for oxygen-15 production for clinical use. *Appl. Radiat. Isot.*, 38, 597–600.

Coenen H.H., Pike V.W., Stöcklin G. and Wagner R. (1987) Recommendation for a practical production of [2-^{18}F]fluoro-2-deoxy-D-glucose. *Appl. Radiat. Isot.*, 38, 605–610.

Crouzel C., Langström B., Pike V.W. and Coenen H.H. (1987) Recommendations for a practical production of [^{11}C]methyl iodide. *Appl. Radiat. Isot.*, 38, 601–604.

Crouzel C., Guillaume M., Barré L., Lemaire C and Pike V.W. (1992) Ligands and tracers for PET studies of the 5-HT system — current status. *Nucl. Med. Biol.*, 19, 857–870.

Guillaume M., Luxen A., Nebeling B., Argentini M., Clark J.C. and Pike V.W. (1991) Recommendations for fluorine-18 production. *Appl. Radiat. Isot.*, 42, 749–762.

Luxen A., Guillaume M., Melega W.P., Pike V.W., Solin O. and Wagner R. (1992) Production of 6-[^{18}F]fluoro-L-DOPA and its metabolism *in vivo* — a critical review. *Nucl. Med. Biol.*, 19, 149–158.

Mazoyer B.M., Heiss W.D. and Comar D. (Eds). (1993) *PET Studies on Amino Acid Metabolism and Protein Synthesis.* Kluwer Academic Publishers, Dordrecht, Boston, London.

Mazière B., Coenen H.H., Halldin C., Någren K. and Pike V.W. (1992) PET radioligands for dopamine receptors and re-uptake sites: chemistry and biochemistry. *Nucl. Med. Biol.*, 19, 497–512.

Pike V.W., Halldin C., Crouzel C., Barré L., Nutt D.J., Osman S., Shah F., Turton D.R. and Waters S.L. (1993) Radioligands for PET studies of central benzodiazepine receptors and PK (peripheral benzodiazepine) binding-sites — current status. *Nucl. Med. Biol.*, In press.

Vaalburg W., Coenen H.H., Crouzel C., Elsinga Ph.H., Långström B., Lemaire C. and Meyer G-J. (1992) Amino acids for the measurement of protein synthesis *in vivo* by PET. *Nucl. Med. Biol.*, 19, 227–237.

PET RADIONUCLIDE PRODUCTION

Syed M. Qaim, John C. Clark, Christian Crouzel, Marcel Guillaume, Hans J. Helmeke, Bruno Nebeling, Victor W. Pike and Gerhard Stöcklin

ABSTRACT. Several short-lived positron-emitters are routinely used in PET studies while a few others are of potential interest. A brief review of the decay data and production methods for several of these positron-emitters is given. Special attention is paid to the production of the four major positron-emitters, namely carbon-11, nitrogen-13, oxygen-15 and fluorine-18, which are widely applied in several European PET centres.

1. Introduction

The number of positron-emitting radionuclides is large (*cf.* Lederer and Shirley, 1978; Browne and Firestone, 1986). Some medically relevant short-lived positron-emitters and their decay data are listed in Table 1. Most of the PET studies to date are carried out with organic positron-emitters (^{11}C, ^{13}N, ^{15}O and ^{18}F). Several other radionuclides, for example potassium-38, selenium-73, bromine-75 and bromine-76, also find some applications. There is also considerable interest in copper-62, gallium-68 and rubidium-82, which are obtained via longer-lived generator systems.

The production of useful and potentially useful positron-emitters has been the subject of several review articles and books (Lambrecht, 1971; Clark and Buckingham, 1975; Welch, 1977; Stöcklin and Wolf, 1982, 1983; Vaalburg and Paans, 1983; Qaim, 1986a). Development of a production process involves a study of several aspects such as nuclear data, high current targetry, chemical processing, automation and quality control. A knowledge of nuclear data is essential for calculating thick target yields, estimating levels of radionuclidic impurities and designing suitable target systems. High current targets are needed to produce radionuclides in sufficient quantities. Due to the short half-lives of the useful positron-emitters the chemical separation and subsequent labelling procedures have to be fast. The high level of radioactivity calls for remotely controlled and, sometimes necessarily, automated methods. Quality control must be concerned with the radionuclidic, radiochemical, chemical and pharmaceutical quality of the products. This chapter deals mainly with the routine methods of production of commonly used positron-emitters. A brief discussion of less commonly used and generator-produced positron-emitters is also given.

The important production routes, the suitable energy ranges and the theoretically expected thick target yields over these energy ranges are given in Table 1. The yields are in

G. Stöcklin and V. W. Pike (eds.), Radiopharmaceuticals for Positron Emission Tomography, 1–43.

Table 1. Some medically relevant short-lived β^+ emitters and their production routes.

Radioisotope	Decay data				Production data		
	$T_{1/2}$	Mode of decay (%)	E_{β^+} (keV)	Principal γ-rays keV (% abundance)	Nuclear reaction	Energy range (MeV)	Theoretical thick target yield MBq (mCi)/μAh
^{11}C	20.4 min	β^+(99.8) EC (0.2)	960	511(199.6)	$^{14}N(p,\alpha)^{11}C$	13 → 3	3820 (103)
					$^{11}B(p,n)^{11}C$*	10 → 0	3400 (92)
					$^{10}B(d,n)^{11}C$*	10 → 0	2479 (67)
^{13}N	10.0 min	β^+(100)	1190	511(200)	$^{12}C(d,n)^{13}N$	8 → 0	1961 (53)
					$^{13}C(p,n)^{13}N$*	10 → 0	4440 (120)
					$^{16}O(p,\alpha)^{13}N$	16 → 7	1665 (45)
^{15}O	2.05 min	β^+(99.9) EC (0.1)	1720	511(199.8)	$^{14}N(d,n)^{15}O$	8 → 0	2368 (64)
					$^{15}N(p,n)^{15}O$*	10 → 0	2220 (60)
					$^{16}O(p,pn)^{15}O$	26 → 16	3700 (100)
^{18}F	109.6 min	β^+(97) EC (3)	635	511(194)	$^{20}Ne(d,\alpha)^{18}F$	14 → 0	1110 (30)
					$^{18}O(p,n)^{18}F$*	16 → 3	2960 (80)
					$^{16}O(^3He,p)^{18}F$	41 → 14	481 (13)
^{38}K	7.6 min	β^+(100)	2680	511(200) 2168(99.9)	$^{35}Cl(\alpha,n)^{38}K$	22 → 7	259 (7)
					$^{38}Ar(p,n)^{38}K$*	16 → 12	777 (21)
					$^{40}Ca(d,\alpha)^{38}K$	12 → 0	207 (5.6)†
					$^{40}Ar(p,3n)^{38}K$	32 → 30	192 (5.2)†
^{73}Se	7.1 h	β^+(65) EC(35)	1320	511(130) 361(97)	$^{75}As(p,3n)^{73}Se$	40 → 30	1406 (38)
					$^{75}As(d,4n)^{73}Se$	45 → 33	651 (17.6)
					$^{72}Ge(^3He,2n)^{73}Se$*	23 → 13	55 (1.5)
					$^{70}Ge(\alpha,n)^{73}Se$*	28 → 13	126 (3.4)

* Using highly enriched isotope as target material.

† Experimental yield.

Table 1. Continued...

Radioisotope	Decay data				Production data		
	$T_{1/2}$	Mode of decay (%)	E_{β^+} (keV)	Principal γ-rays keV (% abundance)	Nuclear reaction	Energy range (MeV)	Theoretical thick target yield MBq (mCi)/μAh
^{75}Br	1.6 h	β^+(75.5) EC (24.5)	1740	511(151) 287(92)	$^{76}Se(p,2n)^{75}Br^*$	30 → 22	3700 (100)
					$^{75}As(^3He,3n)^{75}Br$	36 → 25	277 (7.5)
					$^{76}Se(d,3n)^{75}Br^*$	35 → 29	3034 (82)
					$^{75}As(\alpha,4n)^{75}Br$	65 → 54	277 (7.5)
^{76}Br	16.1 h	β^+(57) EC (43)	3900	511(114) 559(74) 657(16) 1854(15)	$^{75}As(^3He,2n)^{76}Br$	18 → 10	11 (0.3)
					$^{76}Se(p,n)^{76}Br^*$	16 → 10	296 (8)
					$^{77}Se(p,2n)^{76}Br^*$	25 → 16	259 (7)
^{62}Zn ↓ (generator)	9.2 h	β^+(93) EC (7)	660	511(186) 41(25.2) 597 (25.7)	$^{63}Cu(p,2n)^{62}Zn$	26 → 21	144 (3.9)
					$^{60}Ni(\alpha,2n)^{62}Zn$	30 → 15	13 (0.35)
^{62}Cu	9.7 min	β^+(98) EC (2)	2930	511(196)			
^{68}Ge ↓ (generator)	271 d	EC (100)			$^{69}Ga(p,2n)^{68}Ge$	22 → 13	0.74 (0.02)†
					RbBr (p,spall)^{68}Ge	800, 500	0.15 (0.004)†
^{68}Ga	68.3 min	β^+(90) EC (10)	1900	511(180) 1077(3)			
^{82}Sr ↓ (generator)	25 d	EC (100)			Mo(p,spall)^{82}Sr	800	3.7 (0.1)†
					$^{85}Rb(p,4n)^{82}Sr$	60 → 40	14.8 (0.4)
					$^{nat}Kr(^3He,xn)^{82}Sr$	90 → 20	1.3 (0.035)
					$^{nat}Kr(\alpha,xn)^{82}Sr$	120 → 20	1.9 (0.05)
^{82}Rb	1.3 min	β^+(96) EC (4)	3350	511(192) 776(13.4)			

*Using highly enriched isotope as target material.
†Experimental yield.

a few cases experimental yields (Lambrecht *et al.*, 1978; Helus *et al.*, 1980; Pao *et al.*, 1981; Loc'h *et al.*, 1982; Robertson *et al.*, 1982; Thomas, 1987), since the excitation functions are either unknown or uncertain. In general, however, the yields were calculated from the reported excitation functions, as follows: carbon-11 (compilation by Keller *et al.*, 1973; Bida *et al.*, 1980b); nitrogen-13 (compilation by Keller *et al.*, 1973; Bair *et al.*, 1981; Sajjad *et al.*, 1986); oxygen-15 (Vera Ruiz and Wolf, 1977; Sajjad *et al.*, 1984, 1985); fluorine-18 (Nozaki *et al.*, 1974; Ruth and Wolf, 1979); potassium-38 (Qaim *et al.*, 1988; Tárkányi *et al.*, 1992); selenium-73 (Mushtaq *et al.*, 1988; Mushtaq and Qaim, 1990); bromine-75 (Paans *et al.*, 1980; Alfassi and Weinreich, 1982; Kovács *et al.*, 1985); bromine-76 (Janssen *et al.*, 1980; Alfassi and Weinreich, 1982; Kovács *et al.*, 1985); zinc-62 (Neirinckx, 1977; Kopecky, 1985); strontium-82 (Horiguchi *et al.*, 1980; Tárkányi *et al.*, 1988, 1990). Several other details of production methods are described below.

2. Commonly used Positron-emitters

The positron-emitters best suited to PET studies are the 'organic' radionuclides, carbon-11, nitrogen-13, oxygen-15 and fluorine-18. Whereas the former three radionuclides can be used only on site, fluorine-18 is suitable for longer lasting studies and for transport to PET centres without a cyclotron ('satellite' centres).

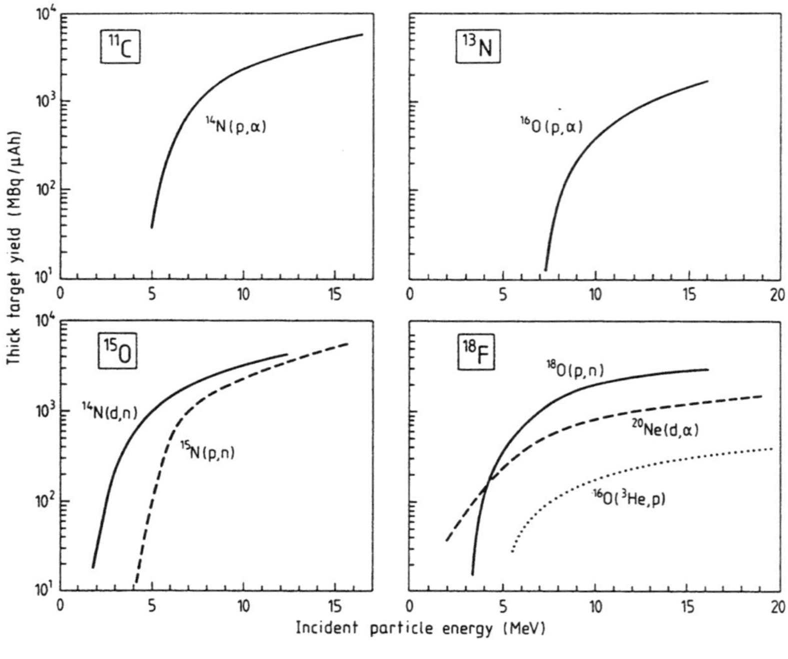

Figure 1. Integrated thick target yields of some commonly used positron-emitters expected from the most common production routes, plotted as a function of incident particle energy. Data were calculated using the measured excitation functions (for reference see text).

The thick target yields of the most common production routes, calculated from the measured excitation functions (Nozaki *et al.*, 1974; Vera Ruiz and Wolf, 1977; Ruth and Wolf, 1979; Bida *et al.*, 1980b; Sajjad *et al.*, 1984, 1985, 1986) are shown in Figure 1 as a function of incident particle energy. The values for nitrogen-13 and oxygen-15 give saturation yields; however, for carbon-11 and fluorine-18 an irradiation time of 1 h was assumed. It is emphasised that the curves should be regarded as approximations since the calculation of the thick target yield from an excitation function showing large fluctuations, as for the light mass nuclei discussed here, is rather uncertain. In Figure 1 no data are shown for the $^{13}C(p,n)^{13}N$ reaction. Due to the very large uncertainty in the excitation function for this process, only the integrated thick target yield for the whole energy range is given in Table 1.

From the data presented in Figure 1 it is evident that, in principle, all four positron-emitters can be produced at a small cyclotron. In practice, however, several important considerations need to be addressed when embarking on a production scheme. State of the art information is summarised below.

2.1. CARBON-11

Over the last two decades a large number of compounds labelled with carbon-11 ($t_{1/2}$ = 20.4 min; $I_{\beta+}$ = 100%; $E_{\beta+}$ = 0.96 MeV) have found application in biomedical and pharmacological studies using PET. With the increasing interest in investigations of receptor-ligand interactions it has become mandatory for radioligands to be prepared in high specific radioactivity. Generally, the starting precursor for radiosyntheses is high specific radioactivity [^{11}C]carbon dioxide. For some radiosyntheses [^{11}C]methane is prepared 'in target' as a precursor to the off-target synthesis of other labelling agents.

Several nuclear reactions can be used to produce carbon-11 (for reviews see Wolf and Redvanly, 1977; Ferrieri and Wolf, 1983). The common reactions are summarised in Table 1. Out of these processes the most convenient and commonly used is the $^{14}N(p,\alpha)^{11}C$ nuclear reaction on a target of nitrogen gas (Blaser *et al.*, 1952; Nozaki *et al.*, 1966; Epherre and Seide, 1971; Jacobs *et al.*, 1974; Casella *et al.*, 1978; Bida *et al.*, 1980b). The experimental production yields are of the order of 3.7–5.2 GBq/μA (100–140 mCi/μA) for proton energies of 16 MeV. Useful activities (0.7–1.2 GBq/μA, 25–31 mCi/μA) can also be produced using lower energies (8 MeV) (*cf.* Wolf and Jones, 1983).

Technical details with regard to achieving an efficient production of [^{11}C]carbon dioxide of high specific radioactivity have been discussed in an EEC Task Group report (Crouzel *et al.*, 1987). Here we give an updated version of that report.

2.1.1. *Target construction.* Pure aluminium or aluminium alloy is a satisfactory material for target construction. Havar™, titanium or stainless steel foils are suitable materials for target windows. Metal gaskets are preferable to rubber 'O' rings. The target should be made as small as possible with respect to beam profile and penetration, in order to achieve high specific radioactivity and fast emptying. For good recoveries of [^{11}C]carbon dioxide, it is recommended that newly constructed targets be carefully washed with 0.1M-phosphoric acid followed by water, and dried under vacuum. It is advised that this process be carried out at each subsequent target maintenance.

2.1.2. *Target material.* The target gas should be of high purity and especially as free as possible from carbon-containing impurities. 'Nitrogen N60' (99.9999% pure, from Air Liquide), 'white spot' nitrogen (nominally 99% from BOC Ltd) and 'CO-free' nitrogen (with < 20 ppb CO and < 50 ppb CO_2, from Linde) are known to be suitable. As a precaution against carbon dioxide contamination, a trap (3 mm x 2 cm) of supported lithium hydroxide, Ascarite^R, molecular sieve (4 Å or 5 Å) or Porapak™ (P or Q) can be inserted into the line that leads from the nitrogen supply to the target. Great care must be taken to prevent any contamination of the target by trap contents. To restrict the entry of carbon dioxide by diffusion, metal (stainless steel or copper) is preferred to nylon or other polymers as the material for the tubing between the gas supply and target. The internal diameter of the tubing should be kept as small as practicable with regard to achieving acceptable flow rates and minimising gas volume.

2.1.3. *Target operation.* Targets are operated only in the batch mode. Both cylindrical and conical targets are used, though the latter is preferred. A conical target is more difficult to construct but gives somewhat higher yields and much higher specific radioactivity, mainly due to the containment of the beam within the gas volume and the smaller volume of the target gas used.

A typical conical target used at the Baby Cyclotron (BC1710) at Jülich (Blessing *et al.*, 1988) is shown in Figure 2. It is 144 mm long, with front and rear parts having diameters

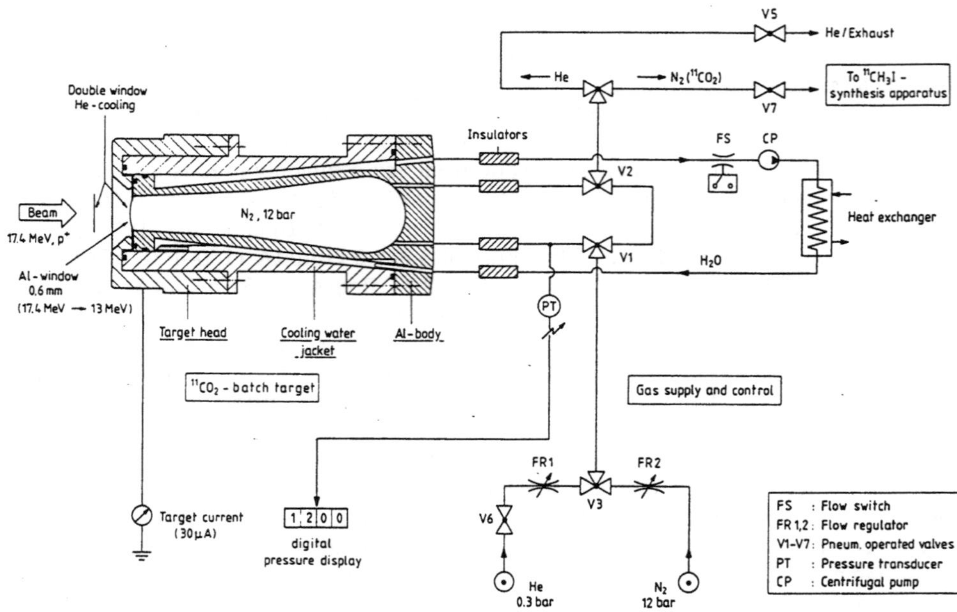

Figure 2. Batch target system used for production of high specific radioactivity [^{11}C]carbon dioxide at KFA Jülich (after Blessing *et al.*, 1988)

of 18 and 44 mm, respectively. The target body is made of aluminium-magnesium alloy containing 3% magnesium (AlMg3). The double window in front of the target consists of a 0.6 mm thick aluminium sheet (closing the target) and a 50 μm thick aluminium foil (separating the cyclotron vacuum). A helium stream (0.8 bar, –7°C) flows through the two foils and cools the window. The target body is cooled by flowing water. The target is filled with 'CO-free' nitrogen gas to a pressure of 12 bar. At a beam current of 45 μA (in a typical production run) the pressure rises to 16 bar. The proton energy range within the gas corresponds to E_p = 13→3 MeV.

2.1.4. *Dose dependence of precursors.* The recoiling carbon-11 atoms undergo hot chemical and radiation chemical reactions in the gas phase, depending on the target fill and the radiation dose (Ache and Wolf, 1968). While using "pure" nitrogen containing traces of oxygen as target gas both [^{11}C]carbon monoxide and [^{11}C]carbon dioxide are formed; the former is favoured at very low doses and the latter at medium and high doses.

From the excitation functions of the competing nuclear reactions on nitrogen, namely $^{14}N(p,\alpha)^{11}C$ and $^{14}N(p,pn)^{13}N$, it is expected that over the optimal energy range for carbon-11 production (E_p = 13→3 MeV) the amount of nitrogen-13 impurity will be small. Experience has shown that the relative amount of [^{13}N]nitrogen is strongly dose-dependent. Results of a radio-GC analysis are shown in Figure 3 (Nebeling *et al.*, 1990). Evidently, very short irradiations lead to relatively high amounts of [^{13}N]nitrogen. Suitable irradiation times for [^{11}C]carbon dioxide production appear to be 30 min or more.

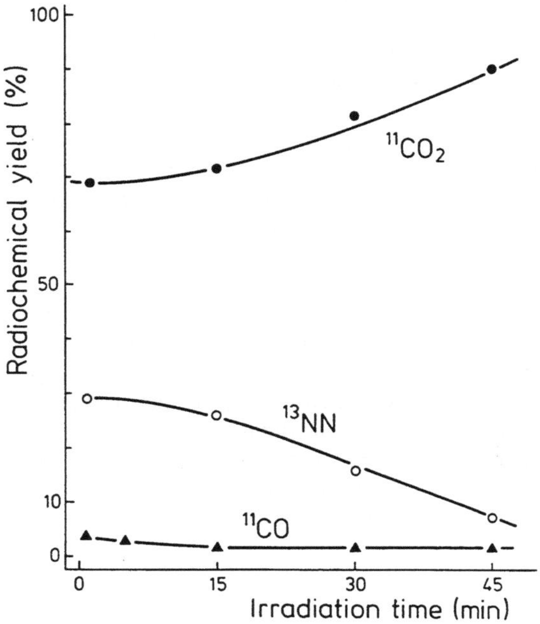

Figure 3. Relative radiochemical yields of some precursors produced by the proton irradiation of nitrogen in a batch target as a function of irradiation time. The proton energy range in the target was E_p = 13→3 MeV and the beam current 30 μA (Nebeling *et al.*, 1990).

2.1.5. *[^{11}C]Carbon dioxide recovery.* [^{11}C]Carbon dioxide should be led from the target to a hot-cell in metal tubing (stainless steel, small diameter) and passed through a column of magnesium perchlorate ($MgClO_4.H_2O$) or granular phosphorus pentoxide to trap out any water from the nitrogen gas. To maintain high specific radioactivity, the [^{11}C]carbon dioxide should be recovered from the target as quickly as possible. Generally, 2 min are required for releasing the target with a flow of 1–2 L/min. Two methods are recommended for [^{11}C]carbon dioxide separation, namely the use of a cryogenic trap or the use of a molecular sieve trap.

a. Use of a cryogenic trap.

[^{11}C]Carbon dioxide is trapped in a small stainless steel tube (40 cm i.d. x 0.2 mm) immersed in liquid nitrogen (b.p., −196°C) or preferably liquid argon (b.p., −186°C), the temperature being maintained using a temperature controller. The [^{11}C]carbon dioxide is recovered simply by passing a slow stream of helium through the trap while it is warmed to room temperature. If liquid nitrogen is used care must be taken to avoid the entrapment of a large quantity of nitrogen which is released vigorously in only a few seconds during delivery. The efficiency of trapping is > 98% and recovery is quantitative. An alternative method uses a cryogenic trap which can be cooled down to −196°C and heated up to 200°C, each temperature in this range being set by a temperature controller.

b. Use of a molecular sieve trap.

[^{11}C]Carbon dioxide is collected in a pre-activated column (6 cm x 9 mm i.d.) of molecular sieve (4 Å, 60–80 mesh). The column is pre-activated by heating to 400°C under vacuum, followed by cooling with a through flow of nitrogen. Entrapment of [^{11}C]carbon dioxide is > 98% efficient. The [^{11}C]carbon dioxide may be recovered in a small volume of nitrogen within 2–3 min by heating the trap to > 230°C, with a through flow of nitrogen (20 mL/min). The recovery of [^{11}C]carbon dioxide is about 90%.

2.1.6. *Yield and purity.* For the target system shown in Figure 2 an irradiation at 45 μA for 0.7 h leads typically to a [^{11}C]carbon dioxide batch yield of > 2 Ci (> 74 GBq). Analysis of the decay curve showed that the activity is more than 99.9% carbon-11 for E_p = 13→3 MeV. The specific radioactivity of [^{11}C]carbon dioxide was found to be about 1100 GBq/μmol (30 Ci/μmol).

2.1.7. *Considerations for the production of [^{11}C]methane.* [^{11}C]Methane can be produced in targetry identical to that used for [^{11}C]carbon dioxide and under similar irradiation conditions except that the target is filled with 5% hydrogen in high purity nitrogen. The yield and specific radiaoctivity are also similar. The [^{11}C]methane may be trapped from the target gas in a Porapak™ Q trap cooled with liquid argon. [^{11}C]Methane is recovered by passing helium or nitrogen at about 100 mL/min through the trap while warmed to room temperature. This process may be repeated to obtain the [^{11}C]methane in a small volume (*ca* 2 ml) of inert gas (see Landais and Crouzel, 1987).

2.2. NITROGEN-13

Nitrogen-13 ($t_{1/2}$ = 10 min; $I_{\beta+}$ = 100%; $E_{\beta+}$ = 1.19 MeV) has found limited application in biological studies (for an earlier comprehensive review see Cooper *et al.*, 1985). The most commonly used ^{13}N-labelled tracer in PET is [^{13}N]ammonia; however, [^{13}N]nitrate, for example, has also found application in plant physiology (*e.g.* Wieneke and Nebeling, 1990).

Both these chemical species can be produced easily using a water target.

Out of several nuclear processes which lead to the formation of nitrogen-13 (see Ferrieri and Wolf, 1983; Table 1), the $^{13}C(p,n)^{13}N$ and $^{16}O(p,\alpha)^{13}N$ reactions are most useful. The optimal energy range for the $^{16}O(p, \alpha)^{13}N$ reaction is $E_p = 16 \rightarrow 7$ MeV, and this process is thus ideally suited to a 'baby' cyclotron. This route offers the advantage of the use of a water target, though the yield is the lowest of the three reactions listed in Table 1. At a small cyclotron (with $E_p \approx 11$ MeV) the nitrogen-13 yield from the $^{16}O(p,\alpha)^{13}N$ reaction is rather low; the alternative at such a low energy cyclotron is the $^{13}C(p,n)^{13}N$ process (Bida *et al.*, 1986) using highly ^{13}C-enriched powder saturated with natural water (*i.e.* a slurry target). Since a natural water target constitutes the standard method for nitrogen-13 production (*cf.* Vaalburg *et al.*, 1975; Parks and Krohn, 1978; Lindner *et al.*, 1979; Slegers *et al.*, 1980), we describe it below in detail.

2.2.1. *Target hardware.* Target bodies made of nickel or titanium have been used. A typical target, as used at Jülich, is shown in Figure 4. It is exactly the same as that employed in [^{18}F]fluoride production via the $^{18}O(p,n)^{18}F$ reaction on ^{18}O-enriched water (see below).

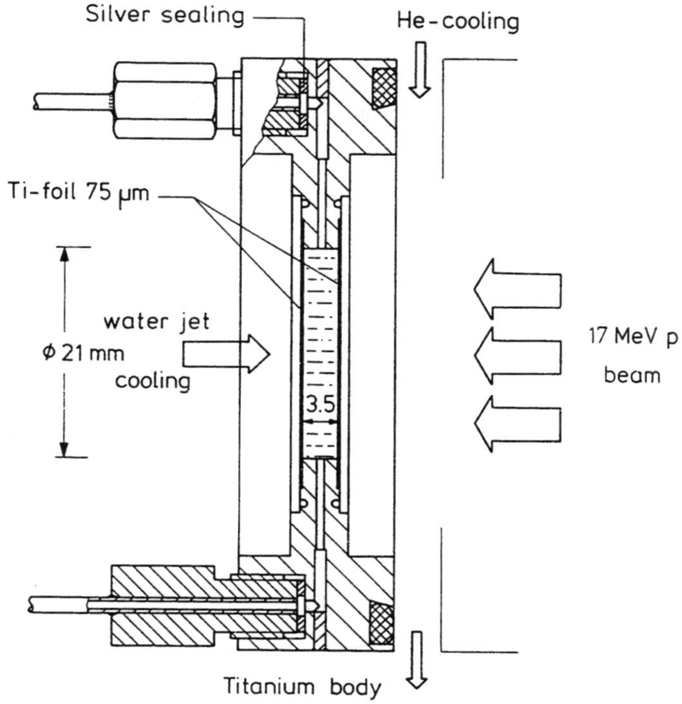

Figure 4. Sectional view of the electron-welded titanium target (internal volume, 1.3 mL) in use at KFA Jülich for nitrogen-13 production via the $^{16}O(p,\alpha)^{13}N$ reaction on natural water. An identical target is used for fluorine-18 production via the $^{18}O(p,n)^{18}F$ reaction using ^{18}O-enriched water.

The target consists of a titanium body, electron beam-welded to two titanium foils (75 µm thick), which act as front and back window. The inner diameter of the target is 21 mm with a water thickness of 3.5 mm. The target takes 1.3 mL of water with no expansion space. Two 1/16" stainless steel tubes, leading to a multi-port valve are connected via screws that are sealed with silver washers. During irradiation, the back window is water-cooled, typically to 8–10°C, and the front window is helium-cooled to –7°C.

2.2.2. *Target operating conditions.* The target is normally operated with a 30 µA beam of 17 MeV protons. The pressure in a routine production run is between 10 and 15 bar.

2.2.3. *Liquid handling and transfer system.* The target can be remotely loaded with water using the filling unit described below for [^{18}F]fluoride production. A polyethylene-polypropylene copolymer tube with an i.d. of 0.8 mm and a helium drive pressure of 1.3 bar is considered a reliable transfer system. Transfer over 40 m through this tubing from the target to the nearest hot-cell by a helium drive pressure of 1.3 bar takes only 2 min.

2.2.4. *Dose-dependence of ^{13}N-labelled precursors.* The major chemical species observed in the irradiated water are [^{13}N]nitrate, [^{13}N]nitrite, [^{13}N]ammonium ion and [^{13}N]hydroxylamine. Dose effects were observed in several studies (Parks and Krohn, 1978; Tilbury and Dahl, 1979; Root and Krohn, 1981). In general, with increasing dose, the proportion of the higher oxidation state increases at the expense of the lower oxidation states. A typical result is shown in Figure 5 (*cf.* Patt *et al.*, 1991). Effects of dose rate are observed only in the low dose region. The highest [^{13}N]nitrate yield in pure water is 85 ± 5% in the high dose region.

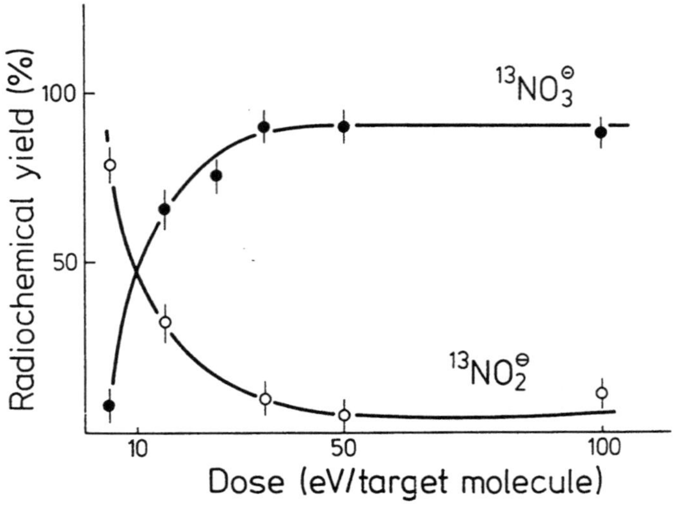

Figure 5. Dose dependence of ^{13}N-labelled precursors in a natural water target. The proton energy range in the target was E_p = 16→3 MeV and the beam current 15 µA (Patt *et al.*, 1991).

2.2.5. *Production of [^{13}N]nitrate.* The irradiated water (1.3 mL, 99.99% ^{16}O-enriched to avoid ^{18}F impurity) is passed through an ion exchange column containing 200 mg of Dowex 50W-X8 (50–80 mesh) and connected to the end of the polyethylene-polypropylene tube. The by-products, [^{13}N]ammonium ion and vanadium-48 (from the activation of titanium), are adsorbed on the column. Sulphuric acid (30%; 100 µL) is then added to the eluted target water and the mixture boiled to decompose nitrous acid and to expel it as nitrogen oxides. Quality control on the residual [^{13}N]nitrate solution is performed by radio-HPLC on a Nucleosil™ 5SB column (250 x 4 mm) eluted with 50mM-perchloric acid adjusted to pH 3.8 with potassium hydroxide (Wieneke and Nebeling, 1990).

A 10 min irradiation with 17 MeV protons at 30 µA leads to about 20.4 GBq (550 mCi) of [^{13}N]nitrate. The radiochemical purity of the [^{13}N]nitrate is > 99.8%. An alternative procedure consists of separation of the [^{13}N]nitrate by preparative chromatography using a Nucleosil™ 10 SB column (250 x 10 mm) and the aforementioned eluent. The same results can be achieved by this method.

2.2.6. *Production of [^{13}N]ammonia.* There are two methods for the production of [^{13}N]ammonia (Figure 6).

A. Classical reduction wih DeVarda's alloy

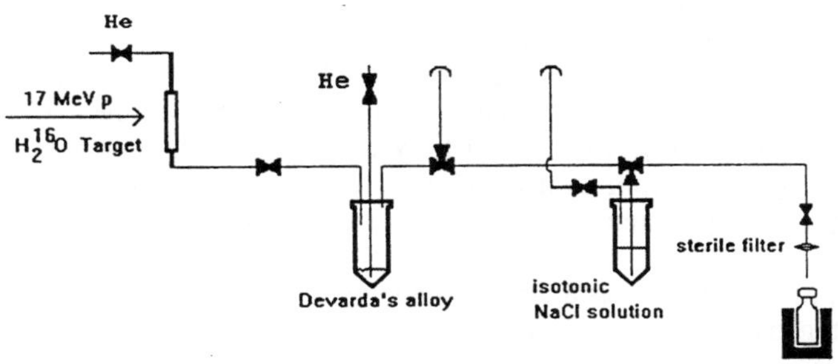

B. On-line reduction *in situ*

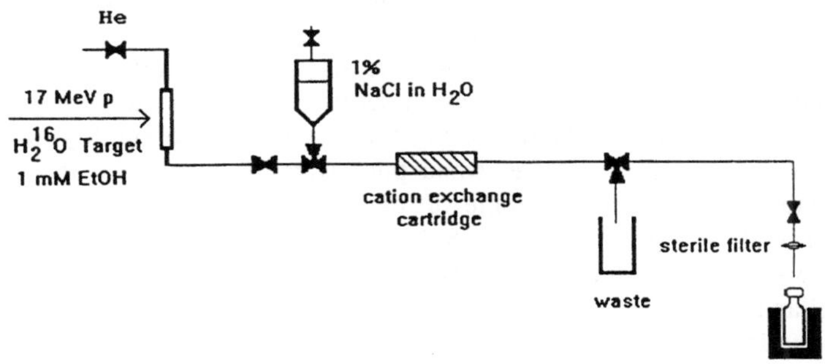

Figure 6. Schemes for the synthesis of [^{13}N]ammonia (A) via classical reduction with DeVarda's alloy and (B) via on-line reduction *in situ*.

In the first method, which is the more classical, the irradiated water is transferred to a vessel containing DeVarda's alloy (*cf.* Vaalburg *et al.*, 1975; Slegers *et al.*, 1980). On reduction of the [^{13}N]nitrate and [^{13}N]nitrite to [^{13}N]ammonia, the gaseous [^{13}N]ammonia is swept by a stream of helium into saline solution. After sterile filtration the product is ready for use. In a new method oxidation is prevented *in situ* (Wieland *et al.*, 1991). Ethanol is added, as scavenger for oxidising radicals, to the distilled and degassed water to give a 1mM-solution. After an irradiation for 10 min at 20 μA, the target volume is transferred to a cation exchange cartridge connected to the end of the transfer line to trap [^{13}N]ammonium ion. The [^{13}N]ammonia is then eluted with an isotonic solution of sodium chloride solution. After final sterile filtration the product is ready for use.

2.3. OXYGEN-15

Oxygen-15 ($t_{1/2}$ = 2.05 min; $I_{\beta+}$ = 99.9%; $E_{\beta+}$ = 1.72 MeV) is extensively used in simple chemical forms to study oxygen metabolism, blood flow and blood volume in man with PET. Methods for the production of oxygen-15 and the preparation of [^{15}O]oxygen, [^{15}O]carbon dioxide, [^{15}O]carbon monoxide, [^{15}O]water and *n*-[^{15}O]butanol are well established. Most of the production aspects were described earlier (Clark *et al.*, 1987). Here we give only a summary of the important features and discuss some of the recent developments regarding this radionuclide.

Methods for the production of oxygen-15 are summarised in Table 1 (*cf.* Clark and Buckingham, 1975; Beaver *et al.*, 1976; Vera Ruiz and Wolf, 1977; Sajjad *et al.*, 1984, 1985; Ruth, 1985; Strijckmans *et al.*, 1985; Welch and Kilbourn, 1985; Krohn *et al.*, 1986; Berridge *et al.*, 1990). The ^{15}N(p,n)^{15}O reaction on highly enriched nitrogen-15 is used only when low energy protons are available ($E_p \approx$ 11 MeV). The use of ^{15}N-enriched nitrogen gas to produce [^{15}O]oxygen for both bolus and steady state metabolic studies has been demonstrated using a 4 mL gas target irradiated with a very well regulated 8–11 MeV proton beam (Wieland *et al.*, 1986b).

The ^{16}O(p,pn)^{15}O process has a threshold energy of 16.6 MeV and is applied when a medium-sized proton only cyclotron is available. The tendency is to use this method of production only when others are inaccessible (Beaver *et al.*, 1976; Ruth, 1985; Krohn *et al.*, 1986). Pure oxygen is used as the target gas and copious amounts of ozone are produced during irradiation. This ozone is removed together with small amounts of [^{13}N]nitrogen oxides and [^{11}C]carbon dioxide using active carbon and soda lime flow-through purifiers. Use of the purified product as [^{15}O]oxygen, suitably diluted to safe physiological levels, is straightforward. However, the conversion of pure oxygen into water by reaction with hydrogen, although feasible, requires great care to control the highly exothermic reaction! A much more attractive route to [^{15}O]water, using this reaction, is to employ an [^{16}O]water target (Mulholland *et al.*, 1990). Here, when pure water is irradiated, the predominant ^{15}O-labelled product is [^{15}O]water. Some nitrogen-13 is produced via the ^{16}O(p,α)^{13}N reaction together with traces of fluorine-18 from the ^{18}O(p,n)^{18}F reaction on natural abundance [^{18}O]water. These impurities may be removed using mixed-bed ion exchange columns (Mulholland *et al.*, 1990).

The production of [^{15}O]carbon dioxide (Beaver *et al.*, 1976) and in particular [^{15}O]carbon monoxide using pure oxygen targets poses many practical problems and, in the case of carbon monoxide, insurmountable problems relating to toxic levels (Krohn *et al.*, 1986). Preliminary studies with water targets to produce high specific radioactivity

[^{15}O]oxygen and hence [^{15}O]carbon monoxide are encouraging (Link *et al.*, 1991).

The ^{14}N(d,n)^{15}O reaction is the most widely used process. The energy of the deuterons incident on the nitrogen target gas should be adjusted to about 8–10 MeV. This energy should minimise the production of the longer lived radionuclidic impurities, nitrogen-13 ($t_{1/2}$ = 10.0 min) and carbon-11 ($t_{1/2}$ = 20.4 min) generated by the ^{14}N(d,t)^{13}N (threshold energy, 4.9 MeV) and ^{14}N(d,αn)^{11}C (threshold energy, 5.8 MeV) reactions, respectively.

2.3.1. *Target design and gas delivery tubes.* The target vessel used to contain the nitrogen during irradiation is usually made of aluminium alloy. The pressure is usually determined by the diameter and length of the radioactive gas delivery pipe. Typically tubes with internal diameters from 1.5 to 2 mm and 50 m length are used; in exceptional cases tubes of a few hundred metres length have also been found to be practicable. Stainless steel, PTFE™ and polypropylene tubes have been used satisfactorily. A titanium beam entry window 25–50 µm thick and 25–30 mm in diameter is fitted with a nitrile, Viton™ or metal sealing ring to a 30–50 mm diameter cylindrical vessel some 100–50 mm long, filled with nitrogen gas between 5 and 6 bar, respectively. As with all gas target and accelerator beam windows, provision must be made for their cooling. This is achieved with air or preferably helium jets with flow rates of 10–20 L/min at 1–1.5 bar, with recirculation in the case of helium.

In recent years conically shaped targets used in batch mode have found increasing application. The target system shown in Figure 2, for example, was adapted at Jülich to irradiations with 10 MeV deuterons.

2.3.2. *Target gases.*

a. [^{15}O]Oxygen production.

In-target production of [^{15}O]oxygen is achieved by irradiating nitrogen containing 0.2–0.5% (vol) oxygen. The lower level is quite critical as the recovered yield of [^{15}O]oxygen falls dramatically when lower concentrations are used, but may be necessary when higher specific radioactivities are required as, for example, in some [^{15}O]carbon monoxide labelling procedures. [^{15}O]Water may also be prepared from [^{15}O]oxygen. [^{15}O]Oxygen production yields of 0.2–0.3 GBq/µAmin (5–8 mCi/µA min) using nitrogen-oxygen (0.5%) as target gas can be achieved at flow rates of 500 mL/min.

b. [^{15}O]Carbon dioxide production.

In-target production of [^{15}O]carbon dioxide is generally preferred to the less efficient chemical conversion of [^{15}O]oxygen using hot activated charcoal. The target gas is nitrogen containing 2–2.5% carbon dioxide. [^{15}O]Carbon dioxide production yields of 0.2–0.3 GBq/µA min (5–8 mCi/µAmin) using nitrogen-carbon dioxide (2.5%) as target gas can be achieved at flow rates of 500 mL/min.

2.3.3. *Target gas supply.* Target gas mixtures are generally purchased and are either certified mixtures, such as 0.2% oxygen in nitrogen 6.0, or made from medical grade gases [mixtures of N45 (99.995%)], depending on the requirements of the local regulating authorities.

2.3.4. *Target operation.* Deuteron beam currents of up to 50 µA have been found to be practicable, the target windows being the principal limitation. It is possible to use the same target vessel for [^{15}O]oxygen and [^{15}O]carbon dioxide production provided that adequate evacuation or flushing of the target and its supply pipes is achieved between irradiations. For [^{15}O]carbon monoxide production, the risk of accidental inclusion of oxygen or carbon dioxide with the inherent risk of producing high levels of carbon monoxide precludes the use of a common target in this case.

The batch targets are more suitable for bolus studies with [^{15}O]water and *n*-[^{15}O]butanol.

2.3.5. *Processing and purification.*

a. [^{15}O]Oxygen, [^{15}O]carbon monoxide and [^{15}O]water.

The main chemical and radiochemical impurities ozone, nitrogen oxides and [^{15}O]carbon dioxide are removed using two adsorber columns in series. The first (25 mm diameter x 120 mm) is filled with sodalime and a second similarly dimensioned column is filled with granules (1.5 mm) of activated charcoal.

When [^{15}O]carbon monoxide is produced by passing previously purified [^{15}O]oxygen into a column of dried activated charcoal (60 mesh; 250 x 15 mm) at 1000°C, the presence of oxygen carrier inevitably leads to the production of potentially hazardous quantities of carbon monoxide. For example if a nitrogen target containing 0.25% oxygen is used, stable carbon monoxide at levels of at least 0.5% are produced. Under these conditions a yield of [^{15}O]carbon monoxide of 37 MBq/μA min (1 mCi/μA min) can be achieved and by 20-fold dilution a carbon monoxide concentration of 0.025% can be administered safely for periods of up to 15 min. On the other hand methods are being developed which are directed towards reducing the stable carbon monoxide content in [^{15}O]carbon monoxide and hence ensuring patients' safety (*cf.* Votaw *et al.*, 1986).

[^{15}O]Water is readily prepared by the palladium-catalysed reaction of [^{15}O]oxygen with hydrogen (*cf.* Clark and Buckingham, 1975; Meyer *et al.*, 1984; Clark and Tochon Danguy, 1992). A flow of purified [^{15}O]oxygen in nitrogen is mixed with hydrogen and passed over a few pellets of palladium-alumina catalyst, the resulting water vapour is trapped by bubbling the nitrogen carrier through sterile isotonic saline.

The catalyst also generates a small amount of ammonia which causes the pH of the saline to rise to 9. Consequently, the use of a physiological buffer may be desirable for some applications. Batches of over 3.7 GBq (100 mCi) can be readily prepared with deuteron beam currents of 20 μA. Two alternative methods for the preparation of [^{15}O]water have been described, one involving the exchange reaction between [^{15}O]carbon dioxide and water (Welch and Kilbourn, 1985) and the other employing in-target reaction of oxygen-15 atoms with hydrogen in a nitrogen-5% hydrogen target gas (Vera Ruiz and Wolf, 1978). However, very little experience of these techniques exists.

b. [^{15}O]Carbon dioxide.

During the irradiation of nitrogen-carbon dioxide (2–2.5%) the chemical and radiochemical impurities, carbon monoxide and [^{15}O]oxygen, are observed. Earlier attempts to reduce these have now been shown to be unreliable. The use of an oxidising column composed of a mixture of copper and iron oxides supported on kaolin reduces the [^{15}O]oxygen and carbon monoxide to < 0.02% and < 10 μL/L respectively (Strijckmans *et al.*, 1985). Nitrogen-13 will inevitably be present in all systems that employ carbon dioxide in the target gas because of the ^{12}C(d,n)^{13}N reaction (threshold energy, 0.4 MeV). For applications where > 0.5% [^{13}N]nitrogen cannot be tolerated the less efficient low temperature combustion of activated charcoal with [^{15}O]oxygen must be employed. The use of the copper-iron oxide column after the carbon furnace is recommended. Another approach to the production of

[^{15}O]carbon dioxide and [^{15}O]oxygen from a common target source is to carry out catalytic interconversion of [^{15}O]carbon dioxide and [^{15}O]oxygen in a flow system using metal oxide catalysts (*e.g.* Hopcalite™-II) (Iwata *et al.*, 1988).

c. n-[^{15}O]Butanol.

This appears to be a very promising agent for regional cerebral blood flow studies. Its production and quality control are described in the chapter on Automation (Crouzel *et al.*, this volume).

2.3.6. *Analysis of gaseous products.* A radio-GC is employed to analyse the chemical and radiochemical 'atmospheric gas' impurities (see Clark and Buckingham, 1975; Meyer, 1982). Typically a dual column instrument, equipped with a thermal conductivity detector for stable gas analysis plus a small sensitive volume flow-cell radioactivity detector for radioactive gas analysis, is used. The two columns most commonly used are:

(a) Porapak™-Q (80–100 mesh, 1500 x 4 mm, pre-conditioned at 250°C)

(b) Molecular sieve 5Å (80–100 mesh 3000 x 4 mm, pre-conditioned at 350°C).

These columns when operated in combination between 25 and 80°C with a helium carrier gas flow rate of about 10 mL/min provide adequate separation of [^{15}O]oxygen [^{13}N]nitrogen, [^{15}O]carbon dioxide, [^{15}O]nitrous oxide and [^{13}N]nitrous oxide.

The chemical analysis of the noxious gases, ozone, nitrogen dioxide, and carbon monoxide, down to the levels necessary for safety prior to the administration of a radioactive gas to man, cannot be carried out satisfactorily by GC. In the case of ozone classical iodometric analysis is recommended. For nitrogen dioxide colorimetric estimation is acceptable.

More details on the quality control of radioactive gases are given in the chapter on Quality Assurance and Quality Control (Meyer *et al.*, this volume).

2.4. FLUORINE-18

For fluorine-18 ($t_{1/2}$ = 109.6 min, $I_{\beta+}$ = 97%; $E_{\beta+}$ = 0.64 MeV), perhaps for more than any other radionuclide, success in labelling depends on factors that are determined by radionuclide production. The following section of this chapter is mainly based on a report of a recently sponsored EEC Task Group (Guillaume *et al.*, 1991) and specifically discusses production.

2.4.1. *Main sources of fluorine-18.* Fluorine-18 can be reached by a variety of well-documented (Qaim 1982, 1986a; Qaim and Stöcklin, 1983; Gandarias-Cruz and Okamoto, 1988) routes (for a recent summary see Guillaume *et al.*, 1991). Of these, the ^{20}Ne(d,α)^{18}F and ^{18}O(p,n)^{18}F reactions are of major practical interest, in view of their requirement for only a moderate projectile energy and a moderate beam current to give a useful yield (Figure 1). Hence, even simple cyclotrons, such as those classified by Wolf and Jones (1983) as Level I (< 10 MeV p or d) and Level II (< 20 MeV p, plus perhaps other particles), are capable of useful fluorine-18 production. The ^{20}Ne(d,α)^{18}F and ^{18}O(p,n)^{18}F reactions are mainly applied to prepare c.a. molecular [^{18}F]fluorine and n.c.a. [^{18}F]fluoride, respectively. Currently, nearly all fluorine-18 radiochemistry stems from these cyclotron products, either through their direct use as labelling agents or via their conversion into others (for reviews see Berridge and Tewson, 1986b; Coenen, 1989; Kilbourn, 1990).

Table 2. Typical conditions and production parameters for the cyclotron production of [^{18}F]fluorine by the ^{20}Ne(d,α) reaction at different centres. (Data from Guillaume *et al.*, 1991, with permission).

Centre		BNL	MRCCU Hammersmith	Jülich	Liège
Target body	(type; mL)	Honed Ni; 50	Polished Ni-201; 100	Ni; 38	Ni; 206
	(internal size, cm)	2.5 i.d. x 10	2.5 i.d. x 20	2.2 i.d. x 10	
Target gas	(% F_2 in Ne)[a]	0.1	0.12-0.15	0.18	0.17
	(μmol F_2)[b]	50-60	88[c]	60	220
Pressure	(beam off, atm)	25.8	13.5	18	12.3
	(beam on, atm)	32.5	23	30	15
Window	(material, μm)	Al, 810-Ni, 25	Havar, 50-Ni, 25	Nb, 25-Havar, 50	Al, 80-Ni, 20
	(seals)	Metal O-ring	Lead	Metal joints	Indium O-rings
E (Incident)	(MeV)	14-9.4	13.8	11.25	12
Irradiation	(μA x h)	15 x 2	15 x 1.67	40 x 1	10 x 1
Recovery of	(GBq)	13.6	9.25	18.5	4.4
^{18}F at EOB	(mCi)	367	250	500	120
	(% of theoretical)[d]	55	43	50	51
Yield	(MBq/μAh at EOB)	463	343-370	444	370-555
	(mCi/μAh at EOB)	12.5	9-10	12	10-15
Specific activity	(MBq/μmol at EOB)	259-370	41	130	29.6-44.4
	(mCi/μmol at EOB)	7-10	1.1	3.5	0.8-1.2
Reference		Casella *et al.*, 1980	Clark *et al.*, 1990	Blessing *et al.*, 1986	Guillaume *et al.*, 1990

a) Nominal value.

b Calculated from target volume and nominal filling parameters.

c) Experimentally determined as 194-242 μmol recovered, under conditions in which the fill-line contributes fluorine.

d Theoretical yields were calculated according to Casella *et al.* (1980).

The $^{16}O(^{3}He,p)^{18}F$ reaction is also occasionally used for [^{18}F]fluoride production. The yield is low (Table 1 and Figure 1); the only advantage is that natural water rather than ^{18}O-enriched water is used. However, the cost of the required helium-3 is also significant.

2.4.2. *Production of c.a. [^{18}F]fluorine by the $^{20}Ne(d,\alpha)^{18}F$ reaction.* The bombardment of high pressure neon (up to 25 bar) containing a low percentage (0.1–0.2%) of molecular fluorine with moderate energy deuterons (Lambrecht *et al.*, 1978a; Casella *et al.*, 1980) is a well-established method for producing c.a. molecular [^{18}F]fluorine. Table 2 shows experimental conditions and typical data for the production of [^{18}F]fluorine via the $^{20}Ne(d,\alpha)^{18}F$ reaction at a few centres. Several factors must be taken into account to achieve satisfactory routine production, as follows.

a. Target design and construction.

Target bodies have been described formerly (*e.g.* Casella *et al.*, 1980; Blessing *et al.*, 1986). Nickel and Monel™, machined or welded, appear to be the optimal metals for the target body. Stainless steel (316) is also convenient but needs longer passivation with fluorine (*vide infra*). Inconel™ also requires longer passivation and gives lower recovery of fluorine-18 (Casella *et al.*, 1980; Blessing *et al.*, 1986). Nickel plating on stainless steel deteriorates after a few runs (Blessing *et al.*, 1986). Generally, target bodies are 10 to 20 cm long and are fabricated from 1.5 to 2.5 cm i.d. tube with gas connections through stainless steel weld fittings. Swagelok™ fittings are recommended for this purpose. The target must be chemically clean before installation.

The window is preferably made from 25 or 50 µm Havar™ foil (Hamilton Precision Metals). Aluminium or Havar™, having a thick layer (*e.g.* 20–25 µm) of nickel on the side exposed to fluorine, nickel, niobium and titanium have also been used. Several methods may be used to seal the beam-entry window to the target body. Those that are satisfactory include the use of a copper ring (Leybold) a gold crush seal, an indium wire or a flat washer made from thick (0.5 mm) lead sheet. Cooling of the foil, preferably with helium is recommended.

b. Target gas.

The neon should be 99.998% pure as obtainable from Air Liquide or Messer Griesheim, in order to recover the radioactivity mainly as molecular [^{18}F]fluorine (*vide infra*) (Bida *et al.*, 1980a; Casella *et al.*, 1980; Dahl and Schlyer, 1985). The pressure regulator should be all metal and designed for use with high purity gases.

In pure neon, nucleogenic fluorine-18 diffuses to the target wall and is chemically adsorbed. When a low (0.1–0.2%) proportion of carrier fluorine is present, exchange of nucleogenic fluorine-18 can compete with surface adsorption and recovery of most of the radioactivity from the target becomes possible (Lambrecht *et al.*, 1978a; Bida *et al.*, 1980a; Casella *et al.*, 1980). Corrosion of target and anciliary components is not a significant problem if only dilute (*e.g.* < 2%) mixtures of fluorine in neon are used. A mixture of 2% fluorine in neon, with certificate of analysis, can be obtained from Union Carbide, Air Liquide or Matheson. The pressure regulator is specially prepared for use with fluorine mixtures by the gas supplier. Alternatively, a mixture of 2% fluorine in helium, as prepared for lasers, can also be used as the source of fluorine gas. This is supplied by Matheson or Air Liquide with a full Monel™ delivery system.

c. Target gas handling.
Given the highly hazardous nature of fluorine, it is emphasised that a safe facility is required to dilute the stock fluorine mixture with further neon to achieve the composition desired within the target.

Stainless steel and Swagelok™ fittings are recommended for transport lines, since surface fluorination (passivation) lasts longer at room temperature than for the alternatives of nickel and Monel™. Teflon tubing, though chemically resistant, is unsuitable as it becomes permeable to fluorine with use (Casella *et al.*, 1980). Stainless steel bellows (Hoke, Nupro) valves are reliable in service. A piezoresistive, low dead-volume pressure transducer (Kistler) is recommended to monitor target pressure before and during irradiation. Great care should be taken to avoid any ingress of air into the gas handling facility and target. Flow purging rather than evacuation of air is thus preferred. It is preferable to dedicate a line for filling the target and to dedicate another low volume line for recovering radioactivity. The fill/empty stoichiometry of this arrangement can be highly reproducible.

d. Target operating conditions.
The main factor that determines [^{18}F]fluorine recovery is the chemical state of the target surface (Bida *et al.*, 1980a; Casella *et al.*, 1980). Passivation (prefluorination) of the surface is necessary before bombardment to avoid a significant loss of fluorine-18 along with fluorine carrier. Two passivation methods have been proposed, namely 'thermal' passivation and 'beam-induced plasma' passivation. Thermal passivation requires the target to be heated for 1–3 h to between 100 and 200°C, when filled to a low pressure (a few bar) with dilute fluorine in neon. Beam-induced plasma passivation is achieved by deuteron bombardment of the target when filled to at least the same partial pressure of fluorine as used in production. Two or three irradiations, using about 10 μA of deuterons for 30 min, are carried out successively, with the contents of the target discarded after each irradiation. Recoil passivation is most easy to operate routinely. In general, the requirement to repeat passivation is more likely the longer a target has not been in use. It is considered that a good passivation is achieved when 75 to 80% of the fluorine-18 can be recovered in a production run. Water-cooling of the target during irradiation is not usually necessary, so simplifying target construction.

e. Chemical forms of the recovered fluorine-18.
The chemical form of the recovered fluorine-18 depends critically on the purity of the target gas (Bida *et al.*, 1980a; Casella *et al.*, 1980; Dahl and Schlyer, 1985). The neon should be as free as possible from nitrogen and carbon oxides, as these incorporate substantial proportions of the fluorine-18 into inert substances namely, nitrogen [^{18}F]trifluoride and carbon [^{18}F]tetrafluoride, respectively. Contamination by fluorocarbons should also be avoided. Under such conditions the fluorine-18 is mainly obtained as molecular [^{18}F]fluorine (Bida *et al.*, 1980a; Dahl and Schlyer, 1985).

The following reaction is useful to monitor the chemical activity of the available fluorine-18, as well as its specific radioactivity (Blessing *et al.*, 1986):

$$^{18}F_2 + Me_3SnPh \xrightarrow[CFCl_3,\ -78^\circ C]{} Ph^{18}F + Me_3Sn^{18}F$$

The amount of [^{18}F]fluorobenzene in the freon solution of labelled products is determined by radio-GC. From measurement of the total recovered activity the reactive fraction of recovered fluorine-18 (presumed to be molecular [^{18}F]fluorine), and its specific radioactivity can be calculated. Blessing *et al.* (1986) found the total organic radiochemical yield to be 51 ± 2% and the fluorobenzene yield to be 36 ± 2% over 30 runs under the production conditions described in Table 2.

It should be noted that deuteron irradiation of neon containing a low percentage (< 15%) of hydrogen has been used by several groups to produce n.c.a. fluorine-18 (Clark *et al.*, 1973; Winchell *et al.*, 1976; Straatman and Welch, 1977; Lambrecht *et al.*, 1978a; Helus *et al.*, 1979; Clark and Oberdorfer, 1982; Dahl *et al.*, 1983; Ehrenkaufer *et al.*, 1983; Blessing *et al.*, 1986). Various means have been used to recover the radioactivity, including removal from the heated target with a stream of hydrogen (Winchell *et al.*, 1976; Clark and Oberdorfer, 1982; Dahl *et al.*, 1983; Blessing *et al.*, 1986), recirculation of the irradiated neon-hydrogen mixture over a basic trap (Clark *et al.*, 1973) and water-washing of the target after irradiation (Helus *et al.*, 1979; Blessing *et al.*, 1986). Removal from the heated target in a stream of hydrogen is invariably described as giving n.c.a. hydrogen [^{18}F]fluoride. Water washing of the target recovers a high proportion (90%) of the radioactivity as aqueous [^{18}F]fluoride with a high specific radioactivity of 370 GBq/μmol (10 Ci/μmol) (Blessing *et al.*, 1986). However, these neon-hydrogen targets are relatively inconvenient to operate and difficult to maintain and so are not widely used.

f. Specific radioactivity.

The effect of systematically varying fluorine content on activity recovery and specific radioactivity has been examined (Blessing *et al.*, 1986). Between 0.10 and 0.18% (60 μmol F_2) of fluorine carrier, [^{18}F]fluorine recovery increased but specific radioactivity did not change. The optimal composition for recovery yield and specific radioactivity seems to be 0.18% fluorine.

The volume of the target is an important factor. It was found that for a collimated (1 cm diameter), defocussed and wobbled beam, the optimal target size is 2.2 cm diameter x 10 cm length giving a total fluorine content of 60 μmol for the target, leading to a specific radioactivity of 55.5–111 GBq/mmol (1.5–3.0 Ci/mmol) in production (Blessing *et al.*, 1986).

The specific radioactivity of molecular [^{18}F]fluorine can be measured via titration of the iodine liberated on passing the target output into potassium iodide solution (Casella *et al.*, 1980). However, in principle, this method does not distinguish between the several oxidising chemical forms of fluorine-18 (such as ^{18}F-labelled OF_2, HOF, NFH_2 or NF_2H) that might arise in the target if there is any contamination by air. A misleading result might therefore be obtained. Preferably, specific radioactivity is measured via the reaction with trimethylphenyl tin (*vide supra*), which is expected to be more selective for fluorine-18 in the form of molecular fluorine (Blessing *et al.*, 1986).

2.4.3. *Production of n.c.a. [^{18}F]fluoride by the $^{18}O(p,n)^{18}F$ reaction on ^{18}O-enriched water.*
The proton irradiation of ^{18}O-enriched water is now the most effective method for the production of n.c.a. [^{18}F]fluoride. Under optimal conditions, greater than 20 GBq (several hundreds of mCi) of aqueous [^{18}F]fluoride are easily available from an 11 MeV proton cyclotron, in a bombardment time of less than 1 h. At a 'baby' cyclotron with $E_p \approx 17$ MeV, batch yields of about 74 GBq (2 Ci) are available. Table 3 summarises typical experimental data on the production of [^{18}F]fluoride from ^{18}O-enriched water targets, as developed in several laboratories.

Table 3. Typical data for [^{18}F]fluorine produced at different centres from ^{18}O-enriched water targets. (Data reproduced from Guillaume *et al.*, 1991, with permission).

Centre	St. Louis	Sendai	Villigen	Turku	Jülich	Hammersmith	Liège
Material insert	SS & Ti	Ti	Ag	Ag	Ti	SS316 & Ti	Ni
Water width (mm)	3, 5, 7	3, 4, 5	5	1.5	3.5	3	3.4
Foils	Havar or Ti	Al/Ti & Ag	Ag	Ni	Ti	Al/Ti & SS316	Ti
Seal	O-ring	O-ring	Ag	Metal	Weld & Ag	Metal to metal	O-ring
Cooling (°C)	Water (10)	Coolant (0)	Water (30)	Coolant (10)	Water (10)	Water (10)	Water (10)
^{18}O-Enrichment of H_2O (%)	97	20	98	98	97	20	5
Volume (mL)	1.2, 2.0, 2.8	2.5	4.5	0.195	1.3	2.0	1.8
Pressure (atm)	1	Open or circulated (Pd)	Open	Open	15-25	2	2-3
E (MeV)	15	16	16	12	16.5	16	22.6
Irradiation (μA x min)	15-20 x 80	20 x 60	20 x 60	10 x 60	20-35 x 60	20 x 60	10 x 60
Yield (GBq/μAh at EOB)	2.22	0.33	2.07	1.11	2.41	0.407	0.11-0.12
(mCi/μAh at EOB)	*ca* 60	9	56	30	70	11	3-3.2
Sp. Act. (TBq/μmol EOB)	1.85	0.148	nca	5.18	7.4	11.1×10^{-3}	0.37
(Ci/μmol at EOB)	*ca* 50	4	nca	140	200	0.3	10
Reference	Kilbourn *et al.*, 1985	Iwata *et al.*, 1987	Huszar & Weinreich, 1985; Vogt *et al.*, 1986	Solin *et al.*, 1988	Qaim *et al.*, 1987; Nebeling *et al.*, 1990	Clark *et al.*, 1990	Guillaume *et al.*, 1990

a. Target systems.

Many different [^{18}O]water targets have been described (Wieland and Wolf, 1983; Kilbourn *et al.*, 1984, 1985; Huszár and Weinreich, 1985; Berridge and Tewson, 1986a; De Jesus *et al.*, 1986; Keinonen *et al.*, 1986; Vogt *et al.*, 1986; Wieland *et al.*, 1986a; Iwata *et al.*, 1987; Qaim *et al.*, 1987; Solin *et al.*, 1988; Berridge and Kjellstrom, 1989; Mulholland *et al.*, 1989; Steinbach *et al.*, 1990). The primary consideration in design has been to consume as little of the costly ^{18}O-enriched water as possible during production. The requirement for small target volume in turn means that target thickness has to be selected carefully for effective use of the beam. Also radiolysis and boiling of the water become important considerations, if impure water is used for irradiation. These can cause significant loss of target water in open targets (Kilbourn *et al.*, 1984; Berridge and Tewson, 1986; Iwata *et al.*, 1987) or unacceptable pressure build up in closed targets, with adverse effect on yield. Effective target cooling of the front window by helium and the back side with water is mandatory.

The decision to operate a low pressure or high pressure target is fundamental, since it bears on target construction and the strategy for coping with the adverse effects of radiolysis and heat. Experience has shown that the most efficient water target is simply composed of a cavity for the target water, bounded by two rigid metallic foils, the rear foil being efficiently cooled by a suitable fluid. Targets requiring only 0.4–2.5 mL of water can be constructed on this basis. Other parameters of importance are the type of target seals, the chemical nature of the metallic insert and foils, the type of transfer tubing (Iwata *et al.*, 1987) and the facility for recovery of the ^{18}O-enriched water, as these potentially bear on the reactivity and the specific radioactivity of the generated [^{18}F]fluoride.

For labelling by nucleophilic substitutions the [^{18}F]fluoride is required to be essentially free of water, *i.e.* to be 'naked' n.c.a. [^{18}F]fluoride. Several procedures have been described for the recovery of n.c.a. [^{18}F]fluoride in a reactive form from ^{18}O-enriched water (*e.g.* Brodack *et al.*, 1986; Schlyer *et al.*, 1987, 1990; Jewett *et al.*, 1988, 1990, 1991a,b; Alexoff *et al.*, 1989; Hamacher *et al.*, 1990). These deliver the [^{18}F]fluoride in natural enrichment water or organic solvent. Generally, the strategy for generating reactive [^{18}F]fluoride is dissolution of the [^{18}F]fluoride with a large counter-ion (*e.g.* K^+, Cs^+, Rb^+, Bu_4N^+ or K^+-Kryptofix™) in a polar aprotic solvent. Where required, water (or other solvent) is removed by distillation from an added base (*e.g.* KOH, K_2CO_3, Rb_2CO_3, Et_4NOH, Bu_4NOH or K_2CO_3-Kryptofix™) and the [^{18}F]fluoride salt dried by, for example, azeotropic distillation with acetonitrile, or even by microwaves. This salt is then resolubilised in the solvent containing the substrate for nucleophilic attack. Resolubilisation efficiency is affected by the reaction vessel, solvent and perhaps other factors such as metal ion contamination (Brodack *et al.*, 1986). The intrinsic reactivity of the [^{18}F]fluoride is affected by several factors, including cation and anion contaminants whose level are largely determined by the materials of target construction and operation (Nickles *et al.*, 1986). Below we describe and discuss examples of reliable target assemblies designed for low and high pressure operation.

b. Example of a reliable low pressure target system.

In the low pressure mode of operation, without taking appropriate precautions, radiolysis and boiling can cause a significant loss of ^{18}O-enriched water, and render the use of high beam currents impractical for high yield. Provision for effective venting (Wieland and Wolf, 1983; Berridge and Tewson, 1986a; Iwata *et al.*, 1987) or for the catalytic recombination of radiolytically generated oxygen and hydrogen (Iwata *et al.*, 1987) must always therefore be considered. Recirculation of the water during irradiation is also advantageous for some targets (Iwata *et al.*, 1987; Keinonen *et al.*, 1987), but results are not necessarily consistent (Iwata *et al.*, 1987). A low pressure target, in use at the MRC Cyclotron Unit at Hammersmith Hospital, is described here as an example of a reliable system.

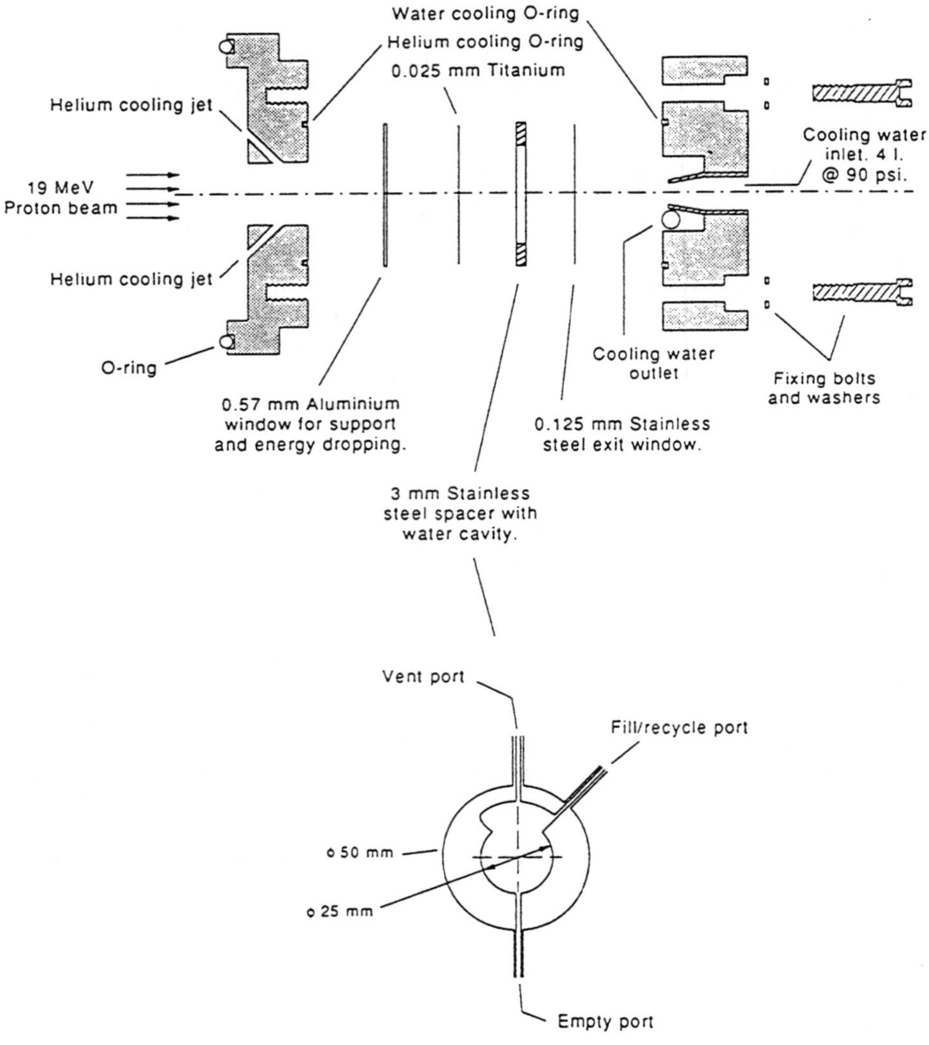

Figure 7. An exploded schematic view of the target (internal volume, 2 mL) in use at the MRC Cyclotron Unit (Hammersmith Hospital) for [^{18}F]fluoride production via the $^{18}O(p,n)^{18}F$ reaction on ^{18}O-enriched water.

The target (Figure 7) is fabricated from 25 mm diameter stainless steel (316) and titanium for the proton irradiation of 20% ^{18}O-enriched water (97% ^{18}O-enriched water from Isotec diluted with sterile HPLC grade water). The front window is aluminium (155 mg/cm^2, 0.57 mm thick) backed on the water side by a titanium foil (12.4 mg/cm^2, 25 μm thick). This maintains a flat front surface to the target and degrades the 19 MeV beam to 16 MeV. The water thickness is determined by a 3 mm thick stainless steel spacer. The back of the target is made from 125 μm thick stainless steel (316) foil which is water-cooled. The foils and spacer are clamped together metal to metal. Hence, no 'O' rings are in the target-water cell. The target cell has three 1/16" stainless steel tubes inserted through the spacer, fixed and sealed with Locktite retainer 601, the joints having been pretreated with Locktite Activator T (Cat. No 74736). A small pellet of palladium catalyst (Engelhard Model D) is supported in an external gas space to recombine any radiolytically-generated hydrogen and oxygen that might otherwise cause excessive internal pressure.

The target is normally operated with an incident beam of 19 MeV protons (20 μA, 20 mm diameter, spun at 45–50 Hz). The target is 45 m from the nearest hot cell in which the fluorine-18 can be used. Teflon™ lines (1/16" o.d., 0.030" bore) are used with a neon drive pressure of 2 bar and flow regulator. The transfer yield for 1–2 mL target water is currently > 95% while the recovery of [^{18}F]fluoride is typically between 95 and 98%, within 5 min from EOB. Though, at the end of irradiation approximately 65% of the radioactivity is nitrogen-13 ($t_{1/2}$ = 9.96 min) from the $^{16}O(p,\alpha)^{13}N$ reaction, this is not a problem for radiosyntheses with the [^{18}F]fluoride which generally take more than one hour. Final products are devoid of nitrogen-13.

A procedure, based on those described by Schlyer *et al.* (1987, 1990) and Hamacher *et al.* (1990), has been adopted for the recovery of [^{18}F]fluoride and for the recycling of ^{18}O-enriched water. Carbonate form ion exchange resin (100–200 mesh AG 1X 8; 90 mg) is made into a column (28 mm x 3 mm). ^{18}O-Enriched water is forced from the target through the column by low neon pressure (2 bar). Finally, neon is blown through the column to extract the last traces of liquid. The recovered water is pooled into 10 to 20 mL batches and distilled under reduced pressure using a microrotary evaporator. The degree of ^{18}O-enrichment is measured with mass spectrometry (Waters, 1990). Bacterial contamination of the ^{18}O-enriched water must be avoided by sterile millipore filtration into clean sterile glass vials (Pierce). The [^{18}F]fluoride is recovered from the anion exchange column by elution with potassium carbonate solution. The procedure is highly efficient with respect to recovery of [^{18}F]fluoride and to recycling of the ^{18}O-enriched water.

The [^{18}F]fluoride is used routinely for the production of 2-^{18}FDG (2-[^{18}F]fluoro-2-deoxy-D-glucose), according to Hamacher *et al.* (1986). Generally, over 90% of the radioactivity reacts in the first stage of the radiosynthesis, the displacement of the triflyl group, if performed in a glassy carbon vessel. If the reaction is performed in a glass vessel, incorporation is typically 60%.

c. Example of a reliable high pressure target system.

Targets without an expansion volume are operable at beam currents up to 30 μA, due to the pressure build up in the target by radiolysis, depending on the purity of the water (Wieland *et al.*, 1986a) which, as a diagnostic, can be monitored during irradiation. A target (Figure 4) in use at Jülich is described here as an example of a system which has functioned reliably, even after reaching an integrated beam current of 3000 μAh.

The target consists of a titanium body electron beam-welded to two titanium foils (75 μm thick), which act as front and back window. The dimensions of the target are exactly the same as those described above for nitrogen-13 production. The target takes 1.3 mL of ^{18}O-enriched water with no expansion space. Two 1/16" stainless steel tubes lead from each end of the target to a multi-port valve (Figure 8) and are connected via screws that are sealed with silver washers.

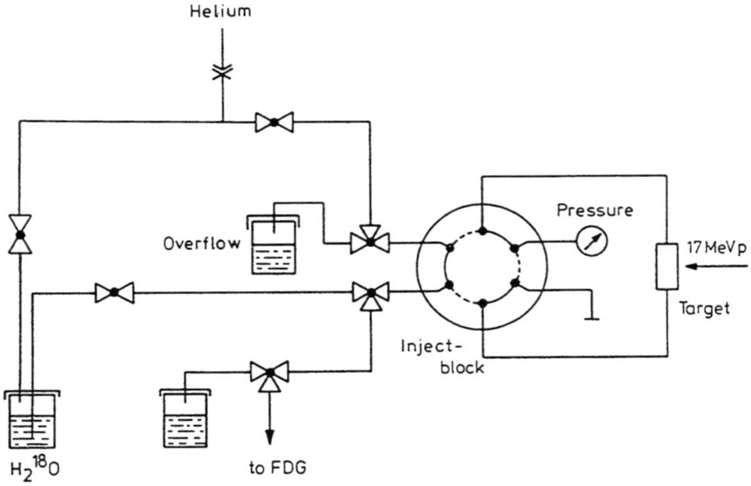

Figure 8. Scheme of the remotely loaded filling unit for the ^{18}O-enriched water target used at KFA Jülich.

The purity of the ^{18}O-enriched water used in high pressure targets is of major concern. It is found that high chemical purity is needed to avoid excessive pressure build-up. For large-scale production, greater than 90% ^{18}O-enrichment is needed to avoid the generation of excessive [^{13}N]nitrogen, which may pose radiation protection problems. Organic impurities must be absent as these can prevent recombination of radiolytically generated oxygen and hydrogen atoms, causing the target to burst. In order to eliminate traces of organic solvents after use, the ^{18}O-enriched water is purified by reflux with potassium permanganate and potassium hydroxide, and finally double distillation. Purity is assessed by capillary GC with an FID detector operating at highest sensitivity.

The target is normally operated at a beam current of 20–30 µA of 17 MeV protons, depending on the purity of water. The maximum current tested was 35 µA. The pressure in a routine production run is in the range 15–25 bar. The yield of aqueous [^{18}F]fluoride is linear with beam current up to 30 µA and irradiation times up to 1 h.

Filling of the target with ^{18}O-enriched water is achieved with a motor-driven syringe through 3-way valves (Asco 368) and 6-way valves (Valco AC6W), which are connected by polyethylene-polypropylene tube. The target is locked by the 6-way valve and the pressure is monitored by a piezoresistive pressure transducer with very low dead volume. A polyethylene-polypropylene copolymer tube with an inner diameter of 0.8 mm and helium drive pressure of 1.3 bar is considered a reliable transfer system. Transfer over 30 m through this tubing from the target to the nearest hot-cell takes only 2 min.

The ^{18}O-enriched water is recovered by retrieving the [^{18}F]fluoride on a carbonate form ion exchange resin (Hamacher *et al.*, 1990). The water can be recycled 4 or 5 times, unless the enrichment of water falls below 90%, as measured by mass spectrometry and by measuring the amount of nitrogen-13 from a production run.

Cation and anion contaminants (Solin *et al.*, 1988) have generally been considered to influence the reactivity of n.c.a. [^{18}F]fluoride. If Havar™ foils are used for the target the contaminants are mainly Fe, Cr and Co ions in concentrations ranging from 0.2 to 3 ppm as assessed by atomic absorption spectroscopy. Use of titanium foils results in a decrease in these ions and therefore can be recommended as the least contaminating metal to use as insert and window foil. Contamination of the ^{18}O-enriched water with vanadium-48 was found to be 6.9 kBq (0.187 µCi) after irradiation for 10 min with a 20 µA beam producing 10 GBq (270 mCi) of fluorine-18. An advantage of the [^{18}F]fluoride recovery system is that cationic species are not co-recovered. Over 90% of the recovered [^{18}F]fluoride reacts in the first stage of the synthesis of 2-^{18}FDG described by Hamacher *et al.* (1986), when a glassy carbon vessel is used. The target delivers [^{18}F]fluoride with specific radioactivities up to 7400 GBq/µmol (200 Ci/µmol) as measured by a fluoride selective electrode.

2.4.4. *Fluorine-18 from the $^{18}O(p,n)^{18}F$ reaction on [^{18}O]oxygen gas.* The $^{18}O(p,n)^{18}F$ reaction is of considerable interest for producing [^{18}F]fluorine in centres having a proton-only cyclotron. Nickles *et al.* (1984) first described the production of [^{18}F]fluorine-18 from an oxygen-18 gas target using a two-step irradiation process. Nickel is used as material for the target body, and nickel and Havar™ foils for the windows. The target is conically shaped and has a volume of 15 mL. After irradiating pressurised ^{18}O-enriched (98%) oxygen gas, fluorine-18 gets deposited on the target walls, and the oxygen-18 is recovered cryogenically. A second and short irradiation of 1% fluorine (75 µmol) in krypton is needed for isotopic exchange of the adsorbed fluorine-18 and the recovery of more than 50% of the total fluorine-18 activity (Sunderland *et al.*, 1989). Target performance is determined by the level of fluorine passivation. Passivation with molecular fluorine at 200°C for several hours gives the best results. The [^{18}F]fluorine can be titrated by well known methods (Casella *et al.*, 1980) and has been converted into acetyl [^{18}F]hypofluorite, which was then used for the synthesis of L-6-[^{18}F]fluoro-DOPA (Sunderland *et al.*, 1990). Chirakal *et al.* (1992) have also produced fluorine-18 in this manner for the direct radiofluorination of dopamine. Solin and Bergman (1986) used a similar process, but substituted fluorine in neon for fluorine in krypton. They recovered up to 25% of the total radioactivity. Half of the radioactivity was recovered in the ^{18}O-enriched oxygen. Given the experience with nickel targets, such variations in recovered activity are not unexpected.

Wieland *et al.* (1989) described a one step proton irradiation of a mixture of helium, fluorine and ^{18}O-enriched oxygen. A gold-plated copper body with a conical bore was used as target and no attempt was made to recover the ^{18}O-enriched oxygen. Also, no aggressive passivation was used to precondition the target. Preliminary results appeared encouraging. For example, Wieland *et al.* (1989) were able to produce more than 37 GBq (1 Ci) of fluorine-18 radioactivity from a 1 h irradiation with 30 µA beam of 10.4 MeV protons on a target containing only 19 µmol of carrier fluorine. The achieved specific radioactivity is close to 1.85 GBq/µmol (50 mCi/µmol), and thus much higher than that usually achieved via the deuteron irradiation of a neon-fluorine mixture (Table 2).

These results have to be reproduced routinely. Especially the radioactive product has to be tested regularly for its suitability in, for example, the preparation of acetyl [^{18}F]hypofluorite, and in turn of a radiopharmaceutical such as L-6-[^{18}F]fluoro-DOPA, before either a one or a two step process with the $^{18}O(p,n)^{18}F$ reaction on [^{18}O]oxyen can be recommended for the production of fluorine-18.

3. Production Limits of Short-lived Organic Positron-Emitters at Low Energy Accelerators

In recent years considerable effort has been devoted to developing very high intensity small accelerators for the production of common positron-emitters, mainly on hospital sites [*cf.* the detailed presentations at Targetry Workshops in Vancouver (1989) and Villigen (1991)]. The major stipulated advantages of such accelerators include small size, a low activation of components, a low neutron background, and hence almost no requirement for shielding. In general three concepts and designs have been projected:

— Deuteron accelerating cyclotron, 3.6 MeV d^+, 70 μA, for producing exclusively oxygen-15 via the $^{14}N(d,n)^{15}O$ reaction on nitrogen gas
— Tandem cascade accelerator, 3.7 MeV p^- or d^-, 1 mA, for producing oxygen-15 via the $^{14}N(d,n)^{15}O$ reaction and fluorine-18 via the $^{18}O(p,n)^{18}F$ reaction
— ^{3}He Radiofrequency quadrupole accelerator, 8 MeV ^{3}He, 15 mA, for producing nitrogen-13 via $^{12}C(^3He,d)^{13}N$, oxygen-15 via $^{16}O(^3He,\alpha)^{15}O$ and fluorine-18 via $^{16}O(^3He,p)^{18}F$ reactions

In principle all three concepts appear to be promising, although the use of the helium-3 beam may be associated with more difficulties. In practice, however, only technology that withstands the stringent test of reliability and simplicity will be acceptable, especially in a hospital environment.

We consider the production of the two major PET radioisotopes oxygen-15 and fluorine-18 at a low energy accelerator in more detail (*cf.* Qaim, 1992). The excitation functions of the commonly used reactions, $^{14}N(d,n)^{15}O$ and $^{18}O(p,n)^{18}F$, are shown in Figure 9 (reproduced from Vera Ruiz and Wolf, 1977; Ruth and Wolf, 1979; Sajjad *et al.*, 1984, 1985). A calculation of the integral oxygen-15 yield for an 'on-gas' deuteron energy of 3.2 MeV leads to a value of 222 MBq/μA, (6 mCi/μA) which is 6.7% of the yield with 10 MeV deuterons. Evidently, to obtain an initial oxygen-15 activity of about 11 GBq (300 mCi), a beam current of about 50 μA on the nitrogen gas target is mandatory. This is achievable with the present day technology; indeed the routine production of oxygen-15 with a small accelerator has now been demonstrated at Hammersmith Hospital. In the case of fluorine-18, on the other hand, the integral yield at E_p = 3.7 MeV amounts to 33 MBq/μAh (0.9 mCi/μAh) and corresponds to only 1.15% of the yield at 15 MeV. Beam currents of about 500 μA are needed to obtain a batch of about 10 GBq (270 mCi) of fluorine-18. The production of intense beams is not a great problem; however, the construction of a target system capable of withstanding such intense beams involves a new dimension in targetry. A thin film of ^{18}O-enriched water cooled at the back by liquid nitrogen, as suggested in one concept, may be promising but practical utility and cost-effective economics have yet to be demonstrated.

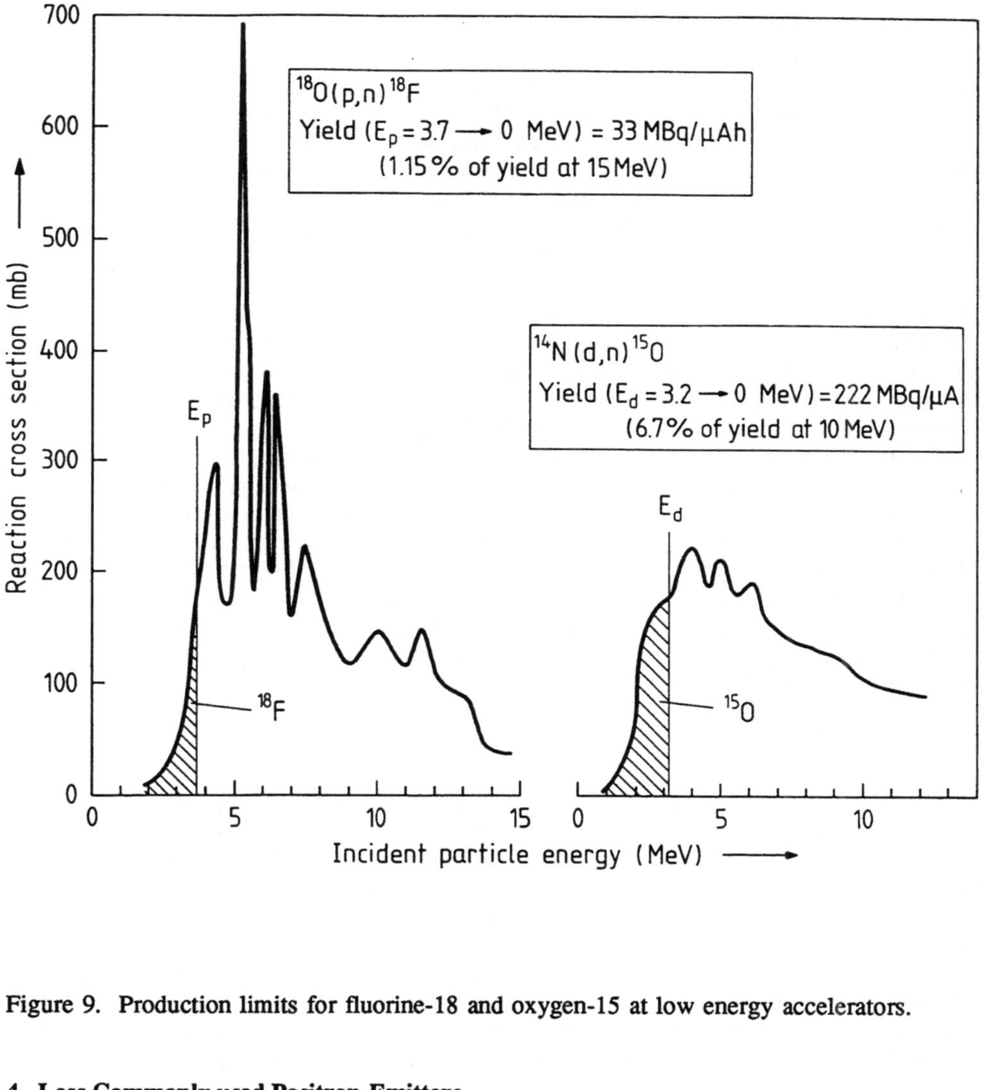

Figure 9. Production limits for fluorine-18 and oxygen-15 at low energy accelerators.

4. Less Commonly used Positron-Emitters

The less commonly used positron-emitters for PET studies include potassium-38, selenium-73, bromine-75 and bromine-76. Furthermore, the positron-emitters, phosphorous-30, manganese-52^m, iron-52, copper-64, krypton-77, rubidium-81 and rubidium-82^m have also found limited applications. Rubidium-82^m ($t_{1/2}$ = 6.2 h) may be of special interest as a longer-lived substitute for generator-produced rubidium-82 ($t_{1/2}$ = 1.3 min), although the radiation dose is somewhat high (see Kovács *et al.*, 1991). In this section we limit ourselves to a description of the production methods of the first four of the aforementioned positron-emitters (Table 1).

4.1. POTASSIUM-38

Potassium-38 ($t_{1/2}$ = 7.6 min; I_{β^+} = 100%; E_{β^+} = 2.7 MeV) has found application in myocardial blood flow studies using PET, although three other competing agents, [^{13}N]ammonia, [^{15}O]water and $^{82}Rb^+$, are more widely used because they are easier to produce with low energy cyclotrons or via a generator system. Among the various methods suggested for the production of potassium-38 (Meyers, 1973; Lambrecht *et al.*, 1978b; Helus *et al.*, 1980; Tilbury *et al.*, 1980; Vandecasteele *et al.* , 1981; Yagi and Amano, 1981; Daube and Nickles, 1985; Guillaume *et al.*, 1988; Qaim *et al.*, 1988; Blessing and Qaim, 1990) the ^{35}Cl(α,n)-process at a medium energy cyclotron is most convenient, the optimal energy range being (E_α = 22→7 MeV). Irradiation of a sodium chloride pellet with α-particles at beam currents of about 10 μA leads to sufficient quantities (500 MBq; 14 mCi) for one patient study. The irradiated pellet has simply to be dissolved in water and, after sterile filtration, is ready for human application. The level of long-lived radioactive impurities like sodium-22 ($t_{1/2}$ = 2.6 a) is very small (< 10^{-4}%).

In an attempt to produce potassium-38 at a small cyclotron, Tárkányi *et al.* (1992) recently investigated the ^{38}Ar(p,n)-process using 95.7% enriched gas as target material. Determination of the excitation function and the measurement of production yields under high current irradiation conditions revealed that, in the optimal energy range of E_p = 16→12 MeV, the yield from this reaction is an order of magnitude higher than that from the ^{35}Cl(α,n)^{38}K process. The ^{38}Ar(p,n)-process, however, has two drawbacks. Firstly, the highly enriched argon-38 is expensive (one target fill is approximately US $10,000) and secondly, the recovery of argon-38 is more problematic as compared to krypton-82 or xenon-124 (used for producing of ^{81}Rb/^{81m}Kr generators and ^{123}I, respectively).

4.2. SELENIUM-73

Selenium-73 ($t_{1/2}$ = 7.1 h; I_{β^+} = 65%; E_{β^+} = 1.32 MeV) is a potentially interesting sulphur analogue for application in PET. It can be produced via several nuclear processes (Guillaume *et al.*, 1978; Nozaki *et al.*, 1979; Mushtaq *et al.*, 1988; Mushtaq and Qaim, 1990; Plenevaux *et al.*, 1990). Detailed comparative studies (Mushtaq *et al.*, 1988; Mushtaq and Qaim, 1990) have, however, revealed that only the ^{75}As(p,3n)^{73}Se and ^{70}Ge(α,n)^{73}Se reactions (the latter using highly enriched target material) are of practical interest. In the latter case a $Cu_3{}^{70}Ge$ alloy was developed for irradiations with internal beams of 28 MeV α-particles and selenium-73 was separated by thermo-chromatography (Blessing *et al.*, 1992). However, the need for very high beam currents, the necessity of recovering the expensive target material, and the low batch yield of selenium-73 make this process rather unattractive. The method of choice is therefore the ^{75}As(p,3n)^{73}Se process.

The excitation functions of ^{75}As(p,xn)^{72,73,75}Se reactions are shown in Figure 10 (*cf.* Mushtaq *et al.*, 1988). Evidently the energy range E_p = 40→30 MeV is optimal for the production of selenium-73. The expected thick target yield of selenium-73 over this energy range is 1406 MBq/μAh (38 mCi/μAh) and the level of selenium-72/75 impurities < 0.1%. The major drawback of the process is the requirement of relatively high energy protons.

Only low current target materials like arsenic(III) oxide have been used so far for producing selenium-73 via the ^{75}As(p,3n)-process (Mushtaq *et al.*, 1988; Plenevaux *et al.*, 1990). The radioselenium is either separated by anion exchange chromatography or extracted directly into benzene. In the latter case the radioselenium is presumably in the

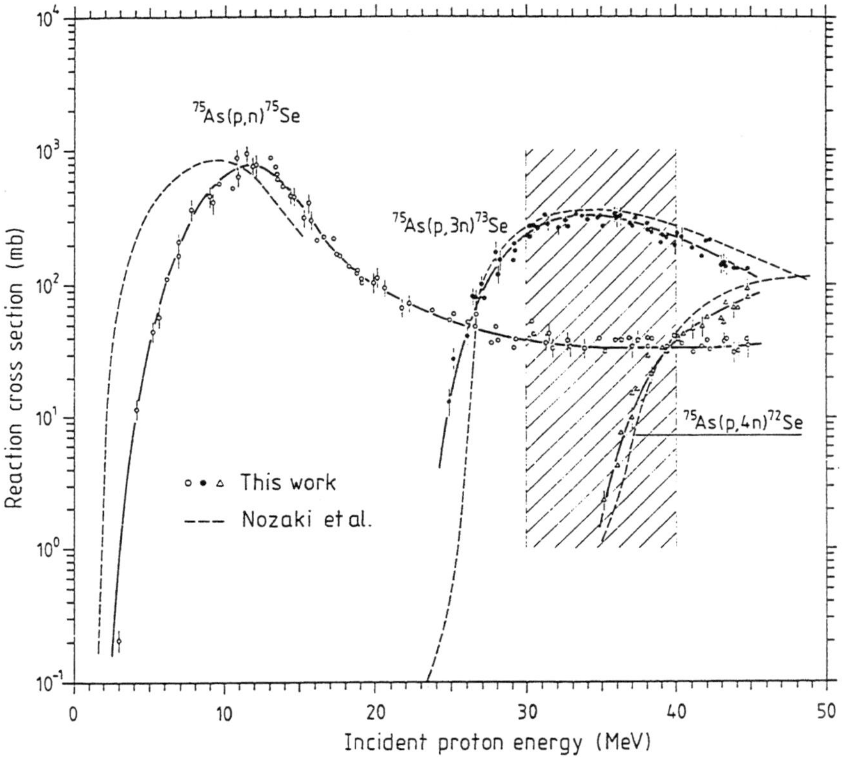

Figure 10. Excitation functions of ^{75}As(p,xn)^{72,73,75}Se reactions. The optimal energy range for the production of selenium-73 is E_p = 40→30 MeV (after Mushtaq *et al.*, 1988).

elemental form and is very suitable for subsequent labelling work (Plenevaux *et al.*, 1990). Attempts to produce large quantities of selenium-73 via development of high current target materials and efficient chemical separation methods are presently underway in several laboratories.

4.3. BROMINE-75

Bromine-75 ($t_{1/2}$ = 1.6 h; I_{β^+} = 75.5%; E_{β^+} = 1.74 MeV) is the most useful radionuclide of bromine for PET studies. For its production several nuclear reactions have been suggested (for reviews see Qaim and Stöcklin, 1983; Qaim, 1986b), out of which two processes, namely ^{75}As(^{3}He,3n)^{75}Br and ^{76}Se(p,2n)^{75}Br, have proved to be most suitable. The thick target yields of bromine-75 expected from those reactions are given in Figure 11 as a function of incident particle energy. The major impurity associated with both the processes is bromine-76; its contributions under the optimal energy ranges are also given in Figure 11. Evidently, the

$^{76}Se(p,2n)^{75}Br$ reaction is more advantageous provided that $E_p \geq 25$ MeV and highly enriched target material are used. The $^{75}As(^3He,3n)^{75}Br$ reaction, on the other hand, makes use of natural arsenic. In both the cases solid targets are used.

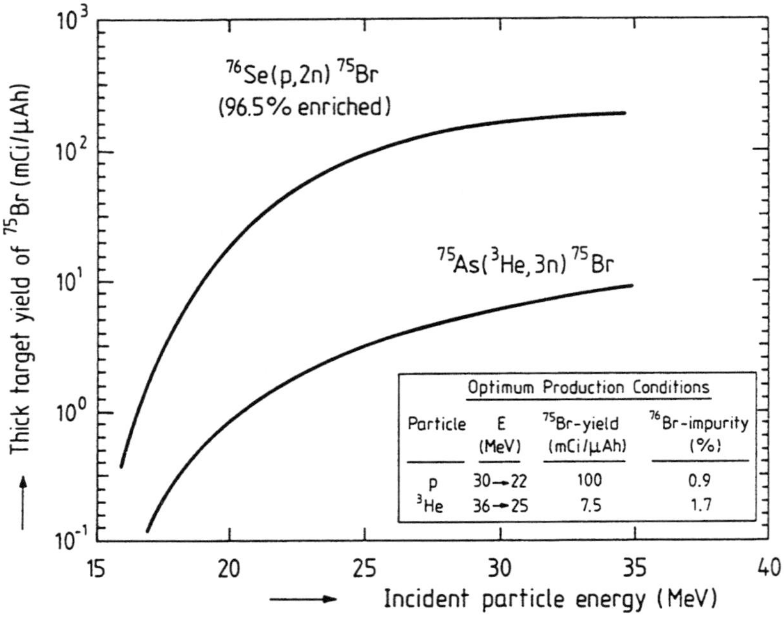

Figure 11. Thick target yields of bromine-75 calculated from the excitation functions (after Qaim *et al.*, 1986b).

In the case of $^{76}Se(p,2n)^{75}Br$ process, a few selenides (like Ag_2Se and Cu_2Se) were found to be suitable for irradiations with beam currents ≤ 7 µA (Paans *et al.*, 1980; Vaalburg *et al.*, 1985). In another approach an external rotating target system was developed (Kovács *et al.*, 1985) where it is possible to irradiate low melting elemental selenium-76 with proton beam currents up to 20 µA. The loss of selenium-76 after a 1 h irradiation amounts to < 1%. The separation of radiobromine from irradiated selenium-76 is effected by thermo-chromatography at 300°C. Radiobromine is taken up in a small volume of hot water. The loss of selenium-76 during the process is about 1% and the target can be reused. The radiochemical yield of bromine-75, however, is only 40%. Due to this reason the process has not found wide application.

The more widely used method for the production of bromine-75 is the $^{75}As(^3He,3n)$-reaction. A Cu_3As-alloy layer on a copper-backing is irradiated in the internal target system of a compact cyclotron with 36 MeV ^3He-particles at beam currents of about 100 µA (Blessing *et al.*, 1982; Blessing and Qaim, 1984). A sketch of the system is shown in Figure 12. The beam falls at an angle of 6.2° and only the back of the target holder is cooled. Radiobromine is separated from the irradiated target material via thermo-chromatography (at 950°C) and is taken up in 1 mL of hot water (*cf.* Blessing *et al.*, 1982). The radiochemical yield of bromine-75 is > 90%. Radiochromatographic analysis shows that bromine-75 is present only as [^{75}Br]bromide . The batch yield of bromine-75 is about 7 GBq (190 mCi). The main disadvantage of the process is the rather high level of bromine-76 impurity (6-8% at EOB).

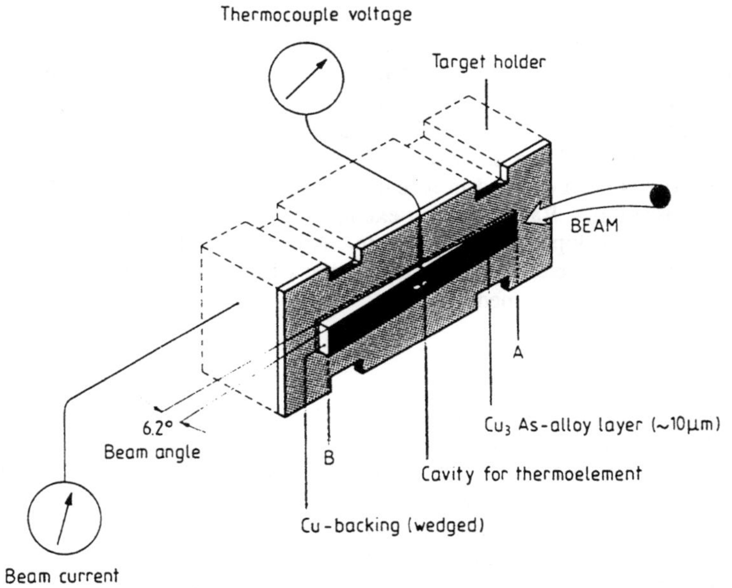

Figure 12. Sketch of the target and target holder used for irradiation with internal beams. The target consists of a thin layer of Cu_3As-alloy on a wedged copper backing. A thermoelement in a cavity in the middle of the target allows the adjustment of the beam (after Blessing and Qaim, 1984).

4.4. BROMINE-76

Bromine-76 ($t_{1/2}$ = 16.1 h; $I_{\beta+}$ = 57%; $E_{\beta+}$ = 3.9 MeV) has found very limited application because it causes a relatively high radiation dose. Nevertheless, this radioisotope seems to be suitable for longer-lasting PET studies, especially on animals (for a review see Mazière and Loc'h, 1986). Its production methods have been reviewed (Qaim, 1986b). The ^{75}As(^{3}He,2n)^{76}Br, ^{76}Se(p,n)^{76}Br and ^{77}Se(p,2n)^{76}Br processes have been suggested, although the latter two methods have not been used practically, mainly due to the difficulty in targetry with highly enriched selenium-76 and selenium-77. The method of choice is the ^{75}As(^{3}He,2n)^{76}Br reaction over the energy range of $E_{^3He}$ = 18→10 MeV, although the yield is low. The production procedure for bromine-76 is the same as for bromine-75 (except for change in the energy range), and quantities up to 1 GBq (27 mCi) have been produced.

Somewhat lesser quantities have been produced via irradiation of elemental arsenic at medium currents, followed by separation of radiobromine via a wet chemical method (Mazière and Loc'h, 1986). The major impurity is bromine-77 ($t_{1/2}$ = 56 h) at a level of < 2%.

5. Generator-produced Positron-emitters

Several generator produced short-lived positron-emitters find application in PET studies at centres without a cyclotron. Their production methods have been reviewed (Lambrecht, 1983; Knapp and Butler, 1984; Clark, 1986; Guillaume and Brihaye, 1986; Qaim, 1987). Of all the systems suggested the ^{62}Zn(^{62}Cu), ^{68}Ge(^{68}Ga) and ^{82}Sr(^{82}Rb) systems are widely used. The decay characteristics of the six radionuclides concerned are summarised in Table 1. Considerable effort has been devoted in recent years to the investigation of chemical aspects of generator preparation. Based on ion-exchange chromatography a large number of generators have been developed for each system. A consideration of all those generators is beyond the scope of this chapter. Here the discussion will be limited to the production of the three parent radionuclides concerned.

5.1. ZINC-62

Copper-62 ($t_{1/2}$ = 9.7 min; $I_{\beta+}$ = 98%; $E_{\beta+}$ = 2.93 MeV) has found application in blood flow studies in heart and brain using PET (Green *et al.*, 1990), especially in chelated form. The parent zinc-62 ($t_{1/2}$ = 9.2 h) is generally produced via the ^{63}Cu(p,2n)-process at a medium-sized cyclotron (see Robinson, 1976; Robinson *et al.*, 1980; Fujibayashi *et al.*, 1989; Green *et al.*, 1990). The optimal energy range for production is E_p = 26→21 MeV. A copper disc or copper-electroplated aluminium sheet is irradiated with protons at high beam currents. After the decay of short-lived radionuclides, copper is dissolved in hydrochloric acid and the solution transferred to an anion-exchange resin column (AG 1X8, 100–200 mesh, Cl^- form). Copper is eluted with 3M-hydrochloric acid, followed by zinc-62 with distilled water. The product is of high radionuclidic purity. The copper concentration in the zinc-62 eluate is < 2 µg/mL (Fujibayashi *et al.*, 1989). The eluate is generally evaporated to dryness and the residue containing zinc-62 is dissolved in 2M-hydrochloric acid. This solution is then loaded onto an anion-exchange generator column for periodic 'milking off' of the copper-62.

The ^{63}Cu(p,2n)^{62}Zn reaction is a high yield process and 15 GBq (400 mCi) quantities of zinc-62 are easily produced (Green *et al.*, 1990). The ^{60}Ni (α,2n)^{62}Zn (Neirinckx, 1977) and ^{64}Zn(γ,2n)^{62}Zn (Yagi and Kondo, 1979) processes give relatively low yields and have therefore not been used for routine production of zinc-62. A direct production route for copper-62 via the ^{62}Ni(p,n)-reaction has also been suggested (Piel *et al.*, 1992). However, it could be of only limited application.

5.2. GERMANIUM-68

Gallium-68 ($t_{1/2}$ = 68.3 min; $I_{\beta+}$ = 90%; $E_{\beta+}$ = 1.9 MeV) is applied for measuring blood-brain barrier integrity as well as for tumour localisation. Furthermore, it is widely used for the attenuation correction of positron tomographs. The parent germanium-68 ($t_{1/2}$ =

271 d) is long-lived and rather difficult to produce. The $^{69}Ga(p,2n)^{68}Ge$ reaction has a high cross section but due to the long half-life of the product radioisotope the yield is low (Pao *et al.*, 1981; Loc'h *et al.*, 1982). Although a high current Ga_4Ni target capable of withstanding proton beams of up to 45 μA was developed (Loc'h *et al.*, 1982), the method has not found wide application due to the very long irradiation times needed. The method of choice is thus the spallation process. This radionuclide is therefore exclusively produced at large accelerators where long irradiations in parasitic positions are possible (see Grant *et al.*, 1982; Robertson *et al.*, 1982). The purification of the product involves several multi-step wet chemical processes. The main impurity is germanium-71 ($t_{1/2}$ = 11.2 d) at a level of 3% at 60 d after EOB.

5.3. STRONTIUM-82

Rubidium-82 ($t_{1/2}$ = 1.3 min; $I_{\beta+}$ = 96%; $E_{\beta+}$ = 3.35 MeV) is mainly used for myocardial blood flow studies and has found rather wide application. The production methods for the parent strontium-82 ($t_{1/2}$ = 25 d) have been reviewed (Waters and Coursey, 1987; Tárkányi *et al.*, 1988, 1990). In principle several processes can be used, for example helium-3- and α-particle-induced reactions on natural krypton (Tárkányi *et al.*, 1988, 1990), (p,4n) reaction on rubidium-85 (Horiguchi *et al.*, 1980; Mausner *et al.*, 1987; Huszár *et al.*, 1989) and, above all, the spallation of molybdenum with high energy protons. In practice, however, the spallation process is the method of choice. The yields in ^{3}He- and α-particle-induced reactions are low and very long irradiations are needed. The (p,4n) reaction is a high yield process but targetry is rather difficult. The major quantities of strontium-82 are therefore presently produced via spallation of molybdenum at high energy accelerators where, similar to germanium-68 production, long parasitic irradiations are possible (see Robertson *et al.*, 1982; Thomas, 1987). Product is purified via multi-step wet chemical separations. The main impurity is strontium-85 ($t_{1/2}$ = 65 d) at a level of about 50% (EOS). On the other hand, the (p,4n) reaction has a great potential, both with regard to strontium-82 yield and strontium-85 impurity.

6. References

Ache H.J. and Wolf A.P. (1968) The effect of radiation on the reactions of recoil carbon-11 in the nitrogen-oxygen system. *J. Phys. Chem.*, 72, 1988–1993.

Alexoff D., Schlyer D.J. and Wolf A.P. (1989) Recovery of [^{18}F]fluoride from [^{18}O]water in an electrochemical cell. *Appl. Radiat. Isot.*, 40, 1–6.

Alfassi Z.B. and Weinreich R. (1982) The production of positron emitters ^{75}Br and ^{76}Br: Excitation functions and yields for ^{3}He and α-particle induced nuclear reactions on arsenic. *Radiochim. Acta*, 30, 67–71.

Bair J.K., Miller P.D. and Wieland B.W. (1981) Neutron yields from the 4–12 MeV proton bombardment of ^{11}B, ^{13}C and ^{18}O as related to the production of ^{11}C, ^{13}N and ^{18}F. *Int. J. Appl. Radiat. Isot.*, 32, 389–395.

Beaver J.E., Finn R.D. and Hupf H.B. (1976) A new method for the production of high concentration ^{15}O-labelled carbon dioxide with protons. *Int. J. Appl. Radiat. Isot.*, 27, 195–197.

Berridge M.S. and Kjellstrom R. (1989) Fluorine-18 production: new designs for O-18 water targets. *J. Label. Compd. Radiopharm.*, 26, 188–189. (Abstract).

Berridge M.S. and Tewson T. (1986a) Effects of target design on the production and utilization of [^{18}F]fluoride from [^{18}O]water. *J. Label. Compd. Radiopharm.*, 23, 1177–1178. (Abstract).

Berridge M.S. and Tewson T.J. (1986b) Chemistry of ^{18}F radiopharmaceuticals. *Appl. Radiat. Isot.*, 37, 685–693.

Berridge M.S., Terris A.H. and Cassidy E.H. (1990) Low-carrier production of [^{15}O]oxygen, water and carbon monoxide. *Appl. Radiat. Isot.*, 41, 1173–1175.

Bida G.T., Ehrenkaufer R.L., Wolf A.P., Fowler J.S., MacGregor R.R. and Ruth T.J. (1980a) The effect of target-gas purity on the chemical form of F-18 during ^{18}F-F_2 production using the neon/fluorine target. *J. Nucl. Med.*, 21, 758–762.

Bida G., Ruth T.J. and Wolf A.P. (1980b) Experimentally determined thick target yields for the $^{14}N(p,\alpha)^{11}C$ reaction. *Radiochim. Acta*, 27, 181–185.

Bida G., Wieland B.W., Ruth T.J., Schmidt D.G., Hendry G.O, Keen K.E. (1986) An economical target for nitrogen-13 production by proton bombardment of a slurry of carbon-13 powder on O-16 water. *J. Label. Compd. Radiopharm.*, 23, 1217–1218. (Abstract).

Blaser J.P., Marmier P. and Sempert M. (1952) Anregungsfunktion der Kernreaktion $^{14}N(p,\alpha)^{11}C$. *Helv. Phys. Acta*, 25, 442–444.

Blessing G. and Qaim S.M. (1984) An improved internal Cu_3As-alloy cyclotron target for the production of ^{75}Br and ^{77}Br and separation of the by-product ^{67}Ga from the matrix activity. *Int. J. Appl. Radiat. Isot.*, 35, 927–931.

Blessing G. and Qaim S.M. (1990) A remotely controlled target and processing system for routine production of ^{38}K via the $^{35}Cl(\alpha,n)$-reaction. *Appl. Radiat. Isot.*, 41, 1229–1232.

Blessing G., Weinreich R., Qaim S.M. and Stöcklin G. (1982) Production of ^{75}Br and ^{76}Br via the $^{75}As(^3He,3n)^{75}Br$ and $^{75}As(\alpha,2n)^{77}Br$ reactions using Cu_3As-alloy as a high-current target material. *Int. J. Appl. Radiat. Isot.*, 33, 333–339.

Blessing G., Coenen H.H., Franken K. and Qaim S.M. (1986) Production of [^{18}F]F_2, $H^{18}F$ and $^{18}F^-_{aq}$ using the $^{20}Ne(d,\alpha)^{18}F$ process. *Appl. Radiat. Isot.*, 37, 1135–1139.

Blessing G. *et al.* (1988) KFA Jülich. *Unpublished results.*

Blessing G., Lavi N. and Qaim S.M. (1992) Production of ^{73}Se via the $^{70}Ge(\alpha,n)$-process using high current target materials. *Appl. Radiat. Isot.*, 43, 455–461.

Brodack J.W., Kilbourn M.R., Welch M.J. and Katzenellenbogen J.A. (1986) N.c.a. 16α–[^{18}F]fluoroestradiol-17ß: the effect of reaction vessel on fluorine-18 resolubilization, product yield, and effective specific activity. *Appl. Radiat. Isot.*, 37, 217–221.

Browne E. and Firestone R.B. (1986) *Table of Radioactive Isotopes*, John Wiley, New York.

Casella V.R., Christman D.R., Ido T. and Wolf A.P. (1978) Excitation function for the $^{14}N(p,\alpha)^{11}C$ reaction up to 15 MeV. *Radiochim. Acta*, 25, 17–20.

Casella V., Ido T., Wolf A.P., Fowler J.S., MacGregor R.R. and Ruth T.J. (1980) Anhydrous F-18 labeled elemental fluorine for radiopharmaceutical preparation. *J. Nucl. Med.*, 21, 750–757.

Chirakal R., Firnau G., Moore W., Nahmias C., Coates G. and Garnett E.S. (1992) [^{18}F]F_2 from ^{18}O gas target for direct electrophilic fluorination: synthesis of 6-[^{18}F]fluorodopamine. *J. Label. Compd. Radiopharm.*, 32, 275. (Abstract).

Clark J.C. (1986) Positrons from generators. In *Progress in Radiopharmacy*, Eds. P.H. Cox, S.J. Mather, C.B. Sampson and C.R. Lazarus. Martinus Nijhoff Publishers, Dordrecht, pp. 67–84.

Clark J.C. and Buckingham P.D. (1975) *Short-lived Radioactive Gases for Clinical Use*, Butterworth, London.

Clark J.C. and Oberdorfer F. (1982) Thermal characteristics of the release of ^{18}F from an Inconel-600 gas target. *J. Label. Compd. Radiopharm.*, 19, 1337–1339. (Abstract).

Clark J.C. and Tochon Danguy H. (1992) MRCCU Hammersmith. *Unpublished results.*

Clark J.C., Goulding R.W., Roman R. and Palmer A.J. (1973) The preparation of fluorine-18 labelled compounds using a recirculatory neon target. *Radiochem. Radioanal. Lett.*, 14, 101–108.

Clark J.C., Crouzel C., Meyer G.J. and Strijckmans K. (1987) Current methodology for oxygen-15 production for clinical use. *Appl. Radiat. Isot.*, 38, 597–600.

Clark J.C. *et al.*, (1990) MRCCU Hammersmith. *Unpublished results.*

Crouzel C., Langström B., Pike V.W. and Coenen H.H. (1987) Recommendations for a practical production of [^{11}C]methyl iodide. *Appl. Radiat. Isot.*, 38, 601–604.

Coenen H.H. (1989) No-carrier-added ^{18}F chemistry of radiopharmaceuticals. In *Synthesis and Applications of Isotopically Labelled Compounds*. Eds. T.A. Baillie and J.R. Jones. Elsevier, Amsterdam, p. 443.

Cooper A.J.L., Gelbard A.S. and Freed B.R. (1985) Nitrogen-13 as a biochemical tracer. *Adv. Enzymology*, 57, 251–355.

Dahl J.R. and Schlyer D. (1985) *Proceedings of First Workshop on Targetry and Target Chemistry*, Heidelberg, pp. 31–43.

Dahl J.R., Lee R., Bigler R.E., Schmall B. and Aber J.E. (1983) A new target system for the preparation of no-carrier-added ^{18}F-fluorinating compounds. *Int. J. Appl. Radiat. Isot.*, 34, 693–700.

Daube M.E. and Nickles R.J. (1985) Development of myocardial perfusion tracers for positron emission tomography. *Nucl. Med. Biol.*, 12, 303–314.

De Jesus O.T., Martin J.A., Yasillo N.J., Gatley S.J. and Cooper M.D. (1986) [^{18}F]Fluoride from a small cyclotron for the routine synthesis of [^{18}F]2-fluoro-2-deoxy-glucose. *Appl. Radiat. Isot.*, 37, 397–401.

Ehrenkaufer R.E., MacGregor R.R., Wolf A.P., Fowler J.S., Ruth T.J., Schlyer D.J. and Wieland B.W. (1983) Production of $H^{18}F$ by deuteron irradiation of a neon hydrogen target. *Radiochim. Acta*, 33, 49–56.

Epherre M. and Seide C. (1971) Excitation functions of ^{7}Be and ^{11}C produced in nitrogen by low energy protons. *Phys. Rev. C.*, 3, 2167–2171.

Ferrieri R.A. and Wolf A.P. (1983) The chemistry of positron emitting nucleogenic (hot) atoms with regard to preparation of labelled compounds of practical utility. *Radiochim. Acta*, 34, 69–83.

Fujibayashi Y., Matsumoto K., Yonekura Y., Konishi J. and Yokoyama A. (1989) A new ^{62}Zn/^{62}Cu-Generator as a copper-62 source for PET radiopharmaceuticals. *J. Nucl. Med.*, 30, 1838–1842.

Gandarias-Cruz D. and Okamoto K. (1988) Status on the compilation of nuclear data for medical radioisotopes produced by accelerators, *IAEA*, Vienna, Report-INDC(NDS)-209/GZ.

Grant P.M., Miller D.A., Gilmore J.S., O'Brien Jr. H.A. (1982) Medium-energy spallation cross sections. I. RbBr irradiation with 800-MeV protons. *Int. J. Appl. Radiat. Isot.*, 33, 415–417.

Green M.A., Mathias C.J., Welch M.J., McGuire A.H., Perry D., Fernandez-Rubio F., Perlmutter J.S., Raichle M.E. and Bergmann S.R. (1990) Copper-62-labeled pyruvaldehyde *bis*(N^4-methylthiosemicarbazonato) copper(II): synthesis and evaluation as a positron emission tomography tracer for cerebral and myocardial perfusion. *J. Nucl. Med.*, 31, 1989–1996.

Guillaume M. and Brihaye (1986) Generators for short-lived gamma and positron emitting radionuclides: current status and prospects. *Nucl. Med. Biol.*, 13, 89–100.

Guillaume M., Lambrecht R.M. and Wolf A.P. (1978) Cyclotron isotopes and radiopharmaceuticals - XXVII. ^{73}Se. *Int. J. Appl. Radiat. Isot.*, 29, 411–417.

Guillaume M., De Landsheere C., Rigo P. and Czichosz R. (1988) Automated production of potassium-38 for the study of myocardial perfusion using positron emission tomography. *Appl. Radiat. Isot.*, 39, 97–107.

Guillaume M. *et al.*, (1990) Liège. *Unpublished results.*

Guillaume M., Luxen A., Nebeling B., Argentini M., Clark J.C. and Pike V.W. (1991) Recommendations for fluorine-18 production. *Appl. Radiat. Isot.*, 42, 749–762.

Hamacher K., Coenen H.H. and Stöcklin G. (1986) Efficient stereospecific synthesis of no-carrier-added 2-[^{18}F]fluoro-2-deoxy-D-glucose using aminopolyether supported nucleophilic substitution. *J. Nucl. Med.*, 27, 235–238.

Hamacher K., Blessing G. and Nebeling B. (1990) Computer-aided synthesis (CAS) of no-carrier-added 2-[^{18}F]fluoro-2-deoxy-D-glucose: an efficient automated system for the aminopolyether-supported nucleophilic fluorination. *Appl. Radiat. Isot.*, 41, 49–55.

Helus F., Maier-Borst W., Sahm U. and Wiebe L. (1979) F-18 Cyclotron production methods. *Radiochem. Radioanal. Lett.*, 38, 395–440.

Helus F., Gasper H. and Maier-Borst W. (1980) Routine production of ^{38}K for medical use. *J. Radioanal. Chem.*, 55, 191–195.

Horiguchi T., Noma H., Yoshizawa Y., Takemi H., Hasai H. and Kiso Y. (1980) Excitation functions of proton induced nuclear reactions on ^{85}Rb. *Int. J. Appl. Radiat. Isot.*, 31, 141–151.

Huszár I. and Weinreich R. (1985) Production of ^{18}F with an ^{18}O-enriched water target. *J. Radioanal. Nucl. Chem. Lett.*, 93, 349–345.

Huszár I., Youfeng H., Jegge J. and Weinreich R. (1989) Development of a production process for ^{82}Sr. *J. Label. Compd. Radiopharm.*, 26, 168. (Abstract).

Iwata R., Ido T., Brady F., Takahashi T. and Ujiie A. (1987) [^{18}F]Fluoride production with a circulating [^{18}O]water target. *Appl. Radiat. Isot.*, 38, 979–984.

Iwata R., Ido T., Fujisawa Y. and Yamazaki S. (1988) On-line interconversion of [^{15}O]O_2 and [^{15}O]CO_2 via metal oxide by isotopic exchange. *Appl. Radiat. Isot.*, 39, 1207-1211.

Jacobs W.W., Bodansky D., Chamberlain D. and Oberg D.L. (1974) Production of Li and B in proton and alpha-particle reactions on ^{14}N at low energies. *Phys. Rev. C*, 9, 2134–2143.

Janssen A.G.M., Van den Bosch R.L.P., De Goeij J.J.M. and Theelen H.M.J. (1980) The reactions ^{77}Se(p,n) and ^{78}Se(p,2n) as production routes for ^{77}Br. *Int. J. Appl. Radiat. Isot.*, 31, 405–409.

Jewett D.M. (1991a) Aqueous carbonic acid: a readily removable electrolyte for the recovery of [^{18}F]fluoride from anion exchange resins. *Appl. Radiat. Isot.*, 42, 410–411.

Jewett D.M. (1991b) Ion exchange reaction of [^{18}F]fluoride with an oxidised carbon surface. *Appl. Radiat. Isot.*, 42, 519–523.

Jewett D.M., Toorongian S.A., Mulholland G.K., Watkins G.L. and Kilbourn M.R. (1988) Multiphase extraction: rapid phase-transfer of [^{18}F]fluoride ion for nucleophilic radiolabeling reactions. *Appl. Radiat. Isot.*, 39, 1109–1111.

Jewett D.M., Toorongian S.A., Bachelor M.A. and Kilbourn M.R. (1990) Extraction of [^{18}F]fluoride from [^{18}O]water by a fast fibrous anion exchange resin. *Appl. Radiat. Isot.*, 41, 583–586

Keinonen J., Fontell A. and Kaireto A-L. (1986) Effective small volume [^{18}O]water target for the production of [^{18}F]fluoride. *Appl. Radiat. Isot.*, 37, 631–632.

Keller K.A., Lange J., Münzel H. and Pfennig G. (1973) *Excitation Functions for Charged-particle Induced Nuclear Reactions*, Volume 5b, Springer-Verlag, Berlin/Heidelberg.

Kilbourn M.R. (1990) Fluorine-18 labelling of radiopharmaceuticals. *Nuclear Science Series NAS-NS3203*, National Academy Press, Washington D.C.

Kilbourn M.R., Hood J.T. and Welch M.J. (1984) A simple ^{18}O water target for ^{18}F production. *Int. J. Appl. Radiat. Isot.*, 35, 599–602.

Kilbourn M.R., Jerabek P.A. and Welch M.J. (1985) An improved [^{18}O]water target for [^{18}F]fluoride production. *Int. J. Appl. Radiat. Isot.*, 36, 327–328.

Knapp Jr. F.F. and Butler T.A., Eds. (1984) *Radionuclide Generators*, ACS Symposium Series, Washington D.C.

Kopecky P. (1985) Proton beam monitoring via the Cu(p,x)^{58}Co, ^{63}Cu(p,2n)^{62}Zn and ^{65}Cu(p,n)^{65}Zn reactions in copper. *Int. J. Appl. Radiat. Isot.*, 36, 657–661.

Kovács Z., Blessing G., Qaim S.M. and Stöcklin G. (1985) Production of ^{75}Br via the ^{76}Se(p,2n)^{75}Br reaction at a compact cyclotron. *Int. J. Appl. Radiat. Isot.*, 36, 635–642.

Kovács Z., Tárkányi F., Qaim S.M. and Stöcklin G. (1991) Production of 6.5 h ^{82m}Rb via the ^{82}Kr(p,n)-process at a low-energy cyclotron - a potential substitute for ^{82}Rb. *Appl. Radiat. Isot.*, 42, 831–834.

Krohn K.A., Link J.M., Lewellen T.K., Risler R., Eenmaa J. and Maier M. (1986) The use of 50 MeV protons to produce carbon-11 and oxygen-15. *J. Label. Compd. Radiopharm.*, 23, 1190–1192. (Abstract).

Lambrecht R.M. (1971) Positron emitting radionuclides — present and future status. In *Radiopharmaceuticals II*, Soc. Nucl. Med., New York, p. 753.

Lambrecht R.M. (1983) Radionuclide generators. *Radiochim. Acta*, 34, 9–24.

Lambrecht R.M., Neirinckx R. and Wolf A.P. (1978a) Cyclotron isotopes and radiopharmaceuticals. XXIII. Novel anhydrous ^{18}F-fluorinating intermediates. *Int. J. Appl. Radiat. Isot.*, 29, 175–183.

Lambrecht R.M., Hara T., Gallagher B.M., Wolf A.P., Ansari A. and Atkins H. (1978b) Production of potassium-38 for myocardial perfusion studies. *Int. J. Appl. Radiat. Isot.*, 29, 667–671.

Landais P. and Crouzel C. (1987). A new synthesis of carbon-11 labelled phosgene. *Appl. Radiat. Isot.*, 38, 297–300.

Lederer C.M. and Shirley V.S. (1978) *Table of Isotopes*. 7th ed., John Wiley, New York.

Lindner L., Helmer J. and Brinkman G.A. (1979) Water "loop"-target for the in-cyclotron production of ^{13}N by the reaction $^{16}O(p,\alpha)^{13}N$. *Int. J. Appl. Radiat. Isot.*, 30, 506–507.

Link J.M., Krohn K.A. and Courter J.H. (1991) Irradiation of water to improve ^{15}O specific activity. *J. Label. Compd. Radiopharm.*, 30, 115–116. (Abstract).

Loc'h C., Mazière B., Comar D. and Knipper R. (1982) A new preparation of germanium-68. *Int. J. Appl. Radiat. Isot.*, 33, 267–270.

Mausner L.F., Prach T. and Srivastava S.C. (1987) Production of ^{82}Sr by proton irradiation of RbCl. *Appl. Radiat. Isot.*, 38, 181–184.

Mazière B. and Loc'h C. (1986) Radiopharmaceuticals labelled with bromine isotopes. *Appl. Radiat. Isot.*, 37, 703–713.

Meyer G.J. (1982) Some aspects of radioanalytical quality control of cyclotron-produced short-lived radiopharmaceuticals. *Radiochim. Acta*, 30, 175–184.

Meyer G.J., Schober O., Bossaller C., Sturm J. and Hundeshagen H. (1984) Quantification of regional extravascular lung water in dogs with positron emission tomography, using constant infusion of ^{15}O-labelled water. *Eur. J. Nucl. Med.*, 9, 220.

Mulholland G.K., Hichwa R.D., Kilbourn M.R. and Moskwa J. (1989) A reliable water target for fluorine--18 production at high beam currents. *J. Label. Compd. Radiopharm.*, 26, 192–193. (Abstract).

Mulholland G.K., Kilbourn M.R. and Moskwa J.J. (1990) Direct simultaneous production of [^{15}O]water and [^{13}N]ammonia or [^{18}F]fluoride ion by 26 MeV proton irradiation of a double chamber water target. *Appl. Radiat. Isot.*, 41, 1193–1199.

Mushtaq A. and Qaim S.M. (1990) Excitation functions of α- and ^{3}He-particle induced nuclear reactions on natural germanium: evaluation of production routes for ^{73}Se. *Radiochim. Acta*, 50, 27–31.

Mushtaq A., Qaim S.M. and Stöcklin G. (1988) Production of ^{73}Se via (p,3n) and (d,4n) reactions on arsenic. *Appl. Radiat. Isot.*, 39, 1085–1091.

Myers W.G. (1973) Radiopotassium-38 for in vivo studies of dynamic processes. *J. Nucl. Med.*, 14, 359–360.

Nebeling B. *et al.* (1990) KFA Jülich. *Unpublished results.*

Neirinckx R.D. (1977) Excitation function for the $^{60}Ni(\alpha,2n)^{62}Zn$ reaction and production of ^{62}Zn bleomycin. *Int. J. Appl. Radiat. Isot.*, 28, 808–809.

Nickles R.J., Daube M.E. and Ruth T.J. (1984) An $^{18}O_2$ target for the production of [^{18}F]F_2. *Int. J. Appl. Radiat. Isot.*, 35, 117–122.

Nickles R.J., Gatley S.J., Votaw J.R. and Kornguth M.L. (1986) Production of reactive fluorine-18. *Appl. Radiat. Isot.*, 37, 649–661.

Nozaki T., Okuo T., Akutsu H. and Furukawa M. (1966) The radioactivation analysis of semiconductor graphite for nitrogen by the $^{14}N(p,\alpha)^{11}C$ reaction. *Bull. Chem. Soc. Japan*, 39, 2685–2690.

Nozaki T., Iwamoto M. and Ido T. (1974) Yield of ^{18}F for various reactions from oxygen and neon. *Int. J. Appl. Radiat. Isot.*, 25, 393–399.

Nozaki T., Itoh Y. and Ogawa K. (1979) Yield of ^{73}Se for various reactions and its chemical processing. *Int. J. Appl. Radiat. Isot.*, 30, 595-599.

Paans A.M.J., Welleweerd J., Vaalburg W., Reiffers S. and Woldring M.G. (1980) Excitation functions for the production of ^{75}Br: a potential nuclide for the labelling of radiopharmaceuticals. *Int. J. Appl. Radiat. Isot.*, 31, 267–272.

Pao P.J., Silvester D.J. and Waters S.L. (1981) A new method for the preparation of ^{68}Ga-generators following proton bombardment of gallium oxide targets. *J. Radioanal. Chem.*, 64, 267–272.

Parks N.J. and Krohn K.A. (1978) The synthesis of ^{13}N-labelled ammonia, dinitrogen, nitrite, and nitrate using a single cyclotron target system. *Int. J. Appl. Radiat. Isot.*, 29, 754–756.

Patt J.T., Nebeling B. and Stöcklin G. (1991) Water-target-chemistry of nitrogen-13 recoils revisited. *J. Label. Compd. Radiopharm.*, 30, 122–123. (Abstract).

Piel H., Qaim S.M. and Stöcklin G. (1992) Excitation functions of (p,xn)-reactions on ^{nat}Ni and highly enriched ^{62}Ni: possibility of production of medically important radioisotope ^{62}Cu at a small cyclotron. *Radiochim. Acta*, 57, 1–5.

Plenevaux A., Guillaume M., Brihaye C., Lemaire C. and Cantineau R. (1990) Chemical processing for production of no-carrier-added selenium-73 from germanium and arsenic targets and synthesis of L-2-amino-4-([^{73}Se]methylseleno)butyric acid (L-[^{73}Se]seleno-methionine). *Appl. Radiat. Isot.*, 41, 829–838.

Qaim S.M. (1982) Nuclear data relevant to cyclotron produced short-lived medical isotopes. *Radiochim. Acta*, 30, 147–162.

Qaim S.M. (1986a) Production of positron emitting radionuclides using cyclotrons. In *Progress in Radiopharmacy*. Eds. P.H. Cox, S.J. Mather, C.B. Sampson and C.R. Lazarus, Martinus Nijhoff Publishers, Dordrecht, pp. 85–98.

Qaim S.M. (1986b) Recent developments in the production of ^{18}F, ^{75,76,77}Br and ^{123}I. *Int. J. Appl. Radiat. Isot.*, 37, 803–810.

Qaim S.M. (1987) Cyclotron production of generator radionuclides. *Radiochim. Acta*, 41, 111–117.

Qaim S.M. (1992) Capabilities of low-energy accelerators for PET. *Annal. Universitatis Turkuensis*, D88, I1-I4. (Abstract).

Qaim S.M. and Stöcklin G. (1983) Production of some medically important short-lived neutron-deficient radioisotopes of halogens. *Radiochim. Acta*, 34, 25–40.

Qaim S.M., Blessing G. and Stöcklin G. (1987) Routinely used cyclotron targets for radioisotope production at KFA Jülich. *Proceedings of Second Workshop on Targetry and Target Chemistry*. Heidelberg, pp. 50–57.

Qaim S.M., Sutisna M.S. and Ollig H. (1988) Production of ^{38}K via the ^{35}Cl(α ,n)-process at a compact cyclotron. *Appl. Radiat. Isot.*, 39, 479–482.

Robertson R., Graham D., Trevena I.C. (1982) Radioisotope production via 500 MeV proton-induced reactions. *J. Label. Compd. Radiopharm.*, 19, 1368. (Abstract).

Robinson Jr. G.D. (1976) ^{62}Cu — a short-lived generator produced positron emitting radionuclide for radiopharmaceuticals. *J. Nucl. Med.*, 17, 559. (Abstract).

Robinson Jr. G.D., Zielinski F.W. and Lee A.W. (1980) The ^{62}Zn/^{62}Cu-generator: a convenient source of ^{62}Cu for radiopharmaceuticals. *Int. J. Appl. Radiat. Isot.*, 31, 111–116.

Root J.W. and Krohn K.A. (1981) Short-lived radionuclides in chemistry and biology. *Advances in Chemistry Series 197*, American Chemical Society, Washington D.C.

Ruth T.J. (1985) The production of [^{18}F]F_2 and [^{15}O]O_2 sequentially from the same target chamber. *Int. J. Appl. Radiat. Isot.*, 36, 107–110.

Ruth T.J. and Wolf A.P. (1979) Absolute cross sections for the production of ^{18}F via the ^{18}O(p,n)^{18}F reaction. *Radiochim. Acta*, 26, 21–24.

Sajjad M., Lambrecht R.M. and Wolf A.P. (1984) Cyclotron isotopes and radiopharmaceuticals XXXIV. Excitation function for the $^{15}N(p,n)^{15}O$ reaction. *Radiochim. Acta,* 36, 159–162.

Sajjad M., Lambrecht R.M. and Wolf A.P. (1985) Cyclotron isotopes and radiopharmaceuticals. XXXVI. Investigation of some excitation functions for the preparation of ^{15}O, ^{13}N and ^{11}C. *Radiochim. Acta,* 38, 57–63.

Sajjad M., Lambrecht R.M. and Wolf A.P. (1986) Cyclotron isotopes and radiopharmaceuticals. XXXVII. Excitation functions for the $^{16}O(p,\alpha)^{13}N$ and $^{14}N(p,pn)^{13}N$ reactions. *Radiochim. Acta,* 39, 165–168.

Schlyer D.J., Bastos M. and Wolf A.P. (1987) A rapid quantitative separation of fluorine-18 fluoride from oxygen-18 water. *J. Nucl. Med.,* 28, 764. (Abstract).

Schlyer D.J., Bastos M.A.V., Alexoff D. and Wolf A.P. (1990) Separation of [^{18}F]fluoride from [^{18}O]water using anion exchange resin. *Appl. Radiat. Isot.,* 41, 531–533.

Slegers G., Vandecasteele C., Sambre J. (1980) Cyclotron production of ^{13}N-labelled ammonia for medical use. *J. Radioanal. Chem.,* 59, 585–587.

Solin O. and Bergman J. (1986) Production of $^{18}F-F_2$ from $^{18}O_2$. *J. Label. Compd. Radiopharm.,* 23, 1202–1204. (Abstract).

Solin O., Bergman J., Haaparanta M. and Reissell A. (1988) Production of ^{18}F from water targets. Specific radioactivity and anionic contaminants. *Int. J. Appl. Radiat. Isot.,* 39, 1065–1071.

Steinbach J., Guenther K., Loesel E., Grunwald G., Mikecz P., Andó L., Szelecsényi F. and Beyer G.J. (1990) Temperature course in small volume [^{18}O]water targets for [^{18}F]F-production. *Appl. Radiat. Isot.,* 41, 753–756.

Stöcklin G. (1988) Spezielle Syntheseverfahren mit kurzlebigen Radionukliden und Qualitätskontrolle. Emissions-Computertomographie mit kurzlebigen Zyklotron-produzierten Radiopharmaka (Hundeshagen H., Ed.) Springer-Verlag, Berlin/Heidelberg, pp. 31–117.

Stöcklin G. and Wolf A.P., Eds. (1982, 1983) Radiochemistry related to life science. *Radiochim. Acta,* 30, 123 and 34, 1. (Combined special issue).

Straatman M.G. and Welch M.J. (1977) Fluorine-18 labelled diethylaminosulphur trifluoride (DAST): an F-for-OH fluorinating agent. *J. Nucl. Med.,* 18, 151–158.

Strijckmans K., Vandecasteele C. and Sambre J. (1985) Production and quality control of $^{15}O_2$ and $C^{15}O_2$ for medial use. *Int. J. Appl. Radiat. Isot.,* 36, 279–283.

Sunderland J.J., De Jesus O.T., Martin C.G. and Nickles R.J. (1989) Electrophilic F-18 from a small proton cyclotron. *J. Nucl. Med.,* 30 (Suppl.), 927. (Abstract).

Sunderland J.J., De Jesus O.T., Solin O. and Nickles R.J. (1990) Radiolabelling of pre-synaptic dopaminergic tracers with electrophilic F-18 from an 11 MeV proton cyclotron. *J. Nucl. Med.,* 31, 901. (Abstract).

Tárkányi F., Qaim S.M. and Stöcklin G. (1988) Excitation functions of ^{3}He- and α-particle induced nuclear reactions on natural krypton: production of ^{82}Sr at a compact cyclotron. *Appl. Radiat. Isot.,* 39, 135–143.

Tárkányi F., Qaim S.M. and Stöcklin G. (1990) Excitation functions of high-energy ^{3}He- and α-particle induced nuclear reactions on natural krypton with special reference to the production of ^{82}Sr. *Appl. Radiat. Isot.,* 41, 91–95.

Tárkányi F., Kovács Z., Qaim S.M. and Stöcklin G. (1992) Production of ^{38}K via the ^{38}Ar(p,n)-process at a small cyclotron. *Appl. Radiat. Isot.,* 43, 503–507.

Thomas K.E. (1987) Strontium-82 production at Los Alamos National Laboratory. *Appl. Radiat. Isot.,* 38, 175–180.

Tilbury R.S. and Dahl J.R. (1979) ^{13}N species formed by proton irradiation of water. *Radiat. Res.,* 79, 22–23.

Tilbury R.S., Myers W.G., Chandra R., Dahl J.R. and Lee R. (1980) Production of 7.6-min potasssium-38 for medical use. *J. Nucl. Med.*, 21, 867–871.

Vaalburg W., Kamphuis J.A.A., Beerling van der Molen H.D., Reiffers S., Rijskamp A. and Woldring M.G. (1975) An improved method for the cyclotron production of ^{13}N-labelled ammonia. *Int. J. Appl. Radiat. Isot.*, 26, 316–318.

Vaalburg W. and Paans A.M.J. (1983) Short-lived positron emitting radionuclides. In *Radionuclides Production II*. F. Helus, Ed., CRC Press, Florida, pp. 47–101.

Vaalburg W., Paans A.M.J., Terpstra J.W., Wiegman T., Dekens K., Rijskamp A. and Woldring M.G. (1985) Fast recovery by dry distillation of ^{75}Br induced in reusuable metal selenide targets via the $^{76}Se(p,2n)^{75}Br$ reaction. *Int. J. Appl. Radiat. Isot.,* 36, 961–964.

Vandecasteele C., Vandewalle T. and Slegers G. (1981) Production of ^{38}K using the $^{35}Cl(\alpha,n)^{38}K$ reaction. *Radiochim. Acta,* 29, 71–74.

Vera Ruiz H. and Wolf A.P. (1977) Excitation function for ^{15}O production via the $^{14}N(d,n)^{15}O$ reaction. *Radiochim. Acta,* 24, 65–67.

Vera Ruiz H. and Wolf A.P. (1978) Direct synthesis of ^{15}O-labelled water at high specific activities. *J. Label. Compd. Radiopharm.,* 15, 185–189.

Vogt M., Huszár I., Argentini M., Oehninger H. and Weinreich R. (1986) Improved production of $[^{18}F]$fluoride via the $[^{18}O]H_2O(p,n)^{18}F$ reaction for no-carrier-added nucleophilic syntheses. *Appl. Radiat. Isot.,* 37, 448–449.

Votaw J.R., Satter M.R., Sunderland J.J., Martin C.C. and Nickles R.J. (1986) The Edison lamp: $[^{15}O]$carbon monoxide production in the target. *J. Label. Compd. Radiopharm.*, 23, 1211–1213. (Abstract).

Waters S.L. (1990) Determination of $H_2{}^{18}O$ enrichment for ^{18}F targetry using a quadrupole mass spectrometer. *Appl. Radiat. Isot.*, 41, 686–688.

Waters S.L. and Coursey B.M., Eds. (1987) The $^{82}Sr/^{82}Rb$ generator. *Appl. Radiat. Isot.*, 38 (3), 171-240. (Special Issue).

Welch M.J., Ed. (1977) Radiopharmaceuticals and other compounds labelled with short-lived nuclides. *Int. J. Appl. Radiat. Isot.,* 28, 1. (Special issue)

Welch M.J. and Kilbourn M.R. (1985) A remote system for the routine production of ^{15}O-radiopharmaceuticals. *J. Label. Compd. Radiopharm.*, 22, 1193–1200.

Wieland B.W. and Wolf A.P. (1983) Large-scale production and recovery of aqueous $[^{18}F]$fluoride using proton bombardment of a small-volume $[^{18}O]$water target. *J. Nucl. Med.,* 24, P122. (Abstract).

Wieland B.W., Hendry G.O., Schmidt D.G., Bida G. and Ruth T.J. (1986a) Efficient small volume O-18 water targets for producing F-18 fluoride with low energy protons. *J. Label. Compd. Radiopharm.*, 23, 1205–1207. (Abstract).

Wieland B.W., Schmidt D.G., Bida G., Ruth T..J. and Hendry G.O. (1986b) Efficient, economical production of ^{15}O-labelled tracers with low energy protons. *J. Label. Compd. Radiopharm.*, 23, 1214–1216. (Abstract).

Wieland B.W., Bida G.T., Padgett H.C. and Hendry G.O. (1989) Current status of CTI target systems for the production of PET radiochemicals. *Proceedings of Third Workshop on Targetry,* Vancouver, Canada, pp. 34–49.

Wieland B., Bida G., Padgett H., Hendry G., Zippi E., Kabalka G., Morelle J.L., Verbruggen R., Ghyoot M. (1991) In-target production of ^{13}N-ammonia via proton irradiation of dilute aqueous ethanol and acetic acid mixtures. *Appl. Radiat. Isot.*, 42, 1095–1098.

Wieneke J. and Nebeling B. (1990) Improved method for ^{13}N-application in short term studies on NO_3^- fluxes in barley and squash plants. *Z. Pflanzenernähr Bodenk.*, 153, 117–123.

Winchell H.S., Wells D.K., Lamb J.F. and Beaudry S.B. (1976) Process for preparing fluorine-18. *United States Patent*, No. 3,981,769. (*Chem. Abstr.*, 85: 590)

Wolf A.P. and Jones W.B. (1983) Cyclotrons for biomedical radioisotope production. *Radiochim. Acta*, 34, 1–7.

Wolf A.P. and Redvanly C.S. (1977) Carbon-11 and radiopharmaceuticals. *Int. J. Appl. Radiat. Isot.*, 28, 29–48.

Yagi M. and Amano R. (1981) Production of carrier-free ^{38}K by means of photonuclear reactions. *Int. J. Appl. Radiat. Isot.*, 32, 225–227.

Yagi M. and Kondo K. (1979) A ^{62}Cu generator. *Int. J. Appl. Radiat. Isot.*, 30, 569–570.

7. Appendix 1. Sources of ^{18}O-Enriched Water

The most popular and effective method of producing fluorine-18 is now by the proton irradiation of ^{18}O-enriched water. Even with efficient recycling of irradiated water, stocks eventually diminish, become contaminated or decrease in enrichment. Reliable continuous production therefore rests on an ample supply of this rather expensive and sometimes elusive material. Known producers and their suppliers are as follows:

7.1. *Isotec Inc.* 3858 Benner Road, Miamisburg OH 45342, USA. Tel. 513 859 1808 and 800 448 9760. FAX 513 859 4878. Telex 288278. Easylink 62014510.

Suppliers:

— Campro Scientific, P.O. Box 316, 3900 AH Veenendaal, The Netherlands. (For Europe) Tel. 31 8385 29437. FAX 31 8385 42181.

— Isotec, 10 Avenue Ampère, B.P. 220, 78051 St. Quentin Cedex, France. Tel. 1 30 45 88 00. FAX 1 30 45 28 89.

7.2. *Iso-Yeda Co. Ltd.* At the Weizmann Institute of Science, P.O. Box 95. Rehovot, Israel.

Suppliers:

— Chemotrade GmbH, Lutzowstrasse 2, 4000 Düsseldorf 30, Germany.

— Medgenix Groups, Deutschland GmbH, 4030 Ratingen 1, Germany.

7.3. *Kernforschungszentrum Karlsruhe GmbH.* Postfach 3640, D-7500 Karlsruhe 1, Germany. Tel. 07247 82 0. FAX 07247/825070. Telex 17724716.

7.4. *Russian sources.*

Suppliers:

— International Chemical Trading Ltd., 17 Royal Parade Mews, Montpellier, Cheltenham, Glos., GL50 ISZ U.K. Tel. 0242 263163. FAX 0242 263303.

— Porfield Ltd., Anglesea Street, Dublin 2, Eire.

7.5. *Miscellaneous suppliers.*

— EG & G Mound Applied Technologies, Stable Isotope Sales, P.O. Box 300, Miamisburg, OH 45343 3000, USA. Tel. 513 865 3501/3502. FAX 513 865 3164.

— Europa Scientific Ltd, Europa House, Electra Way, Crewe, Cheshire CW1 1ZA, U.K. Tel./FAX 0270 589398. Telex 94011165. Easylink 19029480.

— CIL (Cambridge Isotope Laboratories), 20 Commerce Way, Woburn MA 01801, USA. Tel. 1 617 938 0067 (in Mass.) 1 800 322 1174 (Toll free). FAX 617 932 9721. Telex 951935.

— Icon Services Ltd., 19 Ox Bow Lane, Summit NJ 07901, USA. Tel./FAX 201 273 0449.

RADIOCHEMISTRY AUTOMATION FOR PET

Christian Crouzel, John C. Clark, Claude Brihaye, Bengt Långström, Christian Lemaire, Geerd J. Meyer, Bruno Nebeling and Sharon Stone-Elander

ABSTRACT. Methodological approaches to automation for PET radiochemistry are discussed. Detailed examples of automation using i) simple remote control, ii) PLC-operated devices and iii) computer-controlled devices are described for the syntheses of ^{11}C-, ^{15}O- and ^{18}F-labelled radiopharmaceuticals. Approaches to robot-based automation are also discussed and exemplified.

1. Introduction

PET requires compounds labelled with short-lived positron-emitting radioisotopes, such as oxygen-15, nitrogen-13, carbon-11 and fluorine-18 that have half-lives of 2, 10, 20 and 110 minutes, respectively. In order to label the compounds, several steps must often be carried out, ranging from production of the radioisotope as a primary in-target precursor, sequentially through to synthesis of a secondary labelling agent by an on-line or batch procedure, radiolabelling, purification and quality control. This chapter aims to discuss the need to automate these processes and to describe the approaches and methodologies that have been applied.

2. Why Automate?

Only if radiopharmaceutical production is safe, reliable and efficient can PET become a routine clinical tool. In radiopharmaceutical production the short half-lives of the radioisotopes render the total time taken by all the processes a fundamental consideration; it is therefore essential for all steps in each radiosynthesis to be as fast and efficient as possible. The short half-lives also mean that many radiosyntheses are required repetitively. These radiosyntheses must be reliable and easily repeatable for the efficient use of costly PET facilities. Radiosyntheses must usually start from high initial radioactivity but must also be safe to personnel. Automation, within a shielded environment, is increasingly seen as a solution to these key logistical and safety requirements. Furthermore, it must be emphasised that each radiopharmaceutical batch must also meet appropriate quality assurance standards (see Meyer *et al.*, this volume). Significantly, automation can also assist in establishing and complying with all aspects of necessary 'good manufacturing practice' (GMP).

G. Stöcklin and V. W. Pike (eds.), Radiopharmaceuticals for Positron Emission Tomography, 45–89.

3. What to Automate?

In some cases it is preferable to have a simple remotely controlled system rather than a completely automated system, as for example when the radiosynthesis is not very often required or when the radiosynthesis is expected to undergo large modification to increase radiochemical yield. Put simply, full automation should only be applied to radiosyntheses that have reached an adequate degree of refinement and understanding.

For these radiosyntheses all the following processes should be automated or at least remotely controlled:

— Radionuclide production *i.e.*
  - positioning of the target-holder, target cooling and filling with target material.
— Intermediate chemistry *i.e.*
  - production of precursor in-target
  - production of a gaseous labelling agent 'on-line' or of a batch labelling agent.
— Labelling chemistry
— Radiopharmaceutical purification
— Formulation and dispensing.

The following may also be considered for automation:

— Quality control
— Metabolite analysis.

What types of functions can be automated? In order to perform radiosyntheses, the control of reaction temperatures, reaction times, gas flows and pressures is especially important. Furthermore, the automation of all operations, such as radioactivity measurement, reagent additions and extractions, must be considered. These are all amenable to automation of various kinds.

4. How to Automate?

When the radiosynthesis of a certain radiopharmaceutical is selected for automation all the chemical procedures have to be carefully defined with respect to reagents, catalysts, temperatures, feedback parameters, volumes, concentrations, materials and chemicals. This process should take into account the requirement for specific radioactivity. These are the chemical criteria. Two further requirements of automation are ease of operation and ease of maintenance. The setting up of an automated radiosynthesis for operation will involve cleaning and drying and also the changing of reagents, flasks and purification materials. It is particularly important for the system to be easily maintainable to allow a repeat radiosynthesis after a relatively short period.

The process of automation starts by selecting the types of workstation required and their combination. There are four main approaches to automation:

— Remote-control, which may be at various levels of sophistication
— Programmable logic control (PLC) with timed steps, perhaps with feedback control
— Computer-aided automation
— Robotics.

In order to automate, means must be found to measure and control temperatures, to measure radioactivity, to dispense solvents, reagents and to perform purifications, whether by extraction (liquid-liquid, liquid-membrane or solid phase), selective affinity adsorption or chromatography, (such as HPLC). Furthermore, the materials constituting reactors or reaction flasks must be selected taking into account that most radiosyntheses need to be performed with large amounts of radioactivity at high specific radioactivity. Therefore, in any automation, attention must especially focus on:

— Materials in reactors, reaction flasks, tubings, transducers and valves
— Temperature controllers and regulators for reactors, reaction flasks and ovens
— Flow rate controllers and regulators
— Transducers
— Heaters, whether band heaters, heating wires, cartridge heaters (for use in block heaters), heating baths or air heaters (heat guns)
— Dispensing systems for reactors (reaction flasks)
— Extraction hardware (for solid-phase, liquid-liquid, liquid-membrane or gas-membrane extraction)
— Radioactivity detectors.

Specific radiosyntheses, which have been automated by the various non-robotic approaches mentioned above, will be presented. These will give an insight into the solutions that have been found to particular automation problems. This is followed by a general discussion of the robotic approach to automation, with a specific example of a multi-step synthesis. Finally, appendices deal with practical aspects of radioactivity detection (Appendix 1), valve selection (Appendix 2) and sources of glassy carbon reaction vessels (Appendix 3).

5. Examples of Remotely Controlled and Automated Radiosyntheses

5.1. THE REMOTE PRODUCTION OF [1-^{11}C]ACETATE (AS AT HANNOVER)

[1-^{11}C]Acetate is prepared by carboxylation of a Grignard reagent (methylmagnesium bromide) with cyclotron-produced [^{11}C]carbon dioxide (Pike *et al.*, 1982, 1984; Brown *et al.*, 1987; Walsh *et al.*, 1989; Westera, 1991; Meyer *et al.*, 1993). In order to set up [1-^{11}C]acetate production for routine clinical application in heart studies (Pike *et al.*, 1982, 1984; Buxton *et al.*, 1988, 1989; Walsh *et al.*,1989; Kotzerke *et al.*, 1990), a system must be developed which allows repeated synthesis by an easy and remote assembly. The main obstacle to complete automation in the early published procedures (*e.g.* Pike *et al.*, 1982, 1984) is the liquid extraction step that is used to separate [1-^{11}C]acetate from inorganic salts arising from the Grignard reagent. The modification described here is installed at Hannover and avoids this liquid extraction step. It was therefore easy to automate.

5.1.1. *Precursor handling.* After irradiation of nitrogen with protons the target gas is released into a vacuum system, and [^{11}C]carbon dioxide is collected from the target gas in a trap that is cooled in liquid nitrogen. [^{11}C]Carbon dioxide is then distilled into a special glass vessel, to which methylmagnesium bromide (0.1 mmol) in diethyl ether (1 mL) is added.

5.1.2. *Synthetic procedure.* The reaction vessel is connected to the synthesis apparatus shown in Figure 1. When in place the reaction mixture is warmed to 30–40°C for 5 min with a remotely controlled hot-air gun. The radioactive adduct is then hydrolysed by adding water (100 μL) from a pressure-driven dispenser. Organic solvents and decomposition products are removed by

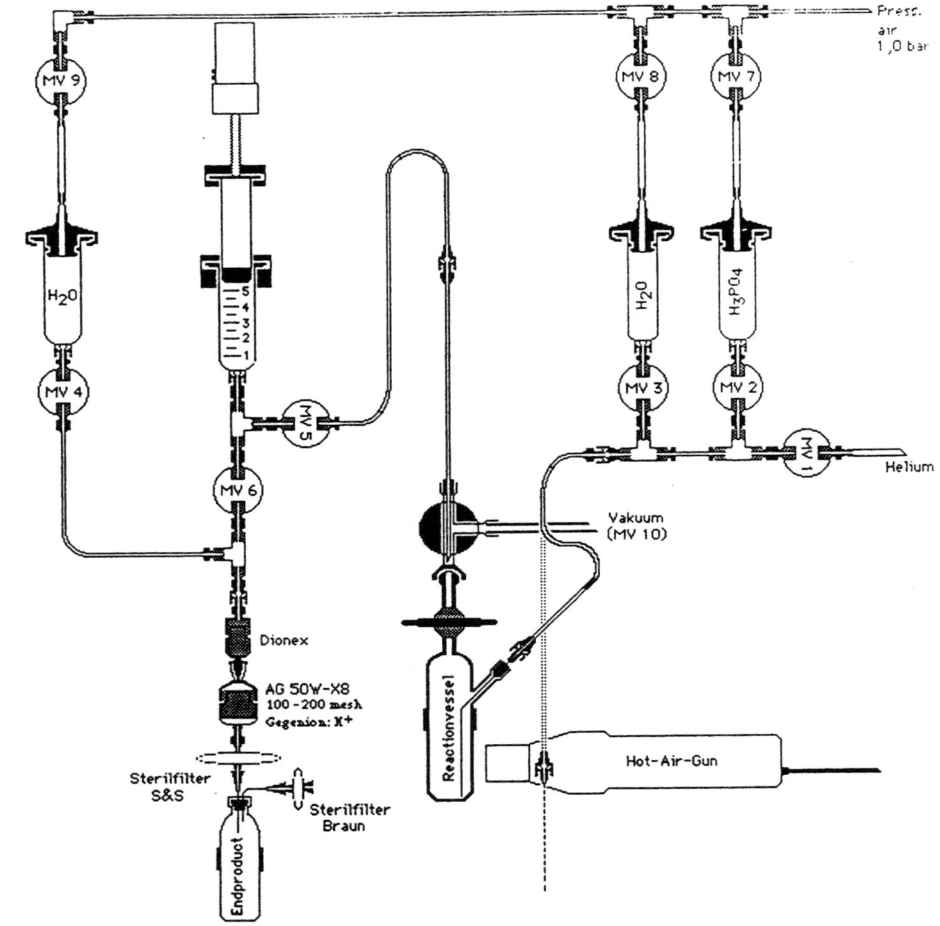

Figure 1. Apparatus for the production of [1-^{11}C]acetate (as at Hannover). MV signifies a solenoid valve.

warming the reaction mixture to 120°C under vacuum. The dry residue is redissolved in dilute phosphoric acid, added from another dispenser. Any free [^{11}C]carbon dioxide is then removed with a stream of helium and by warming to 60°C for 3 min. [1-^{11}C]Acetic acid, in dilute phosphoric acid, is then withdrawn from the reaction vessel into a motor-driven disposable syringe. Bromide and Mg^{2+} ions are removed from the product mixture by passage through a cartridge of silver oxide and cation exchange resin. Washing the purification line with water is performed to improve the radiochemical yield. The solution of purified product is passed through a sterile 0.22 μm filter and enters a sterile vessel containing sufficient sodium hydroxide to neutralise the phosphoric acid. The preparation takes 20 min from EOB. The overall radiochemical yield of [1-^{11}C]acetate is 60%. The radiochemical purity of [1-^{11}C]acetate is found to be > 98% by HPLC.

5.2. REMOTELY CONTROLLED SYNTHESIS WITH CARBON-11 (AS AT ORSAY)

At Orsay remote-control is preferred to full automation for synthesis with carbon-11. This approach is used in several hot-cells and the main advantage is great flexibility. It can be used for many types of synthesis from different labelling agents, including [^{11}C]iodomethane, [^{11}C]formaldehyde, [2-^{11}C]acetone and [1-^{11}C]acid chlorides. The system is based on the use of small pneumatically-powered jacks to move reaction flasks in two dimensions, horizontal and vertical. The jacks are controlled by the operator from a panel located on the front of the hot-cell. The different vials are connected by catheters and can be isolated by remotely operated valves.

5.2.1. *[^{11}C]Carbon dioxide production.* [^{11}C]Carbon dioxide is produced by the $^{14}N(p,\alpha)^{11}C$ reaction on nitrogen (99.9999% purity) and collected in a stainless steel trap immersed in liquid argon. The end of trapping is read from an ionisation chamber. The valves and the cryotrap movements are controlled by the operator.

5.2.2. *Production of labelling agents.* The synthesis of [^{11}C]iodomethane is based on the classical method (Comar *et al.*, 1974; Långström and Lundqvist, 1976), as recommended by Crouzel *et al.* (1987). A two-pot synthesis is used. The syntheses of [^{11}C]formaldehyde, [2-^{11}C]acetone and [1-^{11}C]acid chlorides are based on the methods of Marazano *et al.* (1977), Berger *et al.* (1980) and Luthra *et al.* (1985, 1990), respectively. Heating, cooling and valve-switching are controlled by the operator.

5.2.3. *Labelling.* The labelling agent is distilled into the cold precursor solution with a flow of nitrogen. Maximal transfer of radioactivity is read from an ionisation chamber. For the labelling reaction, the vial is isolated by remotely controlled valves. All stages are controlled by the operator.

5.2.4. *HPLC purification.* The radiopharmaceutical is purified by HPLC. The loop of the injector is filled via a dip-tube from the diluted reaction mixture by applying gas overpressure within the reaction flask. The HPLC eluate containing the labelled product is identified by the operator by monitoring radioactivity and UV absorbance. The labelled product is collected in a flask by manual and remote switching of the fraction collect/waste valve and then heated to evaporate solvent.

5.2.5. *Components of the system.* All the used components are commercially available. The whole unit consists of five sub-units:

— Heating unit: 4 furnaces with fingers resistances (50–250°C)

— Power units and numerical temperature regulators (3 each, all *ex* Vulcanic Co.).

— Pneumatic unit: 7 jacks (6 for vertical displacement, 1 for horizontal displacement) operated by 7 electro-pneumatic units (*ex* Télémécanique Co.).

— Chemistry unit: 2 mL Reacti-vials™ each with a Teflon™-faced silicon septum (3 mm thick) retained by a Quickfit™ cap. The needles are by Becton

Dickinson. The 7 valves with pneumatic actuator are by Rheodyne. They are controlled by 4 electro-pneumatic units. Gas flows are measured by flow meters (Brooks). Radioactivities are monitored by ionisation chambers from Service Development Scientifique (SDS).

— HPLC unit: injection into the HPLC loop is carried out by pressure through a Rheodyne™ valve operated by an electro-pneumatic unit. The HPLC detectors are an ionisation chamber (SDS) for radioactivity and a UV absorbance detector for mass. After evaporation of the solvent, the radiopharmaceutical is dissolved in a physiologically acceptable medium (2–3 mL). This is then transferred into a small evacuated sterile vial using a recovery vial penetrator.

5.2.6. *Performance of the system.* The system is used for the routine production of [*S-methyl*-^{11}C]methionine (Comar *et al.*, 1976), [*N-methyl*-^{11}C]MQNB (Mazière *et al.*, 1982), [*N-methyl*-^{11}C]flumazenil (Mazière *et al.*, 1984) and [*N-methyl*-^{11}C]PK 11195 (Camsonne *et al.*, 1984) from [^{11}C]iodomethane, and several other labelled compounds from other precursors in non-routine production. 3.7–7.4 GBq (100–200 mCi) of each radiopharmaceutical is produced with a specific radioactivity of about 37 GBq/µmol (1 Ci/µmol) at EOS.

5.3. AUTOMATION OF ^{11}C-METHYLATIONS USING A PLC (AS AT HAMMERSMITH HOSPITAL)

Many ^{11}C-labelled compounds of great interest to PET clinical science have now been prepared by the methylation of suitable precursors using [^{11}C]iodomethane and the number continues to grow. At Hammersmith Hospital, in order to respond to the varied needs of a busy clinical research programme, a hot-cell has been successfully equipped with a ^{11}C-methylation facility that can be quickly set up and operated to produce radiopharmaceutical batches for clinical use. The sequence of operations that is needed to achieve each radiosynthesis is controlled in timed steps by a Programmable Logic Controller (PLC). This incorporates a 'plug-in' module that can be programmed to suit each individual radiosynthesis (Clark and Dowsett, 1992).

5.3.1. *[^{11}C]Carbon dioxide production.* [^{11}C]Carbon dioxide is produced by the proton irradiation of high purity nitrogen gas via the ^{14}N(p,α)^{11}C reaction. For labelling operations it is advantageous to concentrate the [^{11}C]carbon dioxide into a few millilitres from a volume of several litres of target gas. An automated cryotrap fabricated from a small coil of stainless steel tubing (20 cm x 1/16" o.d.) cooled in liquid argon is used. The use of liquid argon avoids the problematical co-trapping of significant volumes of nitrogen which occurs if liquid nitrogen is used as the coolant. The valves and cryotrap movement are controlled by the PLC's programme.

5.3.2. *Production of [^{11}C]iodomethane.* The synthesis of [^{11}C]iodomethane using the reaction of [^{11}C]carbon dioxide with lithium aluminium hydride (LAH) and subsequent reaction with hydriodic acid is now widely applied (for a review see Crouzel *et al.*, 1987). The major problem in this radiosynthesis is maintenance of the high specific radioactivity required for ^{11}C-labelled receptor ligands. This can principally be achieved by the use of high quality LAH in small quantities under carefully controlled carbon dioxide-free atmospheres and by working quickly (for a review see Crouzel *et al.*, 1987). The heating, cooling and sequencing of the valves for [^{11}C]iodomethane production are controlled by PLC programme.

5.3.3. *^{11}C-Methylation of precursor.* The conditions under which the precursor is methylated depend critically on the class of compound of interest and the subsequent work-up and purification procedures. An automated reaction vial penetrator is used (see Figure 2). This device allows the relevant precursor to be introduced together with the reaction solvent and base in a septum-sealed vial. [^{11}C]Iodomethane can then be distilled into the precursor solution via a round-tipped side-hole needle, which can be motor-driven through the septum under programme control. The needles can then be withdrawn and the vial lowered into the heating bath. The ^{11}C-methylation takes place for a pre-programmed time. The reaction mixture is extracted by re-inserting the needles and transferred to the loop of an HPLC injection valve. Again this sequence of events is controlled by the PLC.

5.3.4. *HPLC purification.* For some compounds, where the base and/or solvent are detrimental to the performance of the HPLC, sample-enrichment can be included in the programme of operations (see Figure 2). Here an injection loop (10 mL) is loaded with an aqueous wash of the reaction vial and the contents of this loop are then loaded onto a silica C-18 cartridge. This cartridge is washed with water and then back-eluted onto the main silica C-18 column for purification using the chosen eluent. The PLC controls the sequence of operations for the multi-port valves necessary to accomplish these steps. The HPLC eluate that contains the labelled product is identified by the operator by monitoring radioactivity and UV absorbance, and collected in the flask of a rotary evaporator by manual remote operation of the fraction collect/waste valve (see Figure 2).

5.3.5. *Product formulation.* Solvent is removed from the product by evaporation under reduced pressure using a micro-rotary evaporator, modified to allow it to be raised or lowered under the control of the PLC. Finally, under programme control, the formulation solvent is introduced into the flask and the resultant radioactive solution transferred via a millipore filter into a shielded shipping vial outside the hot-cell.

5.3.6. *Components of the system.* Wherever possible commercial components are used with little or no modification. A Toshiba EX40 industrial programmable logic controller, which uses ladder logic was chosen. The programme information is stored on a plug in Electronically Erasable Programmable Read Only Memory (EEPROM) module which can be interchanged readily. The controller contains relays that are suitable for low power (100–240 V a.c.; 2 A) and low voltage (24 V d.c.; 2 A) operations. Most of the valves and motorised drives are controlled directly by these relay outputs. The 240 V operated devices, such as heaters and pumps, are operated via isolating solid state relays. The two- and three-port Teflon™ diaphragm valves for liquid and vapour handling are by Angar Scientific [part nos 3682NC2430 and 368232430 for 24 V and up to 2 bar (30 psi) operation]. They have 1/4" x 28 threads in flat-bottomed ports suitable for use with low pressure chromatography fittings (*e.g.* 'Altex™', 'Omnifit™'). For gas handling the two- and three-port stainless steel valves are by Skinner [Honeywell Lucifer, part nos B2 RX 127 DC-2 and B14 DK 1075 DC-2 operated at 24 V for pressures up to 12 bar (330 psi) and 5.3 bar (80 psi), respectively]. The multi-port rotary valves are by Rheodyne. The low pressure Teflon™/Kel-F™ valve with 1/4" x 28 fittings is a six-port distribution valve with pneumatic actuator (part no 5011P). The HPLC valves are also by Rheodyne and are pneumatically-actuated stainless steel and Vespel™ (Dupont polyimide) rotary valves (part no 7010P). The rotary evaporator is a UV Micro (Heidolph) and has been modified to be raised and lowered pneumatically. The reaction vial for methylation is a Reacti-vial™ (Pierce, 1 mL) with a

Teflon™-faced silicon septum 3 mm thick retained by a Quickfit™ (Corning) SQ 13 cap. The penetration needles are by Hamilton with rounded tips and side holes (part no 100.090.218). The syringe drives and septum penetrator drives are of 'in house' design and manufacture and are 'screw and nut' devices driven by electric motor. The HPLC detectors are by Mini Instruments for radioactivity detection (model 7-10C with a MC10 G-M tube) and by Severn Analytical for UV absorbance detection (model SA 6506).

5.3.7. *Performance of the system.* The system has been used routinely (see Pike *et al.*, 1990) to produce clinical batches of *S*-[*N-methyl*-^{11}C]nomifensine (Ulin *et al.*, 1989) and [*O-methyl*-^{11}C]raclopride (Ehrin *et al.*, 1987). It was also set up to make [*N-methyl*-^{11}C]SCH 23990 (Halldin *et al.*, 1986) for a short period. The production of [*O-methyl*-^{11}C]raclopride in particular benefitted from the sample-enrichment facility. The production parameters for these radiosyntheses are listed below.

a. S-*[*N-methyl-*^{11}C]Nomifensine.*

[^{11}C]Iodomethane is trapped in a solution of *desmethyl-S*-nomifensine (5 mg) in ethanol (400 μL). Then the reaction pot is sealed and heated at 90°C for 5 min. The reaction mixture is purified by HPLC on a μ-Porasil™ column (30 X 0.8 cm i.d.; Waters Associates Inc.) eluted with chloroform-methanol (90:10 v/v) at a flow rate of 3 mL/min. The product is formulated in isotonic saline which is sterilised by millipore filtration. A decay-corrected radiochemical yield of 23% from [^{11}C]iodomethane provides 370–555 MBq (10–15 mCi) of *S*-[*N-methyl*-^{11}C]nomifensine ready for injection with a specific radioactivity of 15 GBq/μmol (405 mCi/μmol at EOS).

b. *[*O-methyl-*^{11}C]Raclopride.*

[^{11}C]Iodomethane is trapped in DMSO (400 μL) containing *desmethyl*-raclopride (2 mg) and sodium hydroxide solution (5M; 10 μL). The reaction pot is sealed and heated at 90°C for 5 min. The reaction mixture is purified by sample enrichment followed by reverse phase HPLC using a μ-Bondapak™ C-18 column (30 x 0.8 cm i.d.; Waters Associates Inc.) eluted with methanol-10mM ammonium dihydrogen phosphate solution (60:40 v/v) at 3 mL/min. The product is formulated in isotonic saline which is sterilised by millipore filtration. A decay-corrected radiochemical yield of 25% from [^{11}C]iodomethane provides 370–555 MBq (10–15 mCi) of [*O-methyl*-^{11}C]raclopride ready for injection with a specific radioactivity of 10 GBq/μmol (370 mCi/μmol at EOS).

c. *[*N-methyl-*^{11}C]SCH 23390.*

[^{11}C]Iodomethane is trapped in acetone (900 μL) containing *desmethyl*-SCH 23390 (1 mg). The reaction pot is sealed and heated at 90°C for 10 min. The acetone is then evaporated off. The reaction mixture is purified by HPLC on μ-Porasil™ column (30 X 0.8 cm i.d.; Waters Associates Inc.) eluted with chloroform-methanol-*aq.* ammonia (90:1:0.1 by vol.) at 3 mL/min. The product is formulated in isotonic saline which is sterilised by millipore filtration. A decay-corrected radiochemical yield of 40% from [^{11}C]iodomethane provides 0.37–1.11 GBq (10–30 mCi) of [*N-methyl*-^{11}C]SCH 23390 ready for injection.

Subsequently a second hot-cell has been equipped with a very similar system to extend the range of routinely available ^{11}C-labelled compounds within each working day, for example, to [*N-methyl*-^{11}C]PK 11195 (Camsonne *et al.*, 1984; Cremer *et al.*, 1992), [*N-methyl*-^{11}C]flumazenil (Mazière *et al.*, 1984) and L-[*N-methyl*-^{11}C]deprenyl (Fowler *et al.*,1987).

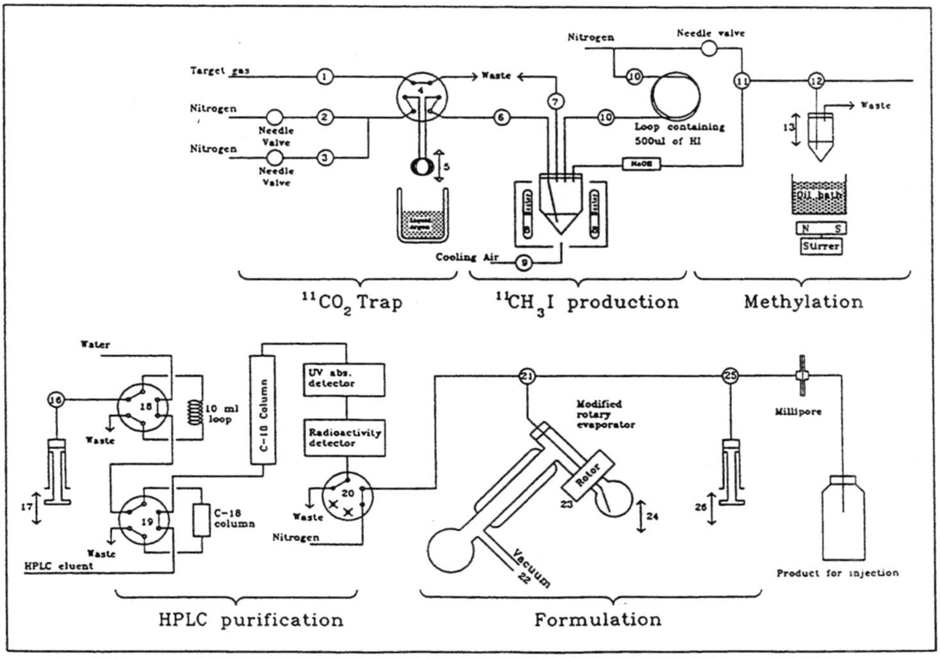

Figure 2. Scheme of PLC-controlled apparatus for labelling radiopharmaceuticals by methylation with [^{11}C]iodomethane (as at Hammersmith Hospital).

5.4. ON-LINE PREPARATION OF [^{11}C]IODOMETHANE AND [^{11}C]METHYL TRIFLATE (AS AT KFA JÜLICH).

5.4.1. *Introduction.* The reliable preparation of [^{11}C]iodomethane with high specific radioactivity and with a significantly reduced requirement for maintenance of the synthesis unit, by avoiding concentrated hydroidic acid as an iodination agent, are major objectives in the construction of a general methylation unit. A very important improvement in the synthesis of [^{11}C]iodomethane is the use of a column of triphenyphosphine di-iodide adsorbed on γ-alumina as the iodination agent (see Holschbach and Schüller, 1993a). An additional on-line column technique, the passage of [^{11}C]iodomethane through an alumina column which is charged with silver triflate, gives n.c.a. [^{11}C]methyl triflate as a highly reactive methylation agent (see Holschbach and Schüller, 1993b). Based on these column techniques, a fully automated unit for methylations with [^{11}C]iodomethane or [^{11}C]methyl triflate, incorporating feedback control and radiochromatography, has been developed in compliance with GMP. The set-up of the system is shown in Figure 3.

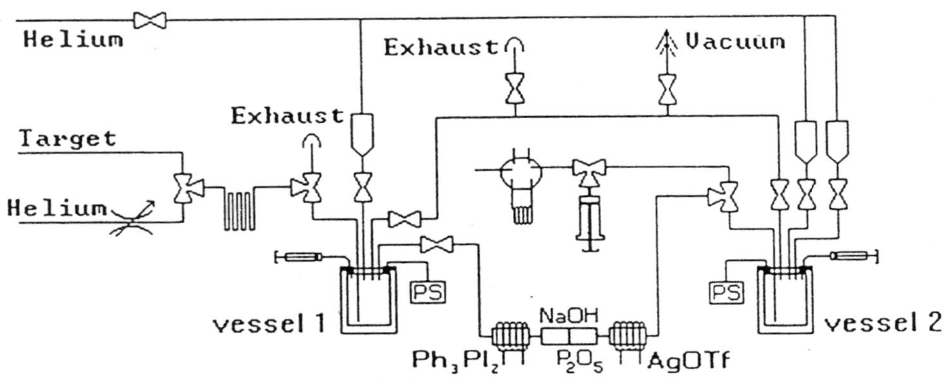

Figure 3. Scheme of the automated on-line preparation of [^{11}C]iodomethane and [^{11}C]methyl triflate (as at KFA Jülich).

5.4.2. *System operation.* The proton-irradiated nitrogen target gas (see Qaim *et al.*, this volume) is passed through a capillary tube at -193°C to -185°C, where the [^{11}C]carbon dioxide is trapped. The trap is temperature controlled from -196°C to 200°C. The [^{11}C]carbon dioxide is then transferred by a flow of helium into reaction vessel 1 and reduced by lithium aluminum hydride. Subsequent addition of a mixture of diethyleneglycol monobutyl ether and water releases [^{11}C]methanol, which is then converted into [^{11}C]iodomethane or into [^{11}C]methyl triflate by a column technique, as described above. ^{11}C-Methylation is performed in reaction vessel 2 by transferring the methylating agent into the precursor solution. Both vessels are temperature controlled from -196°C to 200°C. Also both reaction vessels have pneumatic drives to move the PEEK™ tubings in the vessels.

5.4.3. *System performance.* The preparation of [^{11}C]iodomethane takes 12 min from the end of bombardment and has a radiochemical yield of 90% based on [^{11}C]carbon dioxide. The mean specific radioactivity of the [^{11}C]iodomethane is > 222 GBq/µmol (6 Ci/µmol). HPLC purification of labelled products is performed on-line, including formulation to give an injectable solution.

5.5. AN ADVANCED SYSTEM FOR THE ADMINISTRATION OF [^{15}O]WATER (AS AT HAMMERSMITH HOSPITAL)

5.5.1. *Introduction.* The important blood flow tracer, [^{15}O]water, may be readily prepared by a variety of routes. However, several problems need to be addressed if safe and effective injections or infusions are to be prepared. Of primary concern is that the product should be free from any harmful impurities, both chemical and radioactive, and be sterile and apyrogenic. Due to the short half-life of oxygen-15, quality control of each sample or batch would be impractical. However, most groups carrying out work in this area have evolved safe operating procedures

(SOPs) which have been shown to be capable of maintaining the required standards (for recommendations on QA and QC see Meyer *et al.*, this volume). The measurement and delivery of the prepared doses of [^{15}O]water also requires careful attention both for the administrator and for the recipient. As a typical injected bolus of [^{15}O]water would be 3-3.7 GBq (80–100 mCi) the radiation dose to the administrator is of great concern. Automated injectors and infusers are at advanced stage of development in several laboratories and the commercial exploitation of these devices is anticipated.

5.5.2. *Design and operation of [^{15}O]water infuser.* Figure 4 schematically describes a 'bedside' [^{15}O]water infuser (dubbed 'R2D2') recently developed at the MRC Cyclotron Unit (Hammersmith Hospital) (Clark and Tochon Danguy, 1992). [^{15}O]Water is synthesised in the lead-shielded bedside device by mixing cyclotron-produced [^{15}O]oxygen (in 99% nitrogen-1% oxygen) with 5% hydrogen in nitrogen over a palladium catalyst in an oven at 200°C. The gaseous output is led to a semi-permeable membrane interface (Visking-Medicell International,

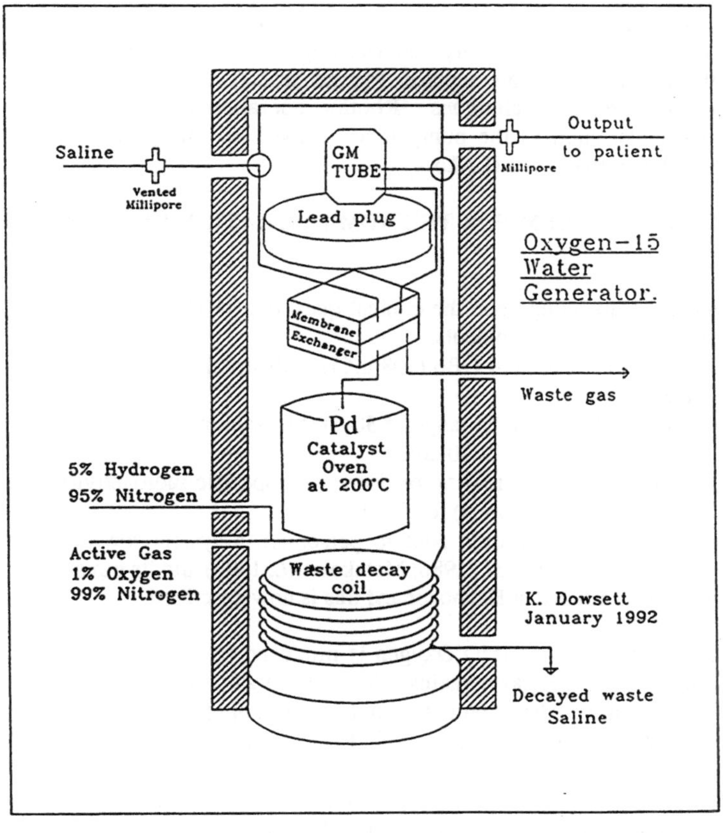

Figure 4. Schematic representation of the bedside [^{15}O]water synthesis apparatus (as at Hammersmith Hospital).

U.K.) sandwiched between Perspex (DWG No 15) blocks. The other side of the interface is flushed with sterile saline. [^{15}O]Water diffuses rapidly across the membrane and is taken up into the sterile saline. This is then infused into the subject for study via a shielded G-M tube and sterile millipore filter, using a pump (IVAC 560) approved for medical application. The fluid handling valves, for control of the infusion parameters, are three-port membrane valves (Angar/Asco, 368, 24 V). 'On-line' radioactivity detection is based on passing the radioactive saline through a loop of Teflon™ tubing (1/16" o.d.) wound around the G-M tube (Philips ZP-1300). The counts are taken into a scaler-ratemeter (Mini Instruments 6-90) modified with adjustable pre-scaler to allow direct calibration as 'mCi infused'. This calibration is routinely checked against a standard ionisation chamber. All controls and power supplies are designed and built to comply with electromedical safety standards. Non-used product is allowed to decay within the unit before discharge into a sterile bag. The device is typically operated to give an infusion for 2 min at a flow rate of 10 mL/min. The amount of radioactivity infused is determined by the mode of operation of the PET scanner (CTI-Siemens Neuro-PET) and is typically 560 MBq (15 mCi) for 'septa out' and 3 GBq (80 mCi) for 'septa in'.

5.5.3. *Infuser maintenance.* Pharmaceutical maintenance involves cleaning and sterilising the membrane exchanger prior to assembly and washing the fluid system with isotonic saline solution while the millipore filters are in place. Pyrogen tests (LAL) and sterility tests are carried out to validate the assembly techniques. Routine operation requires replacement of the disposable components, such as the pump tube, saline bag, millipore filters and infusion catheters, followed by pyrogen tests (LAL).

5.6. AN ADVANCED SYSTEM FOR THE ADMINISTRATION OF [^{15}O]WATER (AS AT HANNOVER)

5.6.1. *Introduction.* Depending upon the clinical question, [^{15}O]water for blood flow studies may be administered by different protocols:

— Bolus injection of up to 4 GBq (108 mCi) with strictly defined and repeatable input function.
— Steady state infusion in the range of 50–300 MBq/min (1.35–8.1 mCi/min) at a flow rate of 2.5 mL/min for 30 min.
— Ramp infusion with increasing or decreasing specific radioactivity in the range of 0.2–1 GBq (5.4–27 mCi) for 5–10 min.

In order to minimise radiation dose to personnel, a system for the fully automated production of [^{15}O]water (Meyer *et al.*, 1986; Matzke *et al.*, 1993) and its infusion or injection by remote control has been installed at Hannover and this is now described.

5.6.2. *[^{15}O]Oxygen production.* [^{15}O]Oxygen is produced by the ^{14}N(d,n)^{15}O reaction in a nitrogen gas target. The target gas contains 0.5% oxygen as carrier and its mean transit time from the target is 2.2 min. The maximal activity at the input of the [^{15}O]water system is 6 GBq/min (160 mCi/min) at a target pressure of 14 bar (210 psi) and a beam current of 30 μA.

5.6.3. *[^{15}O]Water production.* The [^{15}O]water production and infusion system is mounted on a laboratory trolley standing beside the PET camera. All radioactive parts of this system, except the calibration devices, are shielded within a lead box of 20 x 30 x 20 cm inner shape with a 15 x 13 cm lead glass window. The wall thickness of the box is 5 cm. The window has an equivalent shielding factor (see Figure 5). Within the lead box the target gas enters a flow meter. Hydrogen (2 mL/min) is added downstream. The gas mixture passes through a tube oven, filled with about 0.2 g palladium (1%) catalyst on a charcoal support (4–8 mesh) which is held at a reaction temperature of 150–160°C. The resulting [^{15}O]water vapour is trapped in a four-necked flask filled with isotonic saline solution. The level of the saline in the flask is monitored by a set of ten light barriers. With a small gear pump, the [^{15}O]water is pumped out and into the calibration and infusion system. All devices within the lead box are fixed to a mounting plate, which can easily be lifted out of the box for maintenance. Outside the box is a flow meter with a needle valve for the control of the hydrogen gas flow, and also a second gear pump, which withdraws isotonic saline solution from an infusion bottle to fill the absorption flask inside the lead box. The radioactivity levels inside the absorption flask and in the waste line are monitored by two G-M counters and are registered by a pen-recorder.

The whole apparatus is operated under the command of an automatic system, which includes interlock devices in order to prevent mis-operations. For safety reasons all electrical parts which are in contact with the infusion system are driven by 12 V only.

Under maximal radioactivity load (bolus injection), the radiation dose at a distance of one metre from the apparatus is less then 30 μSv/h.

5.6.4. *Bolus injection.* The system for the bolus injection consists of a pneumatically-driven syringe (10 mL), placed in an ionisation chamber and a solenoid valve for switching flow direction. The connection to the patient is by an infusion tube and a sterile filter with a total void volume of 1.7 mL. The amount of [^{15}O]water inside the syringe is monitored by a set of ten pilot lamps at the control unit.

The system is operated in the following manner. The absorption flask is filled to a level of 11 mL. Then [^{15}O]oxygen production is started. When sufficient radioactivity (at least 1.7 times the desired injection radioactivity) is sampled, the labelled water is pumped into the injection syringe. This takes 15 s and gives approximately 1.3 times the injection dose within the syringe. Interlock circuits in the control unit prevent air from pumping into the syringe (minimum level in the absorption flask, 1 mL) and from mistakes in handling the system. Injection is started by pressing a push-button switch when the radioactivity has decayed to 1.2 times the injection dose. It may be stopped immediately at any time. The injection of 10 mL is completed within 7 s.

The whole procedure from start of bombardment to end of injection takes about 10 min, and the next run may be started immediately.

5.6.5. *Constant infusion and ramp infusion.* The radioactivity control unit for the constant infusion and ramp infusion methods is a G-M detector with a calibration loop (0.2 mL). It is connected to the patient by an infusion tube, a three-way valve and a sterilisation filter (void volume, 1.9 mL). In all cases a constant flow rate of 2.5 mL/min is maintained by pump 2.

For steady state infusion the saline volume in the absorption flask is kept constant to 13 mL by pump 1, which is under command of the level control system. The saline flow is started 4 min after the start of [^{15}O]oxygen production. An equilibrium is reached about 10 min later, when the infusion may be started. The radioactivity level of the infusion solution is pre-defined by the beam current and the flow rate of the target gas. The relatively large volume in the absorption flask buffers short deviations in beam current, so that an additional control mechanism for the radioactivity level is unnecessary. A deviation from the saline level in the absorption flask causes an alarm to signal, and both pumps will be switched off by the control unit at differences greater than 15%.

For the ramp infusion, the start procedure is the same as for constant infusion, except that the saline level is low (2 mL) for decreasing, and high (13 mL) for increasing specific radioactivities. When equilibrium is reached, the flow rate of pump 1 is set to a value grater or smaller than 2.5 mL/min. This will result in *e*-function shaped gradients. Linear gradients are realised by continuous variation of the flow rate of pump 1 under the control of an external ramp generator or a computer.

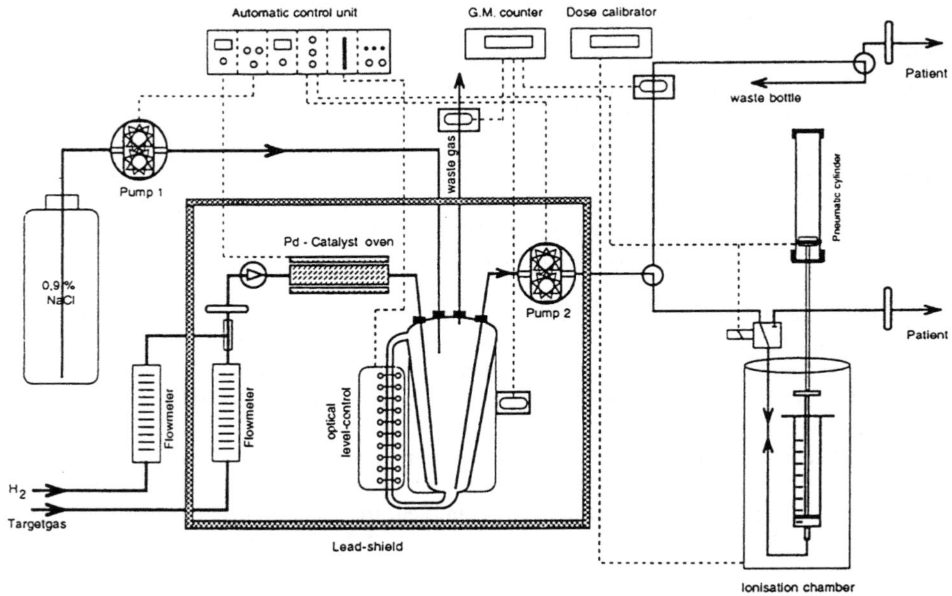

Figure 5. [¹⁵O]Water production system and infusion system, as at Hannover.

5.7. PRODUCTION AND QUALITY CONTROL OF *n*-[¹⁵O]BUTANOL USING A PLC (AS AT KFA JÜLICH)

5.7.1. *Introduction.* *n*-[¹⁵O]Butanol, because of its optimal lipophilicity (Berridge *et al.*, 1991; Walter *et al.*, 1993), is of great interest for measuring regional cerebral blood flow (rCBF) by PET. Labelled *n*-butanol, compared to [¹⁵O]water, is a freely diffusible tracer over a wider range of rCBF (Herscovitch *et al.*, 1987); the use of [¹⁵O]water rather than *n*-[¹⁵O]butanol may underestimate cerebral blood flow in regions with high flow rate (Herscovitch *et al.*, 1983). The efficient and reliable production of *n*-[¹⁵O]butanol, by an automated device that can provide several batches in sterile vials from only one set-up, is a prerequisite for the use of this perfusion tracer in PET.

The synthesis of *n*-[¹⁵O]butanol by reaction of molecular oxygen with tri-*n*-butylborane in tetrahydrofuran was first reported by Kabalka (1984) and by reaction with tri-*n*-butylborane loaded onto an alumina Sep-Pak™ by Kabalka *et al.* (1985) and Takahashi *et al.*, (1986). A procedure to synthesise *n*-[¹⁵O]butanol rapidly and sequentially in sufficient activity and purity for clinical use was soon developed (Berridge *et al.*, 1986). Remotely operated production systems have since been reported (Berridge *et al.*, 1990; Bauer and Wagner, 1991; Goodman *et al.*, 1991; Moerlein *et al.*, 1993).

5.7.2. *Design features.* At Jülich, in order to meet the clinical demand, there was a need for a device operated by a PLC that would be capable of producing up to eight batches of *n*-[^{15}O]butanol, each in four minutes, with built-in quality control (for QA/QC recommendations see Meyer *et al.*, this volume). The schematic form of the device that was built to meet this demand is shown in Figure 6. It was assembled from two 2-position-8-way valves, two pneumatic syringe pumps, two flow controllers, four 2-way diaphragm and six 3-way diaphragm valves. The system contains eight alumina and C-18 cartridges. The [^{15}O]oxygen activity trapped on the alumina cartridge and the activity of the final isotonic solution of the *n*-[^{15}O]butanol are monitored with calibrated G-M tubes. A pneumatic device for dispensing the filtered solution of *n*-[^{15}O]butanol into a shielded sterile and evacuated vial is also used. The system is controlled by a PLC with start, stop and delay push buttons. Up to eight productions of *n*-[^{15}O]butanol in isotonic saline containing 5% ethanol can be performed within a turn-around time of 15 min. For a second set-up of the system, easy replacement of the alumina and the C-18 cartridges is all that is required.

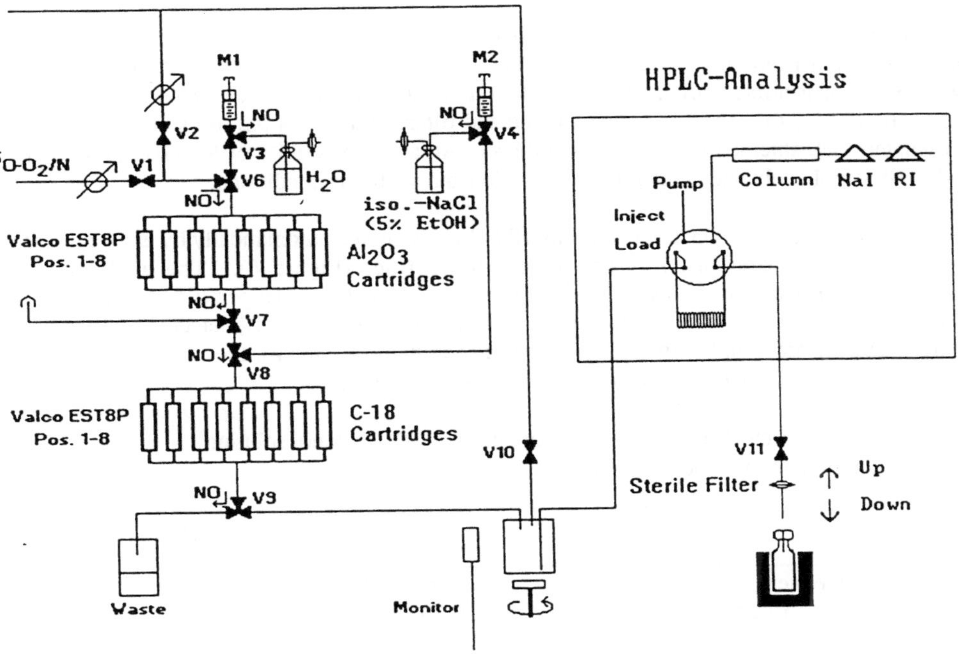

Figure 6. Schematic of the set-up for automated *n*-[^{15}O]butanol synthesis with built-in quality control by HPLC, as at KFA Jülich. VI-VII are diaphragm valves. M1 and M2 are pneumatic syringe pumps.

5.7.3. *System operation.* The production of oxygen-15 *via* the $^{14}N(d,n)^{15}O$ reaction is carried out at either of two cyclotrons, the JSW BC1710 or the CV28 in the Institute of Nuclear Chemistry in Jülich. The high current targets are constructed from aluminum and have a conical shape and a volume of 100 mL; they have as front window, a 50 µm Havar™ foil in the case of the JSW 1710 and a 330 µm aluminum plate to degrade the beam energy from 14 to 10 MeV in the case of the CV 28. The irradiated target gas (0.2% oxygen in nitrogen at a pressure of 5 bar, 75 psi), is typically bombarded with a 22 µA beam of 10 MeV deuterons for 10 min. After irradiation, the target gas is transported over a distance of 40 m through a stainless steel tube of 2 mm inner diameter at a flow rate of 1 L/min and passed for 55 s through an alumina cartridge, pre-loaded with tri-*n*-butyl-borane (80 µL).

$$B(n\text{-}Bu)_3 \xrightarrow{[^{15}O]O_2} B(n\text{-}Bu)(^{15}O\text{-}n\text{-}Bu)(O\text{-}n\text{-}Bu)$$

The hydrolysis of the ^{15}O-labelled *n*-butyl-borane complex with 3 mL of sterile endotoxin-free water takes about 56 s.

$$B(n\text{-}Bu)\text{-}^{15}O\text{-}(n\text{-}Bu)\text{-}O\text{-}(n\text{-}Bu) \xrightarrow{H_2O} n\text{-}Bu^{15}OH + n\text{-}BuOH + B(n\text{-}Bu)(OH)_2$$

The hydrolysed *n*-butyl-borane mixture is then passed into a C-18 cartridge for extraction of the *n*-[^{15}O]butanol from boron compounds. The *n*-[^{15}O]butanol is eluted from the C-18 cartridge with 5 mL of isotonic sodium chloride solution containing 5% ethanol. This procedure takes 73 s. In 45-50 s the eluted volume is mixed and filtered through a 0.2 µm sterile filter into an evacuated vial, shielded by lead (3.5 cm thick). An average activity of 5.5 GBq (150 mCi) of *n*-[^{15}O]butanol is obtained under these irradiation and synthesis conditions.

5.7.4. *Quality control.* Quality control by HPLC is performed automatically by analyzing 20 µL of the solution taken just in front of the sterile filter (Figure 6). The analysis of the *n*-[^{15}O]butanol by radio-HPLC is performed on a C-18 column (Hypersil™, 5 µm, 60 mm x 4 mm) eluted with 15% acetonitrile in water. A sodium iodide [NaI(Tl)] detector and a refractive index detector are coupled in series. Using the short C-18 column, the analysis time is only 1.25 min, just 25 s longer than the time needed for sterile filtration.

Table 1. Retention times and content of the *n*-[^{15}O]butanol solution determined by radio-HPLC, as at KFA Jülich.

	RT (s)	%	Carrier (mg/mL)
[^{15}O]Water	25	0.05 ± 0.02	-
sec-[^{15}O]Butanol	40	0.70 ± 0.2	0.2 ± 0.08
n-[^{15}O]Butanol	49	98.5 ± 0.7	4.8 ± 1.6

Table 1 gives the radioactive components present in *n*-[^{15}O]butanol solution, their HPLC retention times (RT), relative proportions and associated carrier. The radiochemical purity of *n*-[^{15}O]butanol obtained by radio-HPLC is 98.5 ± 0.7%. Only [^{15}O]water and *sec*-[^{15}O]butanol are detected as radioactive impurities. The amount of *n*-butanol carrier varies in the range of 22–28 mg per batch, which represents a chemical yield of about 34 ± 4% based on the starting tri-*n*-butyl-borane. The average specific radioactivity of *n*-[^{15}O]butanol is therefore about 13 GBq/mmol (350 mCi/mmol). The boron impurities, which cannot be determined by HPLC, are analyzed by atomic absorption spectroscopy. The average value is 2.7 ± 1.3 µg/mL. Figure 7 shows chromatograms for eight successive analyses, and their consistency.

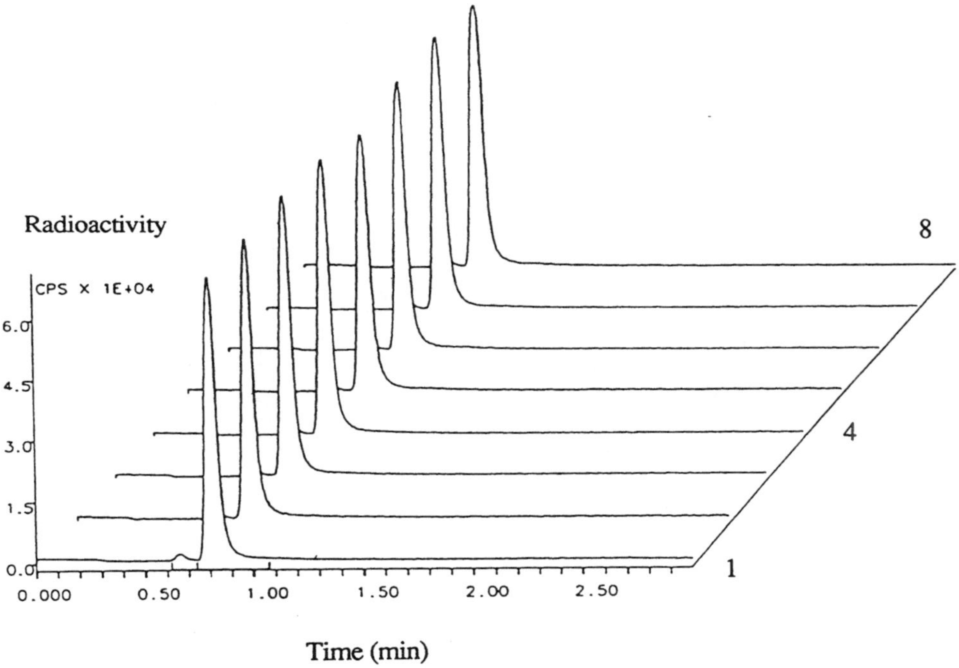

Figure 7. 3-D plot of the radioactivity channel of chromatograms from the quality control of eight successive productions of *n*-[^{15}O]butanol, as at KFA Jülich.

5.8. REMOTELY CONTROLLED SYNTHESIS OF L-6-[^{18}F]FLUORO-DOPA (AS AT HAMMERSMITH HOSPITAL)

5.8.1. *Introduction.* L-6-[^{18}F]Fluoro-DOPA is produced routinely as a marker for central dopaminergic neurons for clinical PET studies at the MRC Cyclotron Unit (Hammersmith Hospital). The radiochemistry used (see Pike *et al.*, 1990) is based on that originally described by Adam *et al.* (1986), as recommended by Luxen *et al.* (1992), namely electrophilic fluorination of a protected L-DOPA derivative [L-ethyl-*N*-acetyl-(β-3-methoxy-4-acetoxyphenyl)-alaninate] with [^{18}F]acetyl hypofluorite, followed by deprotection with hydriodic acid and HPLC separation of the 2- and 6-[^{18}F]fluoro-derivatives of L-DOPA.

5.8.2. *[18F]Fluorine production.* [^{18}F]Fluorine is produced by the deuteron (16.5 MeV; 13–16 μA) irradiation of neon (research grade, BOC Ltd) containing 0.2% v/v fluorine (research grade, BOC Ltd), initially at 200 psi. Target parameters and operating conditions are described in Guillaume *et al.* (1991). At the end of irradiation (90–120 min; 20–32 μAh) the [^{18}F]fluorine is introduced by stainless steel tubing (1/8" o.d.) into a lead-shielded hot-cell through a controllable needle valve (Nupro).

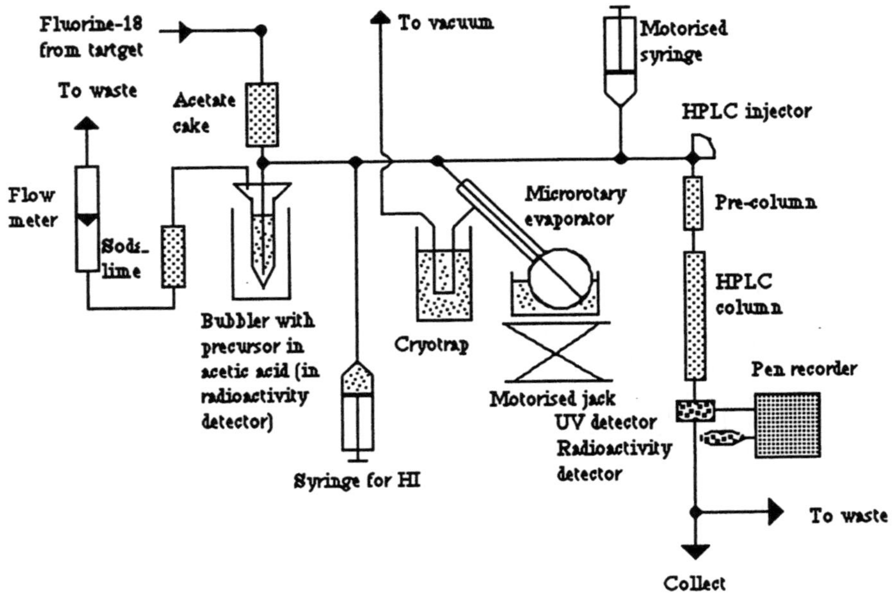

Figure 8. A schematic representation of apparatus for the remote production of L-6-[^{18}F]fluoro-DOPA, as at Hammersmith Hospital.

5.8.3. *Radiochemistry.* The set up of the cell is shown schematically in Figure 8. A stainless steel gauge (Budenberg) is used to monitor gas pressure between the target and needle valve. The fluorine-18 is led in Teflon™ (1/8"o.d.) tubing through a stainless steel cartridge containing sodium-acetate 'cake' and then into a glass bubbler containing a solution of precursor (70–100 mg) in glacial acetic acid (12–15 mL). This sits in a well-counter, thereby enabling the accumulation of radioactivity to be monitored. The outlet of the bubbler is a Teflon™ tube leading the gas to waste through a soda lime trap and flow meter (Meterate OPE RS1, ruby float). Swagelok™ stainless steel fittings are used to connect the tubing to the needle valve and to the cartridge. Altex™ fittings are used to connect the tubing to the bubbler and to the flow meter. The eight three-way switching valves that are used in the system are Rheodyne™ slider valves (model 5301 or 5302) with remotely controlled pneumatic actuators (model 5300). The bubbler is connected to a mini rotary evaporator (Buchi) which has its flask in a silicone oil bath (Heidolph HB140-0) at 165°C. The rotary evaporator is modified to have a liquid nitrogen cooled trap. The oil bath is mounted on a motorised lab-jack which can be raised or lowered by remote control. The acetic acid is taken into the rotary evaporator under reduced pressure through a Teflon™ dip-tube which for most of its length is held straight by a glass tube before finally terminating at the lowest part of the evaporation flask. Acetic acid is then removed from the radiofluorinated product by rotary evaporation. Then hydriodic acid (BDH, 'MAR', 1.5 mL plus hypophosphorous acid, 0.5 mL) is introduced into the rotary evaporator from a plastic syringe on the outside of the cell via Teflon™ tubing (1/16" o.d.). Hydrolysis is performed at 165°C for 20 min. Then the hydriodic acid is rotary evaporated off. Water (*ca* 3 mL) is three times added to the flask and evaporated. Finally 'neutralisation buffer' (KH_2PO_4, 71 g/L plus Na_2HPO_4, 69 g/L; pH 4; 1.5 mL) is added to the flask to dissolve the radioactive product. This is withdrawn into a plastic syringe mounted in a homemade syringe-drive (based on a remotely controlled motorised lead-screw).

5.8.4. *HPLC purification.* The contents of the syringe are injected into a remotely controlled pneumatically-operated HPLC injection valve (Rheodyne 7030, with 5701 actuator) through a vented millipore filter (Sterile Acrodisc, 0.2 µm; Gelman Sciences). The sample is remotely injected onto a preparative HPLC column (Nucleosil™ 5 C 18, 5 µm particle size, 25 cm x 20 mm i.d.) eluted at 6 mL/min with 70 mM-potassium dihydrogen phosphate solution. The eluate is monitored for absorbance at 280 nm and for radioactivity. The peak eluting after L-2-[^{18}F]fluoro-DOPA and with the same retention time as reference L-6-fluoro-DOPA is collected by remote operation of a waste/collect valve and diluted to 10 mL with the same buffer. Finally, this solution is sterilised by millipore filtration (0.22 µm pore size, Millex GS).

5.8.5. *System performance.* The collected product (190–560 MBq; 5–15 mCi) has an average radiochemical purity of 93.8% and an average specific radioactivity of 4–8 MBq/µmol (110–220 mCi/µmol) corrected to EOS. The preparation takes about two hours from EOB.

5.9. COMPUTER-AIDED AUTOMATION OF NUCLEOPHILIC RADIOFLUORINATION (AS AT KFA JÜLICH)

5.9.1. *Introduction.* 2-[^{18}F]Fluoro-2-deoxy-D-glucose (2-^{18}FDG) is currently one of the most important radiopharmaceuticals (see Fowler and Wolf, 1986; Coenen *et al.*, 1987). The increasing demand for 2-^{18}FDG has accelerated the design and construction of remotely controlled or automated procedures as well as laboratory robotic systems for its synthesis. In order to prepare 2-^{18}FDG routinely at Jülich by the favoured method (Coenen *et al.*, 1987) based on Kryptofix™ 2.2.2. (A.P.E. 2.2.2.)-mediated nucleophilic fluorination (Hamacher *et al.*, 1986), a computer-controlled modular apparatus was built. This includes a module for the rapid separation of [^{18}F]fluoride from [^{18}O]water for other nucleophilic fluorinations (Hamacher *et al.*, 1990).

5.9.2. *Computer control unit.* All processes in the synthesis of 2-^{18}FDG are electronically controlled by an IBM PC/AT clone equipped with standard peripherals. The microcomputer is allowed to communicate with an Optomux™ network via an RS 422/485 adapter card, which is plugged in directly and provides up to 4000 V isolation between the PC and the communication link. For standard input/output signals, three Optomux™ digital and one analog brain board with up to 16 I/0 channels are used. Six lines are programmed to read status information from the system, such as temperature, pressure, the level of liquid in the purification unit, and the actual scale of three radioactivity detectors. The temperature is controlled by a 12-bit digital-to-analog converter. A total number of 28 solenoid valves can be operated directly. In the Optomux™ unit an optical coupling is used to prevent any electrical feedback of the valves as they can induce high voltages when they are switched. As a programming language we have chosen Turbo-Pascal™. The run-down in a time-command sequence in the programme and the feedback of intensity factors, such as temperature and pressure, control the procedure of the radiosynthesis. The actual process carried out is described in a menu. Interruption and continuation of the automated process is possible at any time. A report, comprising the date, start and end of radiosynthesis, and the calculation of the radiochemical yield of 2-[18]FDG, is automatically provided.

5.9.3. *Apparatus design.* In accordance with GMP the apparatus is a closed system with helium overpressure. A schematic of the automated system is shown in Figure 9. The modules of the system are combined to achieve the shortest connections and smallest dead-volumes. The tubes are Teflon™ and the valves are air-actuated and Teflon™ membrane valves from Angar Scientific Co. Ltd (Rheodyne™ 7010, type 368 or 190, 24 V d.c.).

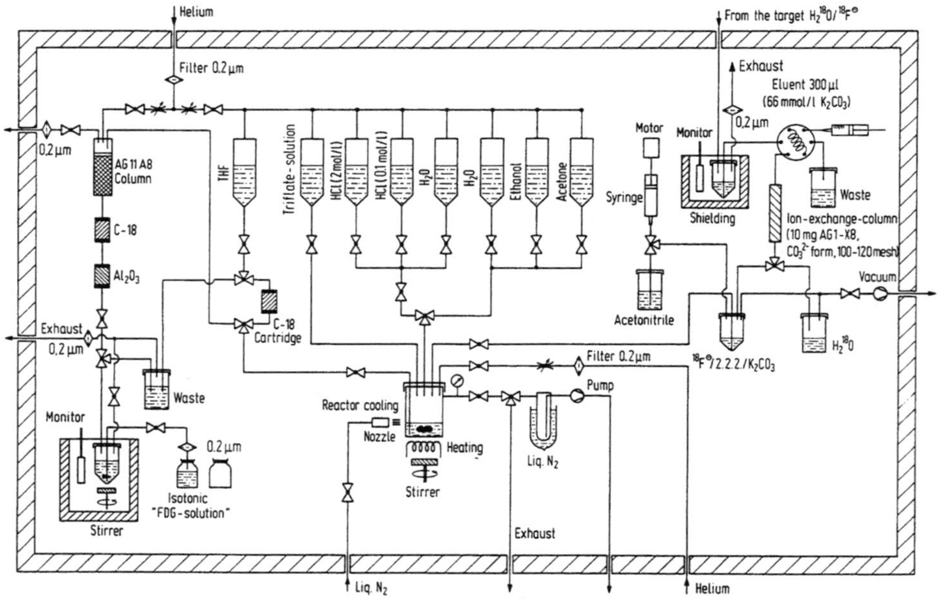

Figure 9. Schematic set-up of the automated system for 2-[18]FDG synthesis including the [^{18}F]fluoride-[^{18}O]water separation unit, as at KFA Jülich. The adjacent solvent reservoirs containing water, ethanol and acetone are only used for the automated cleaning of the apparatus.

5.9.4. *[^{18}F]Fluoride separation.* The fluoride separation unit is connected on-line to the [^{18}O]water target via a polypropylene tube. Before the [^{18}F]fluoride and the [^{18}O]water are separated, the water phase (1.5 mL) is collected in a degassing vessel and the total radioactivity monitored by a System 414 Monitor (Genitron Instruments). This vessel is connected to an air-actuated six-way valve (Valco, AC6W) that is combined with a small ion exchange column (20 x 2 mm) having a G1 Pyrex™ frit and a loop containing potassium carbonate solution. The outlet valve at the column connects to two vials: vial a) to collect the [^{18}O]water after fixation of the fluoride and vial b) to mix, using a motor-driven syringe, the [^{18}F]fluoride containing potassium carbonate solution with the appropriate amount of Kryptofix™ 2.2.2. solubilised in acetonitrile. The transport of the solution through the resin is accelerated by reducing the pressure to about 20 mbar at the end of the column using a vacuum pump.

5.9.5. *Reaction vessel.* The central part of the apparatus is a single unit reactor (Figure 10), for a

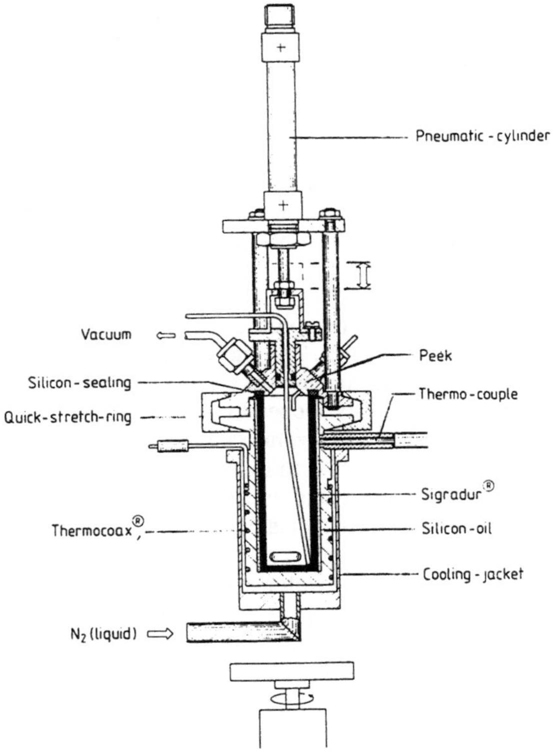

Figure 10. Sectional view of the single unit reactor with a cylindrical reaction vessel (17 x 70 mm) made of glassy carbon, as at KFA Jülich.

one-pot reaction system that contains a single heated reaction vessel combined with a rectangular arrangement of Teflon™ membrane valves and up to nine reagent reservoirs above the reactor. (For the 2-^{18}FDG synthesis only five reservoirs are used). The closed system allows reactions in isothermal and isometric conditions, in the range of ~ 0–2 bar (0–30 psi) as limited by the Teflon™ membrane valves. The cylindrical reaction vessel is made of glassy carbon (Sigradur™, 17 mm in diameter, 2 mm wall thickness and approximately 70 mm in height) surrounded by a copper cylinder with an integrated electric filament (Thermocoax™). The advantage of glassy carbon in comparison with glass is its extreme chemical resistance, low capacity for adsorption and more efficient heat conduction. The top of the glassy carbon vessel is closed by a stainless steel cover which is connected to the cylinder by a 'quick-stretch ring'. The small space between the glassy carbon and the copper cylinder is filled with silicone oil (*ca* 1 mL). Accordingly, the heat capacity is relatively low. The cylinder is surrounded by a steel coat with an inlet for liquid nitrogen at the bottom. (The injection of liquid nitrogen in a closed cooling jacket allows a temperature to be set in the range from 77–500°K, which is of interest in syntheses with [^{11}C]iodomethane).

5.9.6. *Purification unit.* The purification unit consists of a special glass column containing the AG11-A8 resin (Biorad) with a built in liquid level sensor (Honeywell, Dusseldorf) and an eluent reservoir at the top of the resin. The solenoid valves at the top and bottom of the purification column are switched automatically, depending on the signal of the liquid level sensor.

5.9.7. *Filling unit.* All the 2-^{18}FDG produced is collected in a glass vessel with lead shielding and measured by the System 414 Monitor in order to get the radioactivity concentration in MBq or mCi per mL via the computer. After sterile filtration through a millipore filter (0.22 μm) the isotonic 2-^{18}FDG solution is apportioned into evacuated ampoules via pneumatic piloting of a sterile tube cannula. The filling unit is installed below the synthesis device in a separate small lead-shielded box (40 X 40 cm).

5.9.8. *Performance of the system.* The routine production of 2-^{18}FDG has been accomplished several hundred times with excellent reliability. The integrated automatic cleaning programme at the end of radiosynthesis makes it possible to reuse the apparatus within one hour. Nevertheless, it is necessary after each third radiosynthesis to open the reactor and to clean the glassy carbon vessel with a soft tissue. In the course of several radiosyntheses, polymeric side products accumulate which are insoluble in the solvents used for the purification sequence, such as boiling water, ethanol and acetone. Besides the manual purification step, the only manual procedure which has to be performed before running a new radiosynthesis is to fill up the reservoirs and to change the column and the Sep-Pak™ cartridges.

Although some minor problems exist with respect to the decreasing reliability of some membrane valves, especially the three-way valves after 40 radiosyntheses, the automated system is a convenient apparatus for the routine production of high amounts of 2-^{18}FDG. The preparation takes 58 min and gives 2-^{18}FDG in 50 ± 10% radiochemical yield with a radiochemical purity of 98.5 ± 0.5% and a specific radioactivity of > 370 GBq/μmol (10 Ci/μmol). The same device, without any appreciable modification, has been used for the routine production of 2-[^{18}F]fluoro-D-mannose from the epimeric form of the 2-^{18}FDG precursor, and also for the production of 3-*N*-[^{18}F]methylspiperone.

6. Robot-based Automation

6.1. INTRODUCTION

All automation requires standardisation of repetitive procedures. The equipment used is chosen for its compatibility with other components of the system. Personal computers are used to time the execution of pre-programmed operations. The one major feature distinguishing a robot-based system from a dedicated automatic system is that the mechanical operations are performed by a multi-functional manipulator – the robot arm – instead of a series of mono-functional devices.

There are pros and cons to using robots in radiochemical procedures. Once the initial components are chosen and the operator is familiar with the system, a large degree of inherent flexibility is retained since the arm can be re-programmed to perform new operations. As in a dedicated system, the robot-based system can be used to execute a well-optimised procedure in exactly the same way every time. In contrast to dedicated systems, the robot can be programmed to remove contaminated vessels to a shielded waste area, thereby lowering the level of background radiation and increasing accessibility to a shielded work area in a given period. The robot may be used as a developmental tool to optimise the sequences of mechanical operations in a new procedure before building a dedicated system. The same manipulator can potentially perform several different procedures within the same set-up. In high-volume analytical procedures, such as in the analysis of biological samples, the robot always performs the analyses in the same manner, thereby eliminating errors from variations in laboratory techniques. No transcription errors are made since the data are automatically recorded and personnel are freed from time-consuming work.

On the other hand, the cost of the robot alone is often substantially higher than the combined costs of the equipment used in dedicated automated systems. Most glassware and disposable items must be redesigned to a more robot-friendly construction for optimal reliability. Either the shielded work area must be custom-designed to fit the operating and service requirements of the robot or the choice of robot must take into account the limitations of the available work area. Even for commercial robots, custom-made to perform specific tasks, considerable time is usually needed for set up and one or several persons needs to be completely familiar with the function and coding of the control system.

Once the decision has been made that investment in robotics is justified for present and/or future applications, the time required for implementation will depend on the expertise of the personnel working on the project and whether or not the system being considered has previously been optimised for the particular application. Some examples of this developmental procedure are surveyed below, following a specific example of robotic radiosynthesis from the group at Liège. Other laboratories in Europe have experience with robotics, as follows: *France*: Caen and Orsay; *Netherlands*: Groningen; *Russia*: St. Petersburg: *Sweden*: Stockholm and Uppsala. The three main robotic systems to be discussed are summarised in Table 2.

Table 2. Comparison of technical data for the main robots discussed.

	Zymark	**Scanditronix**	**Karolinska**
Robot type	Zymate	(RB-86)Anatech AB	RTX (UMI)
Coordinate system	Cylindrical	Cartesian + linear	Cylindrical
Number of axes	4 + 2	5	7
Operation range	360°	180° - 6 m linear	180°
Programmable speeds	yes	yes	yes
Multiple hands	yes	yes	no
Reach	64 cm		68 cm
Lift capacity	2 kg	10 kg	2 kg
Positioning accuracy	1 mm	0.1 mm	0.5 mm
System controller	Easylab™	IBM PC	IBM PC

6.2. A SPECIFIC EXAMPLE OF ROBOT-ASSISTED RADIOSYNTHESIS — 6-[^{18}F]FLUORO-L-DOPA (AS AT LIÈGE)

6.2.1. *Introduction.* Although, the labelling of radiopharmaceuticals with fluorine-18 by remote-control is feasible, automatic robotic radiosynthesis is more desirable since it appears to be more versatile and therefore more useful for research. In order to demonstrate the potential of such an approach, which avoids excessive radiation exposure to operatives, a robotic system has been developed in the Cyclotron Research Centre of the University of Liège based on the Zymate™ Laboratory Automation System (Zymark Corp.) (Table 2). This was the first robotic system to be used in PET-related procedures and is probably still the most widely used. The robot arm has an operational range of 360°. Easylab™ software and a variety of workstations are available for performing operations often used in laboratory procedures. These may be used as they are, or modified to fit the special vessels and techniques used in PET radiochemistry. It is configured and programmed to prepare a variety of radiopharmaceuticals, such as 6-[^{18}F]fluoro-L-dopa, 2-[^{18}F]fluoro-L-tyrosine, [^{18}F]altanserin and 4-[^{18}F]fluoro-tropapride, all by n.c.a. nucleophilic radiofluorination.

6-[^{18}F]Fluoro-L-dopa and 2-[^{18}F]fluoro-L-tyrosine are produced as tracers of presynaptic dopamine neurons and of cerebral protein synthesis rate, respectively. The n.c.a. enantioselective labelling of 6-[^{18}F]fluoro-L-dopa is based on nucleophilic substitution in 2-trimethylammonium-3,4-dimethoxy benzaldehyde triflate (Lemaire *et al.*, 1992, Lemaire, 1993) and the labelling of 2-[^{18}F]fluoro-L-tyrosine is similarly based on nucleophilic substitution in the corresponding 4-methoxy benzaldehyde. The remaining steps in these multi-step syntheses require conversion of the radiofluorinated aldehydes into the corresponding benzyl iodide [by treatment with di-iodosilane (DIS)], alkylation of *S*-Boc-BMI with this electrophilic agent, hydrolysis and finally HPLC purification (Lemaire *et al.*, 1993). [^{18}F]Altanserin is labelled by nucleophilic substitution in the corresponding nitro compound and purified by HPLC (Lemaire *et al.*, 1991). Its suitability for mapping $5HT_2$ receptors *in vivo* with PET has been demonstrated (Sadzot *et al.*, 1993). Tropapride has been labelled with fluorine-18 at the 4 position of its benzylic group by reductive amination in the presence of 4-[^{18}F]fluorobenzaldehyde and norbenzyl precursor (Damhaut *et al.*, 1992). This molecule exhibits high selectivity and specificity for D_2 receptor sites and appears to be a potential radioligand for the study of the dopaminergic system with PET.

6.2.2. *Components of the system.* The robot used for these radiosyntheses is a Zymate™ II Laboratory Robot (Zymark Corp.), as specified in Table 2. The software control is Easylab Plus™, and routines for several modules were written using this language. Several components were acquired from Zymark, and others modules, more specific to the particular radiosynthesis were designed and fabricated 'in house'. The components were arranged in a 360° arc around the robot arm and were mounted on sectors positioned around the Zymate™ II Core System. All the system was set up on a shielded bench top (150 x 175 cm). Located beneath the robot are the Power and Event Controller as well as the multiplexer, also developed 'in house', which allows the control of 64 outputs for the control of valves and others modules. The controller and the HPLC system are also located beneath the bench top. A block diagram of the Zymate™ system is shown in Figure 11. In the legend the modules marked Zymark were purchased from Zymark Corporation while the modules developed in Liège are marked CRC. Figure 12 shows a photograph of the configured system.

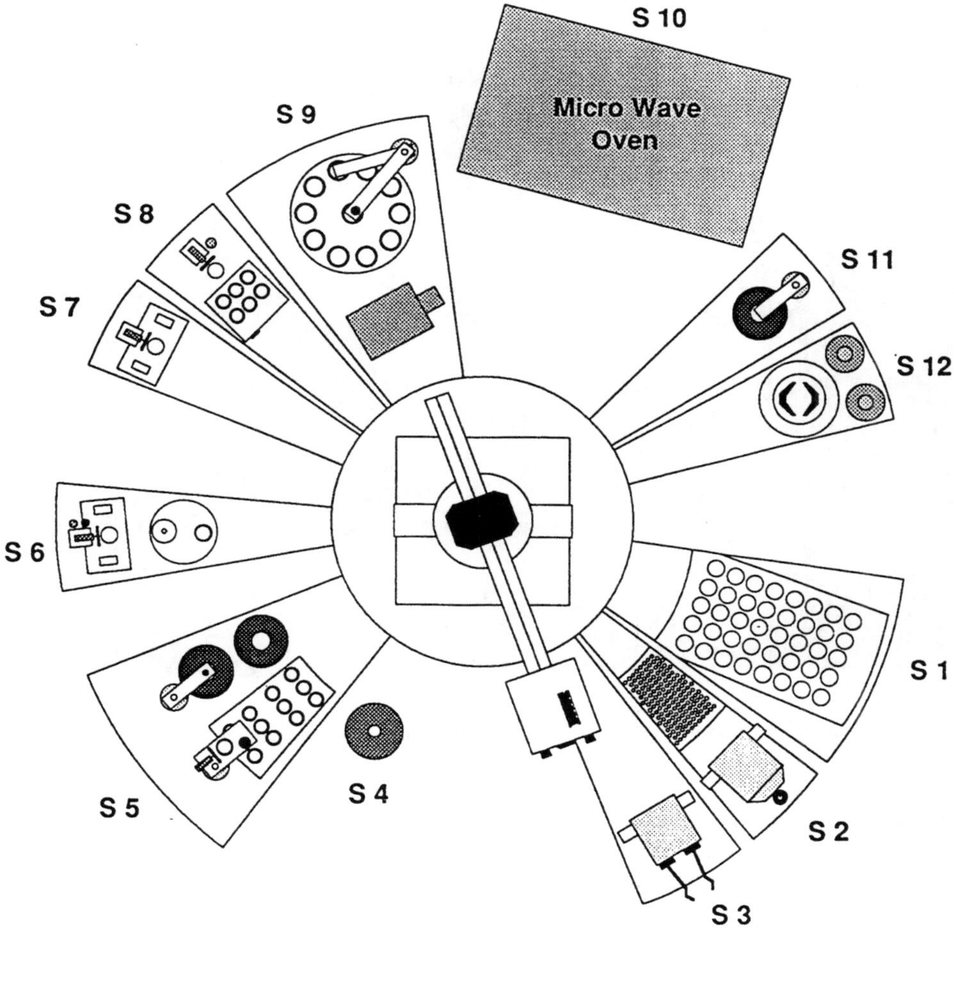

Figure 11. Description of the different sectors (S1–S12) around the Zymate II Core System. S1—Rack containing disposable glass tubes (Zymark). S2—Pipetting Hand and tips (Zymark). S3—General Purpose Seizing Hand (Zymark). S4—Lead pig (CRC). S5—Column for the separation of [^{18}F]fluoride from irradiated water, a rack with capped reagent vials, two ovens, one equipped with an optical level probe (CRC). S6—C-18 Sep-Pak chromatography system (CRC). S7—Sector for formulating the injectable solution (CRC). S8—Homemade silica chromatography system and rack for the preparation of DIS (L-6-[^{18}F]fluoro-Dopa and L-2-[^{18}F]fluoro-tyrosine) (CRC). S9—HPLC injector and fraction collector (CRC). S10—Microwave oven (CRC). S11—Oven for the hydrolysis step (L-6-[^{18}F]fluoro-Dopa and L-2-[^{18}F]fluoro-tyrosine) (CRC). S12—Capping pysection providing capping and uncapping of round, screw cap containers (Zymark).

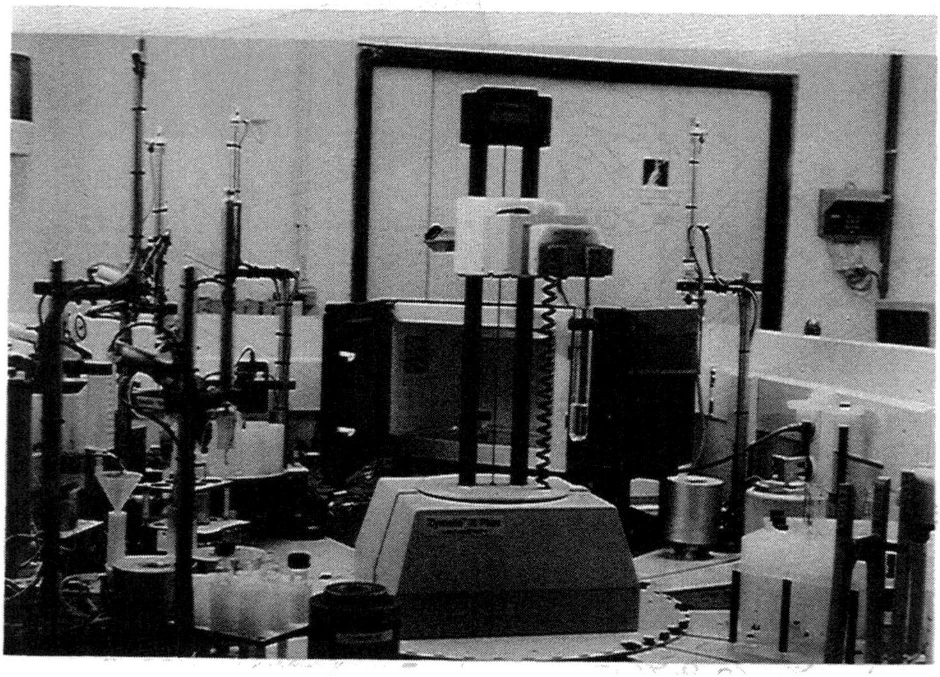

Figure 12. Zymate™ Laboratory System used for the routine production of four ^{18}F-labelled radiopharmaceuticals.

6.2.3. *Labelling of L-6-[^{18}F]fluoro-Dopa as an example.* The radiosynthesis of L-6-[^{18}F]fluoro-Dopa requires many steps in common with the labelling of other radiopharmaceuticals, including production of [^{18}F]fluoride, recovery of ^{18}O-enriched water, evaporation of natural abundance water, resolubilisation of the radioactivity in an aprotic dipolar solvent, labelling in a microwave oven or in an aluminium heating block, Sep-Pak™ pre-purification, HPLC injection and separation, and finally preparation of an injectable solution.

a. Initialisation.

During radionuclide production, the robot initialisation program is loaded into the robot controller and executed. It allows the modules of the robotic system to be loaded with all components (*e.g.* vials, tips, tubes), solvent and reagents necessary for the radiosynthesis. To continue, manual validation of each step of the program with the keyboard, is required. At the end of bombardment, the main program is loaded.

b. Production of [^{18}F]fluoride ion.

No-carrier-added [^{18}F]fluoride is produced in a nickel target by the $^{18}O(p,n)^{18}F$ nuclear reaction on ^{18}O-enriched water (45%). The target is remotely loaded using a syringe pump through a fill entrance at the bottom of the target. A second port at the top of the target is used for venting during loading and irradiation. At the end of bombardment (1 h, 10 μA), the radioactivity (11–13 GBq; 300–350 mCi) is transferred under nitrogen gas pressure (0.67 bar; 10 psi) through Teflon™ tubing (30 m) to the robot room (sector 5, Figure 11).

c. Recovery of n.c.a. [^{18}F]fluoride and ^{18}O-enriched water.
The radioactivity is trapped on a Dowex™ 1X8 anion exchange resin and the ^{18}O-enriched water recovered in a receiving vial placed in sector 5. The end of transfer is detected manually and the command is then entered by keyboard into the robot controller to continue the synthesis. A conical glass vessel containing Kryptofix™ 2.2.2. (22 mg) and potassium carbonate (4.2 mg) is then substituted for the ^{18}O-enriched vial, which is capped in the capping station (sector 12). After distillation, this water is used again for further production. [^{18}F]Fluoride is then eluted from the resin by potassium carbonate solution (7 mg/mL; 400 µL).

d. Labelling reaction.
Conversion of the [^{18}F]fluoride into its potassium-Kryptofix 2.2.2. salt in an anhydrous organic solvent (DMSO) is achieved in the oven in sector 5. The water is evaporated to dryness under nitrogen in an aluminium heating block (120°C). The end of evaporation is detected automatically with an optical probe and a feedback signal is sent to the robot's computer which then allows the synthesis to continue. Therefore, this critical evaporation step can be achieved reproducibly and is highly independent of parameters such as water volume, temperature and nitrogen flow.

The Pipetting Hand, equipped with a tip, is then selected and the [K-Kryptofix 2.2.2.]$^+$[^{18}F]$^-$ salt dried by three successive additions and evaporations of acetonitrile (3 x 100 µL). The precursor (15 mg) in DMSO (900 µL), previously placed in the rack of sector 5, is aspirated in the tip and added to the dry residue. The probe is then moved up. The vial is capped in the capping pysection with the General Purpose Hand and introduced into the second oven in sector 5. After the labelling reaction (10 min, 140°C), the vial is placed either in a lead pig (sector 4, for assessment of radioactivity), or uncapped for subsequent Sep-Pak™ pre-purification.

e. Sep-Pak™ pre-purification.
By using the Pipetting Hand, the DMSO solution is diluted in glass tube number 1 in the rack in sector 1, which contains 20 mL of 0.5M-hydrochloric acid. The labelling vial is rinsed with this solution. With the General Purpose Hand the tube containing the radioactivity is moved from the rack on sector 1, and the solution poured into a pneumatically actuated 50 mL syringe (previously filled with 5 ml of 0.5M-hydrochloric acid). The solution is then pushed through the C-18 Sep-Pak™ cartridge with a slight flow of nitrogen. The level of liquid is detected automatically by measuring the conductivity between two platinum electrodes. Before dryness, the lid is moved up and the support washed with water. The [^{18}F]fluorobenzaldehyde is finally eluted with dichloromethane and dried by passing through a magnesium sulphate column which is rinsed with additional dichloromethane. The final solution is collected in a conical vial and moved from sector 5 into the rack in sector 8.

f. Preparation of DIS and reductive iodination.
In a conical vial containing iodine, phenylsilane is added with the Pipetting Hand. With the General Purpose Hand a Teflon™ lid is placed on the vial and removed after 2 min. The Pipetting hand is selected again and the radiofluorinated aldehyde transferred to the DIS reagent. With the General Purpose Hand the vial containing the [^{18}F]fluorobenzyl iodide is displaced so that the solution is poured onto a silica gel column and eluted with dichloromethane. The purified [^{18}F]fluorobenzyl iodide is collected in another vial and the dichloromethane evaporated.

g. Alkylation and hydrolysis reactions.
After alkylation, which is not presently conducted with the robotic system (under development), the [^{18}F]fluoroalkylated derivative is hydrolysed in the oven in sector 11.

h. HPLC purification.

A homemade fraction collector has been developed (sector 9). Presently robotic controlled injection onto the HPLC is under development. The robotic preparation of L-6-[^{18}F]fluoro-Dopa takes a similar time (120 min) to a remotely controlled preparation and gives a similar radiochemical yield (25 % decay corrected to E.O.B.).

6.2.4. *Other radiopharmaceuticals.* The software written for the L-6-[^{18}F]fluoro-Dopa radiosynthesis can be used for labelling other radiopharmaceuticals with only minor modification. Indeed, the flexibility of the Easilab Plus™ programming language easily allows any modification needed. For the radiosynthesis of L-2-[^{18}F]fluoro-tyrosine all the same homemade workstations are used. For the radiosynthesis of [^{18}F]altanserin the HPLC system is modified to accept an additional C-18 column. The application of robotics is not limited to the routine preparation of these four ^{18}F-labelled radiopharmaceuticals for PET studies. Set up for the labelling and purification of several new radiopharmaceuticals is easily performed the same day with all the hardware presently available on our robotic system.

6.3. A SURVEY OF OTHER APPLICATIONS OF ROBOTICS IN RADIOSYNTHESIS

6.3.1. *At the University of Washington (St. Louis).* The PET group at the University of Washington (St. Louis), first reported the use of the Zymate system in the radiosynthesis of 16α-[^{18}F]fluoroestradiol-17β (Brodack *et al.*, 1985, 1986). This particular radiosynthesis was chosen because the half-life of the radioisotope is adequately long, the operations are compatible with robotic procedures and the long synthesis time and low radiochemical yield require large amounts of starting radioactivity. The procedures performed included conversion of [^{18}F]fluoride into the tetra-*n*-butylammonium salt in anhydrous solvents, handling of air-sensitive solvents, evaporation of solvents to dryness, heating and cooling, liquid-liquid separations and HPLC purification. In addition to the commercially available equipment incorporated in the procedure a number of modifications were introduced by the St. Louis group. These included the use of radiosynthesis-specific reagent and vessel racks, methods for the reproducible placement of the reaction vessels in heating or cooling baths and of specially constructed nitrogen purge lines that allowed the robot to perform other tasks during the evaporation of solvents. The General Purpose Hand was modified for Luer™ adapters to accommodate disposable needles, injections onto the HPLC system, monitoring of the eluate and the collection of fractions. The robotic procedure requires less time than the manual procedure (80 *vs* 90 min) but the radiochemical yields are lower (5–6 *vs* 22%). The major problems reportedly encountered were control of the evaporation time needed for resolubilisation of the [^{18}F]fluoride, lower efficiency in sample extractions than when performed manually and inefficient transfer for injection onto the HPLC system.

Based on their experiences with this first application, the St. Louis group subsequently modified the system to include smaller custom-made workstations and standardised the addition of reagents and the reaction vessels (Brodack *et al.*, 1988b). The robot workspace is more efficiently used. They demonstrated the flexibility of the procedure by performing several radiosyntheses within the same set-up, namely those of 16α-[^{18}F]fluoroestradiol-17β with improved yields, 3-*N*-(ω-[^{18}F]fluoropropyl)spiperone and *n*-[1-^{11}C]butanol. In the new radiolabelling with [^{18}F]fluoride, a rack is simply added for the reagents and for vessels specific to 3-*N*-(ω-[^{18}F]fluoropropyl)spiperone synthesis and the HPLC system is modified to accept an additional silica column. The radiochemical yields of 3-*N*-(ω-[^{18}F]fluoropropyl)spiperone are slightly lower than for the manual procedure (15–18% *vs* 20–28%, EOS) due to the longer synthesis time required (70 *vs* 40 min). A third reagent rack in the same robotic set-up allowed two preparations of *n*-[1-^{11}C]butanol within 25 min of each other without operator intervention (compared to at least 60 min in manual preparations). The time required for the robotic preparation is slightly longer than for the manual-remote preparation (25 *vs* 17 min), but the radioactivity yields are essentially the same.

Using the same reagent and vessel racks already implemented in the previous radiofluorinations, only minor modifications were necessary for the production of 2-^{18}FDG in sufficient activities for clinical PET studies (Brodack *et al.*, 1988a). The resolubilisation station was modified to include a platinum crucible. A new lab-station allowed attachment of a reflux column to a Reacti-vial™. Extraction procedures were performed as previously with columns packed with the appropriate material (silica C-18 and AG11 A8 ion retardation resin). The radiochemical yields and time of preparation are comparable to the manual-remote results: 12–17% *vs* 12–23% and 70 *vs* 60 min, respectively. Since sub-routines already generated in the previous robotic procedures can be used, this new robotic synthesis reportedly requires about one week for implementation.

The St Louis group have recently described the use of an articulated arm produced by CRS PLUS (Hudson Robotics) for 2-^{18}FDG synthesis (Gaehle and Welch, 1992). Total Control Software™ controls the system through an IBM or compatible PC. The system is a space-saving alternative to the Zymark™ system.

6.3.2. *At the University of Washington (Seattle).* Since robotic procedures are normally slower than manual procedures, their primary application has been in labelling with fluorine-18 rather than carbon-11. One additional application of the Zymark system in ^{11}C-labelling has, however, been reported by the PET group at the University of Washington in Seattle (Link *et al.*, 1989), namely the synthesis of the tracer [1-^{11}C]D-glucose. This requires large activities of the labelling agent, [^{11}C]cyanide, to be handled. In addition to manipulations and reagent additions, a sensitive titration of the pH of the reaction mixture is performed by the robot. The total time required for the robot-assisted radiosynthesis is less than 5 min more than the manual-remote procedure and the quantities of radiotracer produced are sufficient for PET studies. The same group has recently reported the use of Zymark robotics for the multi-stage synthesis of [2-^{11}C]thymidine from hydrogen [^{11}C]cyanide (Courter *et al.*, 1992).

6.3.3. *At Brookhaven National Laboratory.* The Zymark system has recently been used by the Brookhaven PET group for measuring the plasma kinetics of total radioactivity and fraction of unmetabolised tracer (Alexoff *et al.*, 1991, 1992), an otherwise time- and personnel-demanding procedure. As demonstrated with blood samples from a PET study with 3-*N*-[^{18}F]methylspiperone, the robot centrifuged, counted and pipetted different samples simultaneously to determine the discrete time-input function. The throughput of the robot is half that of a highly trained technician. Metabolite assays for 3-*N*-[^{18}F]methylspiperone, [*N-methyl*-^{11}C]cocaine and [*O-methyl*-^{11}C]raclopride, based on solid-phase extractions, can also be performed with excellent reproducibility for replicate samples. Not only might the total throughput be increased by this use of robots, but human exposure to radiation and potentially infectious biological materials are minimised. Possible errors due to variations in laboratory techniques are also reduced.

6.3.4. *At Stockholm University-Karolinska Hospital.* For a number of reasons, a PET group may wish to design and implement its own robotics. The reasons may include space limitations, economy, the flexibility of tailoring the system to fit its own needs, and the desire to do basic research in the technique as a whole. In this case, a manipulator with the best performance characteristics (reproducibility, flexibility, strength) is chosen to use the planned work area effectively. If the group of scientists designing the system are competent in computer programming and interfaces, mechanical and electrical engineering and chemistry, a versatile system can be developed.

The system designed by the Stockholm University-Karolinska PET group (Appelquist *et al.*, 1989, 1991, 1993) illustrates such a development. The chosen robot arm is an RTX from Universal Machine Intelligence (Table 2). It is vertically mounted on a rail and can be installed on the back wall of a hot-cell for operation in the semi-circle in front of it. A Multi-Function Editor (MFE) was developed for building and interpreting control sequences for the system. The computer program recognises commands for moving the robot and for operating the equipment used in the syntheses (electrovalves, flow regulators, heating elements, event waits, *etc).* The user-interface of the MFE is based on mouse-activated pull-down menus to provide a user-friendly mode of operation. The robot can be guided through motions in the desired directions by moving the mouse or by coordinates entered from the keyboard. Since simple editing commands and mouse-driven input are used in building the command sequences, the time required for a new user to learn how to program the system is minimised.

Radiosynthesis-specific equipment is fixed on a removable Plexiglas™ tray connected to the base plate of the robot, allowing easy access for service or cleaning but still ensuring reproducible re-positioning. Supporting equipment is installed separately in or around the hot-cell. The glassware is, where possible, selected from common reaction vessels such as Reacti-vials™ or, for special applications, is designed to be robot-friendly and standardised. Flow-line connections via needle stations, heating units, electrovalves, radioactivity monitors, as well as storage stations for reaction vessels have been specifically designed for optimal reliability of the total system. The use of the system as a developmental tool has been demonstrated in the production and applications of [^{11}C]iodomethane and in nucleophilic substitution reactions with [^{18}F]fluoride and [^{11}C]cyanide.

6.3.5. *At Uppsala.* Installation and the time required for the first successful use of robotics may be reduced by choosing a complete commercial radiosynthesis system. One such system, based on the Anatech RB-86 robot (Table 2), has been adapted for PET radiochemical procedures by Scanditronix AB (Kjellström and Lindbäck, 1988). For radiosyntheses, the robot arm is installed on a rail on the back wall of the shielded area. Since it can be moved linearly up to a distance of six metres, it can be used to service separate but adjacent hot-cells. However, to utilise this feature maximally, the working space must be custom-designed for installation of the rail through all the cells from the back side. The robot system is delivered with lab-stations for performing common operations (pipetting, liquid dispensing, solid phase extractions, vortexing, vial capping, heating, cooling, evaporations and millipore filtrations). Additional equipment specific to the radiosyntheses of 2-^{18}FDG and [^{11}C]iodomethane is also available, thereby enabling application of the robotics soon after installation. However, as with all robotic systems, routine operation requires that at least one person is well-versed in the control characteristics of both the robot and the supporting equipment. The system is extendable to alkylations with [^{11}C]iodomethane, other types of syntheses or even analytical procedures associated with PET. The vendor supplies a tool for performing such operations but the applications will require user-design.

6.3.6. *At St Petersburg.* The group at St. Petersburg, in collaboration with Scanditronix AB, have recently reported the use of the RB-86 robot (Anatech AB) with workstations from Scanditronix AB for the synthesis of [1-^{11}C]acetate (Korsakov *et al.*, 1992a) and also for [*S-methyl*-^{11}C]methionine from [^{11}C]iodomethane (Korsakov *et al.*, 1992b).

7. References

Adam M.J., Ruth T.J., Grierson J.R., Abeysekera and Pate B.D. (1986) Routine synthesis of L-6-[^{18}F]fluorodopa with fluorine-18 acetyl hypofluorite. *J. Nucl. Med.*, 27, 1462–1466.

Alexoff D.L., Gatley S.J., Wolf A.P. and Fowler J.S. (1991) Robotic assay of C-11 cocaine and [F-18]N-methylspiroperidol (F-18 NMS) metabolites in plasma. *J. Nucl. Med.*, 32, 1088. (Abstract)

Alexoff D.L., Shea C., Gatley S.J., Fowler J.S. and Wolf A.P. (1992) Development and validation of a robotic solid phase extraction assay for 11C raclopride in plasma. *J. Nucl. Med.*, 33, 853. (Abstract)

Alexoff D.L., Gatley S.J., Wolf A.P. and Fowler J.S. (1993) Robotic determination of discrete time input functions for quantitative PET: measurement of plasma radioactivity concentration. *J. Label. Compd. Radiopharm.*, 32, 514–515. (Abstract).

Appelquist G., Bohm C., Eriksson H., Wang R., Eriksson L., Halldin C., Johnstrom P. and Stone-Elander S. (1989) Evaluation of a versatile process control system for a robot arm. *J. Label. Compd. Radiopharm.*, 26, 474–475. (Abstract).

Appelquist G., Bohm C., Eriksson H., Halldin C. and Stone-Elander S. (1991) A robot-assisted synthesis system applied to ^{11}C-alkylations. *J. Label. Compd. Radiopharm.*, 30, 161–162. (Abstract).

Appelquist G., Bohm C., Eriksson H. and Stone-Elander S. (1993) A robot-based system for the development of production methods for radiotracers for PET. *J. Label. Compd. Radiopharm.*, 32, 184. (Abstract).

Bauer B. and Wagner R. (1991) Improved synthesis of [^{15}O]butanol for clinical use. *J. Label. Compd. Radiopharm.*, 30, 69–71. (Abstract).

Berger G., Maziere M., Prenant C. and Comar D. (1980) Synthesis of carbon-11 labelled acetone. *Int J. Appl. Radiat. Isot.*, 31, 577–578.

Berridge M.S., Franceschini M.P., Tewson T.J. and Gould K.L. (1986) Preparation of oxygen-15 butanol for positron tomography. *J. Nucl. Med.*, 27, 834–837.

Berridge M.S., Cassidy E.H. and Terris A.H. (1990) A routine, automated synthesis of oxygen-15-labeled butanol for positron tomography. *J. Nucl. Med.*, 31, 1727–1731.

Berridge M.S., Adler L.P., Nelson A.D., Cassidy E.H., Muzic R.F., Bednarczyk E.M. and Miraldi F. (1991) Measurement of human cerebral blood flow with [^{15}O]butanol and positron emission tomography. *J. Cerebr. Blood Flow Metab.*, 11, 707–715.

Brodack J.W., Welch M.J., Kilbourn M.R. and Katzenellenbogen J.A. (1985) Application of robotics for the routine production of fluorine-18-labeled radiopharmaceuticals. *Advances in Laboratory Automation Robotics*, Zymark Corp., Hopkington, p. 663.

Brodack J.W., Kilbourn M.R., Welch M.J. and Katzenellenbogen J.A. (1986) Application of robotics to radiopharmaceutical preparation: controlled synthesis of fluorine-18 16α-fluoroestradiol-17β. *J. Nucl. Med.*, 27, 714–721.

Brodack J.W., Dence C.S., Kilbourn M.R. and Welch M.J. (1988a) Robotic production of 2-deoxy-2-[^{18}F]fluoro-D-glucose: a routine method of synthesis using tetrabutylammonium [^{18}F]fluoride. *Appl. Radiat. Isot.*, 39, 699–703.

Brodack J.W., Kilbourn M.R. and Welch M.J. (1988b) Automated production of several positron-emitting radiopharmaceuticals using a single laboratory robot. *Appl. Radiat. Isot.*, 39, 689–698.

Brown M., Marshall D.R., Sobel B.E. and Bergmann S.R. (1987) Delineation of myocardial oxygen utilization with carbon-11-labeled acetate. *Circulation*, 76, 687–696.

Buxton D.B., Schwaiger M., Nguyen A., Phelps M.E. and Schelbert H.R. (1988) Radiolabeled acetate as a tracer of myocardial tricarboxylic acid cycle flux. *Circulation Res.*, 63, 628–634.

Buxton D.B., Nienaber C.A., Luxen A., Ratib O., Hansen H., Phelps M.E. and Schelbert H.R. (1989) Noninvasive quantitation of regional myocardial oxygen consumption in vivo with [1-^{11}C]acetate and dynamic positron emission tomography. *Circulation*, 79, 134–142.

Camsonne R., Crouzel C., Comar D., Mazière M., Prenant C., Sastre J., Moulin M.A. and Syrota A. (1984) Synthesis of *N*-[^{11}C]methyl, *N*-methyl-propyl), (chloro-2-phenyl)isoquinoline carboxamide-3 (PK 11195): a new ligand for peripheral benzodiazepine receptors. *J. Label. Compd. Radiopharm.*, 21, 985–991.

Clark J.C. and Dowsett K. (1992) Automated carbon-11 radiopharmaceutical production. *PSI Proceedings* 92-01, pp. 207–209. ISSN 1019-6447. (Proc. IVth Int. Workshop on Targetry & Target Chemistry, PSI, Villigen, Switzerland, 1991). (Abstract).

Clark J.C. and Tochon Danguy (1992) "R2D2", a bedside [oxygen-15]water infusor. *PSI Proceedings* 92-01, pp. 234–235. ISSN 1019-6447. (Proc. IVth Int. Workshop on Targetry & Target Chemistry, PSI, Villigen, Switzerland, 1991). (Abstract).

Coenen H.H., Pike V.W., Stöcklin G. and Wagner R. (1987) Recommendation for a practical production of [2-^{18}F]fluoro-2-deoxy-D-glucose. *Appl. Radiat. Isot.*, 38, 605–610.

Comar D., Mazière M. and Crouzel C. (1974) Synthese et métabolisme de molecules radiopharmaceutiques marquées au carbone-11. I-iodomethylate de chlorpromazine-^{11}C. *Radiopharmaceuticals and Labelled Compounds*. Vol I. IAEA, Vienna.

Comar D., Cartron J.C., Mazière M. and Marazano C. (1976) Labelling and metabolism of methionine-methyl-^{11}C. *Eur. J. Nucl. Med.*, 1, 11-14.

Cremer J., Hume S.P., Cullen B.M., Myers R., Manjil L.G., Turton D.R., Luthra S.K., Bateman D.M. and Pike V.W. (1992) The distribution of radioactivity in brains of rats given [*N-methyl*-^{11}C]PK 11195 *in vivo* after induction of cortical ischaemic lesion. *Nucl. Med. Biol.*, 19, 159–166.

Crouzel C., Långström B., Pike V.W. and Coenen H.H. (1987) Recommendation for a practical production of [^{11}C]methyl iodide. *Int. J. Appl. Radiat. Isot.*, 38, 601–604.

Courter J.H., Link J.M. and Krohn K.A. (1992) Automation of the synthesis of [2-carbon-11]thymidine. *PSI Proceedings* 92-01, pp. 210–214. ISSN 1019-6447. (Proc. IVth Workshop on Targetry & Target Chemistry, PSI, Villigen, Switzerland, 1991). (Abstract).

Damhaut Ph., Cantineau R., Lemaire C., Plenevaux A., Christiaens L. and Guillaume M. (1992) 2- and 4-[^{18}F]fluorotropapride, two specific D2 receptor ligands for positron emission tomography: n.c.a. syntheses and animal studies. *Appl. Radiat. Isot.*, 43, 1265–1274.

Ehrin E., Gawell L., Högberg T., de Paulis T. and Ström P. (1987) Synthesis of [methoxy-3H]- and [methoxy-11C]-labelled raclopride. Specific dopamine D_2 receptor ligands. *J. Label. Compd. Radiopharm.*, 24, 931–940.

Fowler J.S and Wolf A.P. (1986) 2-Deoxy-2-[^{18}F]fluoro-D-glucose for metabolic studies: current status. *Appl. Radiat. Isot.*, 37, 663–668.

Fowler J.S., MacGregor R.R., Wolf A.P., Arnett C.D., Dewey S.L., Schlyer D., Christman D., Logan J., Smith M., Sach H., Aquilonius S.M., Bjurling P., Halldin C., Hartvig P., Leenders K.L. Lundqvist H., Oreland L., Stålnacke C-G. and Långström B. (1987) Mapping human brain monoamine oxidase A and B with ^{11}C-labeled suicide inactivators and PET. *Science,* 235, 481–485.

Gaehle G.G. and Welch M.J. (1992) Improved automated systems for the production of radiopharmaceuticals. *PSI Proceedings* 92-01, pp. 186–189. ISSN 1019-6447. (Proceedings of the IVth Workshop on Targetry & Target Chemistry, PSI, Villigen, Switzerland, 1991). (Abstract).

Goodman M.M., Devinney J.L., Kabalka G.W., Longford C.P.D., Ladetsky M. and Green J.F. (1991) Computer controlled synthesis of oxygen-15 butanol and water: automated production and dispensing systems. *J. Label. Compd. Radiopharm.,* 30, 166–168. (Abstract).

Guillaume M., Luxen M., Nebeling B., Argentini M., Clark J.C. and Pike V.W. (1991) Recommendations for fluorine-18 production. *Appl. Radiat. Isot.*, 42, 749–762.

Halldin C., Stone-Elander S., Farde L., Ehrin E., Fasth K-J., Långström B. and Sedvall G. (1986) Preparation of ^{11}C-labelled SCH 23390 for the *in vivo* study of dopamine D-1 receptors using positron emission tomography. *Appl. Radiat. Isot.*, 37, 1039–1043.

Hamacher K., Coenen H.H. and Stöcklin G. (1986) Efficient stereospecific synthesis of no-carrier-added 2-[^{18}F]-fluoro-2-deoxy-D-glucose using aminopolyether supported nucleophilic substitution. *J. Nucl. Med.*, 27, 235–238.

Hamacher K., Blessing G. and Nebeling B. (1990) Computer-aided synthesis (CAS) of no-carrier-added-2-[^{18}F]fluoro-2-deoxy-D-glucose: an efficient automated system for the aminopolyether-supported nucleophilic fluorination. *Appl. Radiat. Isot.*, 41, 49–55.

Herscovitch P., Markham J. and Raichle M. E. (1983) Brain flow measured with intravenous $H_2{}^{15}O$. I. Theory and error analysis. *J. Nucl. Med.*, 24, 782–789.

Herscovitch P., Raichle M.E., Kilbourn M.R. and Welch M.J. (1987) Positron emission tomographic measurement of cerebral blood flow and permeability-surface area product of water using [^{15}O]water and [^{11}C]butanol. *J. Cerebr. Blood Flow Metab.*, 7, 527–542.

Holschbach M. and Schüller M. (1993a) A new and simple on-line method for the preparation of n.c.a. [^{11}C]methyl iodide. *Appl. Radiat. Isot.*, In press.

Holschbach M. and Schüller M. (1993b) An on-line method for the preparation of n.c.a. [$^{11}CH_3$]trifluoromethanesulfonic acid methyl ester. *Appl. Radiat. Isot.*, In press.

Kabalka G.W. (1984) Incorporation of stable and radioactive isotopes via organoborane chemistry. *Accts. Chem. Res.*, 17, 215.

Kabalka G.W., Lambrecht R.M., Sajjad M., Fowler J.S., Kunda S.A. and McCollum G.W. and Macgregor R. (1985) Synthesis of [^{15}O]-labelled butanol via organoborane chemistry. *Int. J. Appl. Radiat. Isot.*, 36, 853–855.

Kjellström R. and Lindbäck S. (1988) Automated radiopharmaceutical preparation system utilizing robotics. *J. Nucl. Med.*, 29, 976. (Abstract).

Korsakov M.V., Solovyov D., Horti A.G., Kuznetsova O.F., Nilsson L-E. and Ulin J. (1992a) Robotic synthesis of [1-carbon-11]acetic acid. *PSI Proceedings 92-01*, pp. 218–219. ISSN 1019-6447. (Proc. IVth Workshop on Targetry & Target Chemistry, PSI, Villigen, Switzerland, 1991). (Abstract).

Korsakov M.V., Kisselev M.Y., Solovyov D., Horti A.G., Vasilev D.A., Nilsson L-E. and Ulin J.

(1992b) Robotic synthesis of [carbon-11]methionine. *PSI Proceedings 92-01*, pp. 220–222. ISSN 1019-6447. (Proc. IVth Workshop on Targetry & Target Chemistry, PSI, Villigen, Switzerland, 1991). (Abstract).

Kotzerke J., Hicks R.J., Wolfe E., Herman W.H., Molina E., Kuhl D.E. and Schwaiger M. (1990) Three-dimensional assessment of myocardial oxidative metabolism: a new approach for regional determination of PET-derived carbon-11-acetate kinetics. *J. Nucl. Med.*, 31, 1876–1893.

Långström B. and Lundqvist H. (1976) The preparation of ^{11}C-methyl iodide and its use in the synthesis of ^{11}C-methyl-L-methionine. *Int. J. Appl. Radiat. Isot.*, 27, 357–363.

Lemaire C. (1993) Production of L-[^{18}F]fluoro amino acids for protein synthesis: overview and recent developments in nucleophilic syntheses. In *PET Studies on Amino Acid Metabolism and Protein Synthesis*", Mazoyer B.M, Heiss W.D. and Comar D. (Eds). Kluwer Academic Publishers. pp. 89-108.

Lemaire C., Cantineau R., Guillaume M., Plenevaux A. and Christiaens L. (1991) Fluorine-18 altanserin: a radioligand for the study of serotonin receptors with PET: radiolabeling and in vivo biologic behavior in rats. *J. Nucl. Med.*, 32, 2266–2272.

Lemaire C., Plenevaux A., Comar D. (1992) Feasibility of multimillicurie preparation of L-6-[^{18}F]fluorodopa by nucleophilic asymmetric synthesis. *Eur. J. Nucl. Med.* , 19, 591. (Abstract).

Lemaire C., Plenevaux A., Cantineau R., Christiaens L., Guillaume M. and Comar D. (1993) Nucleophilic enantioselective synthesis of L-6-[^{18}F]fluorodopa via two chiral auxiliaries. *Appl. Radiat. Isot.*, In press.

Link J.M., Courter J.H.and Krohn K.A. (1989) Remote automated synthesis of 1-[^{11}C]-D-glucose for patient imaging with PET. *J. Nucl. Med.*, 30, 928. (Abstract).

Luthra S.K., Pike V.W. and Brady F. (1985) The preparation of carbon-11 labelled diprenorphine: a new radioligand for the study of the opiate receptor system in vivo. *J. Chem. Soc. Chem. Commun.*, 1423–1425.

Luthra S.K., Pike V.W. and Brady F. (1990) Preparation of some NCA [1-^{11}C]acid chlorides as labelling agents. *Appl. Radiat. Isot.*, 41, 471–476.

Luxen A., Guillaume M., Melega W.P., Pike V.W., Solin O. and Wagner R. (1992) Production of 6-[^{18}F]fluoro-L-DOPA and its metabolism *in vivo* — a critical review. *Appl. Radiat. Isot.*, 19, 149–158.

Marazano C., Maziere M., Berger G. and Comar D. (1977) Synthesis of methyl iodide-^{11}C and formaldehyde-^{11}C. *Int. J. Appl. Radiat. Isot.*, 28, 49–52.

Matzke K-H., Meyer G.J. and Hundeshagen H. (1993) An advanced sysytem for the administration of ^{15}O-water. *J. Label. Compd. Radiopharm.*, 23, 1209–1210. (Abstract).

Mazière M., Berger G. and Comar D. (1982) ^{11}C-Radiopharmaceuticals for brain receptor studies in conjunction with positron emission tomography. In *Applications of Nuclear and Radiochemistry*. Eds. Lambrecht R. and Morcos. Pergamon Press, New York. pp. 251–270.

Mazière M., Hantraye P., Prenant C., Sastre J. and Comar D. (1984) Synthesis of ethyl 8-fluoro-5,6-dihydro-5-[^{11}C]methyl-6-oxo-4H-imidazo[1,5a][1,4]benzodiazepine-3-carboxylate (RO 15-1788-^{11}C): a specific radioligand for the in vivo study of central benzodiazepine receptors by positron emission tomography. *Appl. Radiat. Isot.*, 35, 973–976.

Moerlein S.M., Gaehle G.G., Lechner K.R., Bera R.K. and Welch M.J. (1993) A microprocessor-controlled system for the production of multiple batches of oxygen-15 labelled butanol. *J. Label. Compd. Radiopharm.*, 32, 162–163. (Abstract).

Meyer G-J., Osterholz A. and Hundeshagen H. (1986) ^{15}O-Water constant infusion system for clinical routine applications. *J. Label. Compd. Radiopharm.*, 23, 1209–1210. (Abstract).

Meyer G-J., Günther K., Matzke K-H., Harms Th. and Hundeshagen H. (1993) A modified preparation method for ^{11}C acetate, preventing liquid phase extraction steps. *J. Label. Compd. Radiopharm.*, 32, 182–183. (Abstract).

Pike V.W., Eakins M.N., Allan R.M. and Selwyn A.P. (1982) Preparation of [1-^{11}C]acetate—an agent for the study of myocardial metabolism by positron emission tomography. *Int. J. Appl. Radiat. Isot.*, 33, 505–512.

Pike V.W., Horlock P.L., Brown C. and Clark J.C. (1984) The remotely-controlled preparation of a ^{11}C-labelled radiopharmaceutical — [1-^{11}C]acetate. *Int. J. Appl. Radiat. Isot.*, 35, 623–627.

Pike V.W., Kensett M.J., Turton D.R., Waters S.L. and Silvester D.J. (1990) Labelled agents for PET studies of the dopaminegic system — some quality assurance methods, experience and issues. *Appl. Radiat. Isot.*, 41, 483–492.

Sadzot B., Lemaire C., Maquet P., Plenevaux A., Salmon E., Degueldre C., Hermanne J.P., Guillaume M., Cantineau R., Franck G. and Comar D. (1993) Serotonin 5HT2 receptor imaging in the human brain using positron emission tomography and a new radioligand, [^{18}F]altanserin. Results in young normal controls. *J. Cerebr. Blood Flow Metab.*, In press.

Takahashi K., Murakami M., Hagami E., Sasaki H., Kondo Y., Mizusawa S., Nakamichi H., Tida H., Miura S., Kanno I., Uemura K. and Ido T. (1986) Radiosynthesis of ^{15}O-labelled butanol available for clinical use. *J. Label. Compd. Radiopharm.*, 23, 1111–1113. (Abstract).

Ulin J., Gee A.D., Malmborg P., Tedroff J. and Långström B. (1989) Synthesis of racemic (+) and (-)-N-[methyl-^{11}C]nomifensine, a ligand for evaluation of monoamine re-uptake sites by use of positron emission tomography. *Appl. Radiat. Isot.*, 40, 171–176.

Walsh M.N., Geltman E.M., Brown M.A., Henes C.G., Weinheimer C.J., Sobel B.E. and Bergman S.R. (1989) Noninvasive estimation of regional myocardial oxygen consumption by positron emission tomography with carbon-11 acetate in patients with myocardial infarction. *J. Nucl. Med.*, 30, 1798–1808.

Walter H., Kristeva R., Knott U., Schlaug G., Huangy A., Steinmetz H., Nebeling B., Herzog H., and Seitz R. J. (1993) Individual intermodal matching of MEG, PET, and MRI. *J. Cerebr. Blood Flow Metab.*, In Press.

Westera G. (1991) Production and quality control of 11-C acetate. *Proc. 4th Eur. Symp. Radiopharmacy & Radiopharmaceuticals*, May 1st–4th, Baden, Switzerland. (Abstract).

8. Appendix 1. Radioactivity Detectors

8.1. RADIOACTIVITY DETECTORS — GENERAL CONSIDERATIONS

There are several requirements for radioactivity monitoring in automated chemistry for PET. These include the monitoring of processes with radioactive gases, liquids and vapours as, for example, in the distillation of [^{11}C]iodomethane, quantitative detection of radioactive product eluted from HPLC, dose calibration for batch products and continuous dose calibration for bedside infusion systems, such as [^{15}O]water generators. A wide variety of methods of radioactivity detection are in use, each tailored to solve a specific problem. A comprehensive review is not possible here but a small selection of detectors is discussed below.

8.1.1. *Ionisation chambers.* These devices are invariably operated in the d.c. mode. Essentially, the ionisation caused in a gas by the radiation flux of either γ-rays, X-rays or β-particles is collected by electrodes polarised with a potential of 12-600 V. The collected charge is monitored with respect to time either as a rate of change of charge, as a d.c. current or in an integral mode as Coulombs collected in a pre-set sampling time. The currents measured are generally quite small (*e.g.* 0.1–100 pA), but these can be handled adequately with currently available devices such as the Keithley Model 485 or homemade units incorporating operational amplifiers (*e.g*. Teledyne Philbrick 1702).

The geometry of ionisation chambers can take many forms depending on the application. For example, dose calibrators generally employ re-entrant well-type chambers, hot-spot monitors usually use cylindrical or spherical chambers while flow-through chambers, for use with radioactive gases, are usually cylindrical. The filling gas is usually air at atmospheric pressure, the radioactive gas to be monitored or in some cases high pressure argon (20 bar; 300 psi). The latter provides for increased sensitivity to γ-rays as in, for example, the IG12 a re-entrant well-type ionisation chamber (see below).

8.1.2. *Commercial ionisation chambers.* The following commercial devices are useful.

a. Radioactivimeter ionisation chamber.

This is a three channel device with a variety of ionisation chambers for hot-spot monitoring (as used at Orsay) and available from:

Service Development Scientifique
47 Rue Clisson,
75013 PARIS — Tel. 45 82 46 09
France

b. High pressure ionisation chamber, type IG12.

This is suitable for dose calibration (as used at Hammersmith Hospital) and available from:

Centronic Ltd
Centronic House,
King Henry's Drive,
New Addington,
CROYDON CR9 OBH — Tel. (0689) 42121
U.K. — FAX (0689) 4305

c. Autoranging picoammeter model 485.
Available from:

Keithley Instruments
28775 Aurora Road,
Cleveland,
OH 44139 Tel. (216) 248-0400
USA. FAX (216) 248 6168

8.1.3. *Homemade ionisation chambers.* The PET group in Turku (Finland) have described several ionisation chambers designed for specific applications. These include two devices for monitoring flowing gas phase positron-emitters and one for liquid phase positron-emitters *e.g.* chromatography. They are all polarised with 12 V d.c and use a home-assembled current amplifier based on the Teledyne Philbrick 1702 device, avaialble from:

Teledyne Philbrick
Allied Drive at Route 128,
Dedham,
MA 02026
USA.

8.1.4. *Photodiode detectors.* A radiation-sensitive Pin silicon or photodiode may be used with a suitably compact positron-sensitive detector. It is possible to operate diodes in pulse or d.c mode. A preamplifier and nuclear type pulse amplifier are essential and the diode may be polarised with as little as 15 V. The d.c. mode is more attractive for high level measurements and here d.c. currents of 1 pA to 1 nA are measured with commercial or homemade current amplifiers, such as the Devar 529-01-5 integrated optical detector/amplifier, available from:

Devar Inc.
706 Bostwick Ave.,
Bridgeport,
CT 06605 Tel. (203) 368 6751
USA.

8.1.5. *Cadmium telluride detectors.* A range of very compact (*ca* 1 cm^3) cadmium telluride γ-sensitive detectors, that do not yet appear to have been exploited in the PET field, are available from:

Radiation Monitoring Devices Inc.
44 Hunt St,
Watertown,
MA 02171 Tel. (617) 926 1167
USA. FAX (617) 9743.

8.1.6. *Scintillator plus photomultiplier detectors.* This type of detector is classically the most flexible and easiest to operate. The size of the smallest practicable PM tube (Hamamatsu

Type R1460) is now 100 x 20 mm diameter. A variety of scintillators are available, ranging from bismuth germinate for small size γ-sensitive detectors to plastic scintillator NE 102A for tiny β-sensitive detectors, and glass scintillator-packed flow cells for HPLC detectors. This type of detector is usually operated in pulse mode but d.c. operation is also possible. The University of Madison at Wisconsin recently described a detector that operates in count mode for low levels and which changes over to d.c. mode for high levels.

8.1.7. *Geiger-Müller (G-M) tubes.* These are probably the simplest and most flexible detector currently available for hot-spot monitoring in PET chemistry. Very small tubes are readily available commercially. For example, the Philips ZP 1300 is 6 mm in diameter and has a sensitive length of 8 mm and operates on 500 V. Simple circuits are available to convert the G-M pulses into clean logic pulses for feeding into scalers or ratemeters. Alternatively, commercial multi-channel units are available from:

Centronic Ltd
(address above)

Genitron Instruments (for monitor 414 High dose, special model in use at KFA Jülich)
Heerst 149,
D-6000 FRANKFURT 90,
Germany

Mini Instruments
8 Station Industrial Estate,
Burnham on Crouch,
ESSEX CMO 84N — Tel. (0621) 783282
U.K. — FAX (01) 636 0394

Service Development Scientifique
(address above)

8.1.8. *Final comment.* Ionisation chambers and G-M counters appear to be used most extensively in this field and it is hoped that the wider distribution of the information relating to the supply of commercial units will in turn allow the manufacturers to offer economically packaged units if the demand grows!

9. Appendix 2. Selection Criteria for Remotely Operated Valves Used in PET Chemistry

9.1. INTRODUCTION

As most PET radiopharmaceutical syntheses involve small-scale reactions, the dead-volume of valves is of prime importance. Also, as reaction conditions are often quite aggressive, in order to achieve rapid synthesis, valves having inert contact surfaces are also vital. This appendix gives a list of useful valve manufactures, their addresses and telephone numbers and both a description and comment on particular valves used in PET automation. These valves are first discussed generally, according to type.

9.2. VALVE TYPES

9.2.1. *Membrane valves.* Membrane valves can be manufactured to meet the requirements of low dead-volume and inertness. These use fluorinated polymers for the body, such as Teflon™ (*e.g.* the Bürkert Contromatic AG range). The Teflon™ membrane has several major shortcomings. Firstly, Teflon™ is not very elastic and can fracture prematurely. Secondly, radiation can accelerate this process as it causes Teflon™ to become brittle. Furthermore, Teflon™ is quite permeable to solvents, vapours and gases. Thus, for example the exposure of Teflon™ membrane valves to chloride ion can soon lead to premature valve failure through corrosion of the 'non-contacting' parts of the valve (*i.e.* chlorine attack on stainless steel and aluminium). It is of course vital that these valves are provided with low dead-volume port fittings. Most manufacturers offer 1/4" x 28 UNF female ports suitable for use with flanged Teflon™ and 'Altex™' or 'Omnifit™' fittings. 1/8" NPT ports are disastrous for this type of valve, as the NPT fittings can rarely be made to mate without leaving a void of several hundred μL!

One further warning on membrane valves relates to their pressure rating. Most of the valves listed can, the manufacturers claim, operate at up to 2 bar (30 psi) but not necessarily in either direction *cf.* the Bürkert Contromatic AG range. Two- and three-port versions of membrane valves are available but in automated equipment it is recommended that two-port normally-closed (NC) valves are used, as three-port valves will always have a port to port interconnection, whether powered or not!

9.2.2. *Slider valves.* Inert low dead-volume slide valves, for example, the Rheodyne 5301, 5302 and Altex CAV 2031, are alternatives to membrane valves, when higher operating pressures are encountered. Both types of valve can be air-operated.

9.2.3. *Gas control valves.* Valves for controlling inert gases are widely available in, for example stainless steel or Viton™, from, for example, General Valve Corporation and Skinner Precision Industries. In the rather severe conditions involved in handling fluorine for radiochemistry with [^{18}F]fluorine, care must be exercised in selecting suitable valves. Nupro Co. air-operated bellows valves and General Valve Corporation electrovalves have been used satisfactorily, both having stainless steel (316) bodies with Kel-F™/Kalrez™seals.

9.2.4. *Rotary valves.* Where multi-port valves are needed it is wise to look at the wide range of rotary valves that are available. For low pressure applications low dead-volume inert (Teflon™/Kel-F™) valves are available from, for example, Rheodyne Inc. and Hamilton Co.

For high pressure systems, such as HPLC, stainless steel or Vespel™ valves are available from, for example, Rheodyne Inc. and Valco Instruments Co. Remote operation of these valves is achieved using air or electrical power.

9.3. VALVE LISTING

With some care and peer group guidance it is now possible to find suitable valves for all the known problems in PET radiopharmaceutical chemistry. The following is an alphabetical list of valve manufactures, giving their addresses, telephone numbers and details on useful valves. Some comments are made with respect to experience of their application in PET chemistry. A key to the mentioned valve types (coded a- j) is given at the end of this Appendix.

9.3.1. *Altex Scientific Inc.* 1780 4th Street, Berkeley, CA, USA. Tel. (415) 527 5900.

Types CAV 2031 *etc.*, air-operated slider valves (see key a, b, g).

Rated pressure	:	33 bar (500 psi)
Contact parts	:	Kel-F™, Teflon™
Body	:	Delrin™, (Kel-F™ option)
Ports	:	1/4" x 28
Operation	:	Pneumatic

These valves are difficult to maintain in routine use. The Delrin™ body is not acid-resistant. They are also known as Cheminert™ valves.

9.3.2. *Angar Scientific Co. Inc.* 52 Horsehill Road, Cedar Knolls, NJ 07927 2098, USA. Tel. (201) 538 9700. (Angar Scientific Co. Inc. are a subsidiary of Asco).

Types 368-2-xx-24-30, diaphragm valves (see key a, b, c).

Rated pressure	:	2 bar (30 psi)
Contact parts	:	Teflon™
Body	:	Aluminium, stainless steel
Ports	:	1/4" x 28
Operation	:	Electrical

xx denotes valve type. These valves are generally satisfactory. Over-pressure results in (reversible) valve opening. There is no leakage to atmosphere below 6.7 bar (100 psi).

9.3.3. *Bürkert Contromatic AG.* Hardstrasse 95, Postfach 42 CH-4020, Basel, Switzerland. Tel. (061) 425488.

Type 127-A-1, 2-H-TZ 1/4" 28 UNF 24/GR-R-000, diaphragm valves (see key b).

Rated pressure	:	2 bar (30 psi) forward, 0.33 bar (5 psi) reverse
Contact parts	:	Teflon™, Teflon™-coated EPDM
Body	:	Teflon™
Ports	:	1/4" x 28
Operation	:	Electrical

These valves are highly favoured by KFA Jülich.

9.3.4. *Chemcon (Production Techniques Ltd).* 13 Kings Road, Fleet, Hants, U.K. Tel. (0252) 616575. FAX 0252 615818.

Type SV1D-3-11T-1/4-28, diaphragm valves (see key b, c).

Rated pressure	:	2 bar (30 psi)
Contact parts	:	Teflon™
Body	:	Aluminium, Teflon™
Ports	:	1/4" x 28
Operation	:	Electrical

Over-pressure results in rupture of the Teflon™ diaphragm and leakage to atmosphere.

9.3.5. *General Valve Corporation.* 202 Fairfield Road, Fairfield, NJ, USA. Tel. (201) 575 4844.

Type 9-216-90, solenoid valve.

Rated pressure	:	83 bar (1250 psi)
Contact parts	:	Stainless steel, Kalrez™ and Kel-F™
Body	:	316 Stainless
Ports	:	1/8" NPT or 1/4" Swagelok™
Operation	:	Electrical

These valves are suitable for dilute fluorine mixtures.

9.3.6. *Hamilton Co.* P.O. Box 10030, Reno, NV 89520, USA. Tel. (702) 786 7077.

Type HV series valves (see key a-e, g).

Rated pressure	:	33 bar (500 psi)
Contact parts	:	Kel-F™, Teflon™
Body	:	Aluminium
Ports	:	1/4" x 28
Operation	:	Manual (electrical option available)

These are very compact rotary valves with various configurations available from two ports upwards.

Type HVDX and HVLX series valves (f, i, j see key)

These are six- and eight-port versions of the HV series.

9.3.7. *Neptune Research Inc.* 6 Lombardy Place, Maplewood, NJ 07040, USA. Tel. (201) 761 4268.

Series 225 T valves (see key a,b,c).

Rated pressure	:	23 bar (30 psi)
Contact parts	:	Teflon™
Body	:	Aluminium

Ports	:	1/4" x 28
Operation	:	Electrical

This company also makes pinch valves.

9.3.8. *Nupro Co.* 4800 East 345th Street, Willoughby, OH 44094, USA.

Type SS-SS2, needle valves.

Rated pressure	:	133 bar (2000 psi)
Contact parts	:	Stainless steel, Viton™ (Kalrez™ option)
Body	:	Stainless steel
Ports	:	1/8" Swagelok™ (SS-SS1 = 1/16"Swagelok™)
Operation	:	Manual

These are good general purpose needle valves.

Type SS-4 BMW, all stainless steel welded bellows needle valves (suitable for fluorine).

Rated pressure	:	47 bar (700 psi)
Contact parts	:	Stainless steel, (Monel™ option)
Body	:	Stainless steel
Ports	:	1/4" Swagelok™
Operation	:	Manual

Metering needle valve is suitable for low concentrations of fluorine at room temperature.

Type SS-HB S4-C, pneumatically-operated bellows valve (a,b see key).

Rated pressure	:	23.3 bar (3500 psi)
Contact parts	:	Stainless steel, Kel-F™ (Vespel™ option)
Body	:	Stainless steel
Ports	:	1/4 Swagelok™
Operation	:	Air

High pressure valves are used on [^{18}F]fluorine gas targets.

Type SS-HB S4-CM, as SS-HB S4-C but with electrical feedback contacts.

9.3.9. *Rheodyne Inc.* P.O. Box 996, Cotati, CA 94928, USA. Tel. (707) 664 9050. FAX (707) 664 8739.

Types 50xxP, Teflon™ 6-way valves (see key f, h, i)

Rated pressure	:	20 bar (300 psi)
Contact parts	:	Kel-F™, Teflon™
Body	:	Stainless steel and aluminium
Ports	:	1/4" x 28 Swagelok™ (flanged tubes)
Operation	:	Air

xx denotes valve type. These valves feature low dead-volume and electrical feedback of valve position and are available for 1/8" or 1/16" tubing.

Types 5301 and 5302, 3-port slider valves with 5300 actuator (see key c).

Rated pressure	:	6.7 bar (100 psi)
Contact parts	:	Teflon™ and Tefzel™
Body	:	Polypropylene
Ports	:	1/4" x 28 Swagelok™
Operation	:	Air

These valves are low dead volume and generally reliable. The valve face may distort on old valves. The 5301 has 0.030" passages while the 5302 has 0.060" passages.

Type 7010P, HPLC injector valves (see key i).

Rated pressure	:	46.6 bar (7000 psi)
Contact parts	:	Stainless steel and Vespel™
Body	:	Stainless steel
Ports	:	Special Rheodyne™ 1/16"compression
Operation	:	Air

Vespel™ is not recommended for use with strong bases and extremely polar solvents.

9.3.10. *Skinner Precision Industries Inc.* 95 Edgewood Avenue, New Britain, CT 06050, USA. Tel. (203) 225 6421.

Type B2 RX 127-DC2, 2-port valve with push on electrical connections (see key b).

Rated pressure	:	12 bar (180 psi)
Contact parts	:	Stainless steel, Viton™
Body	:	Stainless steel
Ports	:	1/8" NPT taper
Operation	:	Electrical

These valves are large dead-volume. They are useful in low pressure gas-handling systems.

Type B14 DK 1075-DC2, 3-port wire ended (see key c).

Rated pressure	:	5.3 bar (80 psi)
Contact parts	:	Stainless steel, Viton™
Body	:	Stainless steel
Ports	:	1/8" NPT taper
Operation	:	Electrical

This is a three-way valve similar to that above.

9.3.11. *Valco Instruments Co. Ltd.* P.O. Box 55603, Houston, TX, USA. Tel. (713) 688 9345.

Types P, PX, T, TX and related valves (see key a-h, k10, k12).

Rated pressure	:	200 bar (3000 psi)
Contact parts	:	Stainless steel, carbon-filled Teflon™
Body	:	Stainless steel
Ports	:	Compression fittings
Operation	:	Manual (pneumatic or electrical option)

This is an interesting selection of multi-way valves.

9.3.12. *Valcor Scientific.* 2 Lawrence Road, Springfield, NJ 07081, USA. Tel. (201) 467 8400. FAX (201) 467 8382

Types SV-74 and SV-75. Solenoid valves (see key a, b, c).

Rated pressure	:	2.3 bar (35 psi)
Contact parts	:	Teflon™
Body	:	Stainless steel, aluminium
Ports	:	1/4" x 28
Operation	:	Electrical

Pinch valves are also available from this manufacturer.

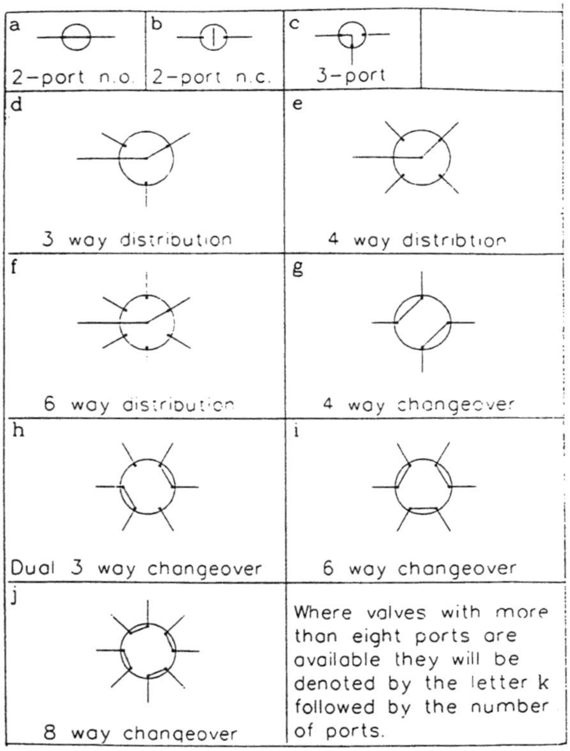

Figure 13. Key to mentioned valve types.

10. Appendix 3. Sources of Glassy Carbon Vessels

Glassy carbon has been found to be an excellent material for performing radiofluorinations from cyclotron-produced [^{18}F]fluoride and is used by many groups in preference to glass or platinum. The following is an alphabetical list of suppliers of glassy carbon vessels.

Cesiwid Electrowärme GmbH
Neumühle 4,
D-8520 ERLANGEN
Germany
Tel. 09131 45000
FAX 09131 450045

Electrocarbonium S.p.A.
Vialle della Liberazione, 18,
I-20124 MILANO
Italy
Tel. 02 67 58 1
FAX 02 66 98 56 25

Electrodenwerk Steeg Ges.m.b.H. and Co.
Postfach 1,
A-4823 STEEG AM HALLSTATTER SEE
Austria
Tel. 06135 8641 0
FAX 06135 864 1202

Hamosands Grafit AB
13 Varvsallen,
Box 223,
S-87125 HAMOSAND
Sweden
Tel. 0611 10530
FAX 0611 19122

L.G.D. Les Graphites Divers S.A.
70–76 rue Edith Cavell,
F-94400 VITRY,
France
Tel. 14 45730431
FAX 14 45730343

Polycarbon Inc.
28176 North Avenue Standford,
VALENCIA CA 91355
USA
Tel. 805 257 0500
FAX 805 257 2755

Ringsdorff-Werke GmbH
Drachenburgstrasse 1,
D-5300 BONN 2
Germany
Tel. 0228 841 0
FAX 0228 841 511

SIGRI Corporation
550 Route 206,
BEDMINSTER NJ 07921
USA
Tel. 201 231 3100
FAX 201 234 1953

SIGRI GmbH
Werner-von-Siemans Str. 18,
Postfach 1160,
D-8901 MEITLINGEN
Germany
Tel. 08271 83 0
Telex 53823
FAX 08271 83 3127

QUALITY ASSURANCE AND QUALITY CONTROL OF SHORT-LIVED RADIOPHARMACEUTICALS FOR PET

Geerd-J. Meyer, Heinz H. Coenen, Stephen L. Waters, Bengt Långström, Robert Cantineau, Karel Strijckmans, Willem Vaalburg, Christer Halldin, Christian Crouzel, Bernard Mazière and André Luxen

ABSTRACT. General guidelines for the quality assurance and quality control of short-lived radiopharmaceuticals for positron emission tomography (PET) are given. Quality assurance and quality control recommendations are also given for a selection of frequently used short-lived radiopharmaceuticals for PET, namely [1-^{11}C]acetate, *S*-[*carbonyl*-^{11}C]CGP 12177, L-[*N-methyl*-^{11}C]deprenyl, [*N-methyl*-^{11}C]flumazenil, ^{11}C-labelled-L-methionines, 3-*N*-[^{11}C]methylspiperone, [*O-methyl*-^{11}C]-raclopride, [^{13}N]ammonia, ^{15}O-labelled gases, *n*-[^{15}O]butanol, [^{15}O]water, [^{18}F]fluoride, 2-[^{18}F]fluoro-2-deoxy-D-glucose, L-6-[^{18}F]fluoro-DOPA and ^{18}F-labelled 3-*N*-alkylspiperones.

1. Foreword

Short-lived radiopharmaceuticals, especially those labelled with positron-emitting radionuclides of less than two hours half-life, call for special safety evaluation, quality assurance (QA) and quality control (QC) procedures. This has recently been acknowledged by the legislative bodies in Germany who have exempted these compounds from the regular testing requirements for pharmaceuticals during phase II and III trials (Bundesministerium der Justiz, 1989). However, special guidelines for the safety, quality assurance and quality control of these compounds have to be formulated. It was the aim of this expert group to help in establishing such guidelines not only for the needs of all users of these compounds in Europe but also for regulatory bodies, especially those within the EEC and member states.

In detail, this task group intended to:

— Formulate and recommend general guidelines for the development and production of safe and efficacious short-lived radiopharmaceuticals

— Formulate and recommend special quality control requirements for those radiopharmaceuticals that have passed from pure research to enter routine production for clinical use at several medical institutions

— Offer its help in formulating monographs and entries in the European and member-state pharmacopoeias for the preparation of these short-lived radiopharmaceuticals.

The focus of this chapter is on short-lived radiopharmaceuticals for use with positron emission tomography (PET).

G. Stöcklin and V. W. Pike (eds.), Radiopharmaceuticals for Positron Emission Tomography, 91–150.

2. General Guidelines for the QA and QC of Short-lived Radiopharmaceuticals for PET

2.1. INTRODUCTION

The special status of short-lived radiopharmaceuticals is based on the fact that they have to be produced within strict time limits near the site of their application and that there is insufficient time between their production and application to perform all currently accepted quality control tests. This holds true not only for tests of sterility and apyrogenicity but also for some tests of chemical quality.

Two further features of short-lived radiopharmaceuticals complicate their quality control measurements. One is the high radioactivity levels that must be dealt with during the production of these compounds. Their short half-lives may require initial radioactivity levels near 100 GBq (2.7 Ci) in order to end up with useful amounts for clinical investigations after perhaps two to four half-lives used for production. This implies a necessity to control all production steps remotely.

The other feature which hampers quality control measurements is the extremely small amount of the compound to be investigated. Most short-lived radiopharmaceuticals are produced in the so-called 'no-carrier-added' range (see Section 2.5.4.), often corresponding to near nanomole quantities. This offers the advantage to measure physiological functions without pharmacodynamic effect as, for example, in the determination of receptor binding sites or in the study of highly toxic materials. However, the analytical methods used for quality control must consequently be driven to their lower limits of detection.

In order to establish production guidelines that should ensure the safety and efficacy of short-lived radiopharmaceuticals, an international group of experts called in by the IAEA recently formulated general aspects and problems of quality control (Vera Ruiz *et al.*, 1990).

2.2. QUALIFICATION OF PERSONNEL

Any adequate quality control and quality assurance system for short-lived radiopharmaceuticals depends on a body of personnel that is highly qualified by virtue of advanced training and experience. Namely, this requires the special expertise of radiopharmaceutical chemists with experience in pharmaceutical practice or radiopharmacists with experience and training in the specialised production control and analysis of short-lived radiopharmaceuticals.

2.3. GENERAL PROCEDURES

According to good manufacturing practice (GMP) (Sharp, 1983; Bryant, 1989; Commission of the European Communities, 1990) the reliable production and quality assurance of (radio)pharmaceuticals has to follow 'documented general procedures' and 'batch protocols'. The documented general procedure must contain detailed descriptions of the:

- Qualitative and quantitative particulars of the developmental pharmaceutical and of all constituents
- Method of preparation
- Control of starting materials
- Control tests on the final product
- Stability tests.

Furthermore, the documented general procedure must contain a 'standardised operating procedure' (SOP) which is a detailed working manual for all individual steps of set-up, production, formulation, analysis, storage and documentation. The documentation should contain a batch protocol, which is an individual checklist to accompany each production run. The batch protocol, which is a crucial part of quality assurance, should include necessary checks on the individual steps as mentioned above.

In the special case of short-lived radiopharmaceuticals, where the quality control of the final product is limited by time, in-process control becomes the dominant factor for quality assurance. The general production philosophy for short-lived radiopharmaceuticals is therefore to establish individually strict production control measurements which, when adhered to, guarantee a certain product quality. This can be achieved by integrating, for example, radio-HPLC and radio-GC into the production process. A further efficient method of 'in-line' production control is the continuous monitoring of the radioactivity from one step of the synthesis to the next. This is likely to identify most problems in synthesis at a very early phase. It is essential to implement such processes during the development of a production procedure.

At the end of the development of a production procedure and with any subsequent substantial change, full quality control on several batches should verify the necessary quality criteria of the radiopharmaceutical.

Although it seems inappropriate to discuss all general quality control parameters in detail (*cf.* Vera Ruiz *et al.*, 1990), the five quality criteria which must be addressed for each individual preparation are discussed briefly in Section 2.5. below.

2.4. CONTROL OF STARTING MATERIALS

As mentioned in Section 2.3., the control of constituents and starting materials is part of GMP. Some general consideration of the often called 'entry control' is given here, since most radiopharmaceutical chemists in the PET field have little background in pharmacy or radiopharmacy and even standard books on nuclear pharmacy or radiopharmacy do not address this topic. Further quality control of short-lived radiopharmaceuticals depends largely on in-process control. This gives the quality of the starting materials special importance.

This topic is discussed in GMP rules (Sharp, 1983; Commission of the European Communities, 1990, 1991). In each country there might be special instructions for pharmaceutical industry, for example in Germany, the Betriebsverordnung für pharmazeutische Unternehmer (1985).

'Starting materials' means all constituents of a pharmaceutical product including the container, the septum *etc.* The Annex to Council Directive 75/318/EEC (Commission of the European Community, 1991) expressly states that target materials must be included as starting materials for radiopharmaceuticals. For each batch of starting material, identity and quality must be ensured and documented. After 'entry control', the batches of product must be labelled and the lot numbers later documented on the production control forms. Instructions for testing protocols and the description of the analytical methods, like final quality control, must be established. When the constituents are described in a pharmacopoeia, a detailed reference is sufficient. If the testing methods are not mentioned in a pharmacopoeia, they must be validated and quality requirements must be proven. If the starting materials are not in a pharmacopoeia, which is often true for precursors for PET radiopharmaceuticals, they must be described in a monograph. This will include name (IUPAC), methods of identification, description of purity tests, stability (maximal period of storage) and physico-chemical characteristics.

Whenever possible, certified materials from pharmaceutical manufacturers or the 'in-house' pharmacy should be purchased. Here, only identity tests are necessary and much time and documentation can be saved. This consideration is important to the generally small radiopharmaceutical chemistry groups.

2.5. QUALITY CRITERIA

2.5.1. *Radionuclidic purity.* Radionuclidic purity may be defined as '*the fraction of total radioactivity that is present as the specified radionuclide*'. Radionuclidic impurities may be isotopic or non-isotopic, and shorter or longer-lived than the specified radionuclide. Impurities may therefore 'decay out' or 'grow in'; hence the time between radionuclide production and administration must always be considered.

The primary determinant of the possible types and levels of radionuclidic impurities is the method of radionuclide production. Radionuclidic impurities may arise from undesired nuclear reactions induced in the target isotope, or a non-target isotope and by recoil reactions and sputtering in targets (body materials and especially window foils).

The need for radionuclidic purity in a radiopharmaceutical is primarily to avoid unnecessary radiation dose to the subject of the study, to avoid degradation of the image quality and to limit errors on measurements *in vivo*. Any requirement on radionuclidic purity should therefore be 'sufficient for the intended use', rather than systematically severe *i.e.* it should take into account any real inconveniences that might result to the subject and to the intended measurement.

2.5.2. *Chemical purity.* The chemical purity of a radiopharmaceutical may be defined as '*the fraction of compound in the formulated radiopharmaceutical that is in the desired molecular form*'. As for normal pharmaceutical preparations, appropriate chemical purity is mandatory in radiopharmaceuticals to avoid adverse reactions in human application, and pharmacological or toxic effects.

The first requirement in terms of chemical purity is the verification of the chemical identity of the labelled compound. This includes verification of the stereoisomeric purity of the compound, whenever this has to be considered. Because of the low chemical mass of cyclotron-produced radiopharmaceuticals, which sometimes prohibits or hinders the use of standard analytical procedures, chemical identity is often established by comparison with standards. Most often this is achieved by chromatographic methods that compare the mobility of the labelled compound with non-radioactive reference material. The necessary reference compounds include not only the desired compound, but also its stereoisomers. This method requires advanced experience in chromatography and their detectors, with both radioactive and non-radioactive materials, in order to select suitable operating conditions. These should be optimised for the separation of the reference compound from known and possible derivatives, precursors and likely impurities. In order to minimise errors by this identification procedure, at least two different and independent chromatographic procedures should be applied.

The second requirement in establishing chemical purity calls for the absence of any undesired chemical compound in the preparation. A small amount of chemical impurity, even below that which produces a clinically detectable response, can interfere with the efficacy of the diagnostic procedure at the molecular level. Contaminants may compete for active transport mechanisms and enzyme- or receptor-binding.

In cases, where there is no interference with the physiological process to be measured, higher amounts of a by-product may be tolerable. Since the starting material, or a closely related derivative produced during the synthesis, is the most likely chemical contaminant from any labelling procedure, it is advantageous to have a method of preparative chromatography that will elute the starting material after the low mass of radiopharmaceutical. In cases where this is not possible, peak tailing can lead to considerable contamination.

For administration by intravenous injection, the final preparation must be a clear, colourless and particulate-free solution.

2.5.3. *Radiochemical purity.* Radiochemical purity may be defined as '*the fraction of a specific radionuclide that is present in the desired chemical form and in the specified molecular position*'. Since PET is a technique which is capable of delivering quantitative measurements, it demands radiopharmaceuticals of the highest achievable radiochemical purity.

Radiochemical impurities may originate from radionuclide production, from subsequent chemistry (*e.g.* through incomplete reactions, side reactions, reactions with impurities or solvents, or incomplete removal of protecting groups), from failed or incomplete preparative separation or as a result of chemical change during storage (*e.g.* radiation-induced). Because of time limitations, routine quality assurance is usually based on chromatography with sensitive radioactivity detection.

Radio-HPLC is most applicable to the routine quality control of the radiochemical purity of labelled compounds, since it can combine high speed, high resolution and high sensitivity. Accurate quality control has to be performed by independent analysis on the separated end-product, preferably as closely before administration *in vivo* as possible. Analytical data, taken from the preparative HPLC separation of the labelled compound only, cannot reveal errors in peak collection or poor resolution of impurities. The latter problem is compounded by the intrinsically lower selectivity of preparative HPLC compared to analytical HPLC. Pitfalls are best avoided by regular calibration of the analytical procedure with appropriate standards. However, a virtue of HPLC is that the use of a suitable detector for stable compounds in series with the radioactivity detector also provides for simultaneous measurement of chemical purity and specific radioactivity. In special cases other techniques can be applicable to the determination of radiochemical purity including radio-GC, radio-TLC and enzyme assays.

2.5.4. *Specific radioactivity.* Specific radioactivity refers to the '*amount of radioactivity per mass of a radiopharmaceutical*' and is usually expressed as Bq per µmol. It should be stated on the label of the individual dose with respect to a specified time. In certain applications, as in the preparation of glucose derivatives, amino acids, fatty acids and other tracers, which have physiologically abundant counterparts, a representative measurement of the specific radioactivity is sufficient. Contamination of the radiopharmaceutical with compounds of similar biological activity (such as precursors, analogues and derivatives) will reduce the *apparent* or *effective* specific radioactivity *in vivo*.

In the past the term 'carrier-free' has seldom been used in its most rigorous sense and examples of the direct measurement of specific radioactivity, where no carrier dilution was found, have been rare. Therefore it has been proposed (*cf.* Wolf, 1981) to establish three categories of specific radioactivity: 1) carrier-free, 2) no-carrier-added, and 3) carrier-added. According to these categories the term 'carrier-free' should only be used for compounds where analytical verification of a carrier-free state has been established.

2.5.5. *Pharmaceutical quality.* In the production of radiopharmaceuticals with short-lived radioisotopes the assurance of sterility, apyrogenicity, isotonicity, acceptable pH and a predefined stability rests predominantly on the maintenance of an adequate production procedure. Tests on these criteria should be carried out to ensure that the products meet the requirements of the local pharmacopoeia.

a. Sterility.

Sterilisation refers to the destruction and/or removal of bacteria and organisms. It should be mentioned here that no radiopharmaceutical is self-sterilising due to its own radiation. If the solution for injection is sterilised by autoclaving, an additional assurance is given by recording the temperature of the autoclave with time. However, the stability of the radiopharmaceutical to autoclaving must be confirmed beforehand.

Due to the short half-life of most cyclotron-derived radiopharmaceuticals that are used in-house and due to the fact that many of them are heat-labile compounds, sterilisation is generally achieved by sterile filtration (0.22 μm). For each radiopharmaceutical for human use, the effectiveness of sterilisation should be confirmed independently by a qualified professional using accepted procedures.

b. Apyrogenicity.

Pyrogens are materials that cause fever. Typically, they are bacterial by-products and the term pyrogen is used interchangeably with bacterial endotoxin. Pyrogens are not removed by simple boiling of the solution and are not removed by microporous membrane filtration. It is recommended that pyrogen-free aqueous solutions, reagents and glassware be used. In syntheses which require the hydrolytic removal of protecting groups with mineral acids, additional safety may be achieved, since the heating of solutions at $pH < 1$ above $80^{o}C$ for more than 10 min destroys pyrogens quite effectively. On the other hand, separation and purification steps that use ion exchange material or a gel material like Sephadex™, which are potential carriers of pyrogens, call for special attention.

Verification of the apyrogenicity of a product from a particular production procedure should be confirmed by independent testing of a portion by a qualified professional using accepted procedures. These tests should be performed not only during the set-up phase but at regular intervals during routine production. Given the unusually demanding circumstances under which short-lived radiopharmaceuticals are prepared from cyclotron-produced radioisotopes it is strictly recommended to perform the Limulus test. In the Limulus test the product meets the requirements of the bacterial endotoxin tests, the limit of endotoxin content being not more than 175/V USP endotoxin unit per mL of the injection in which V is the maximal recommended total dose in mL at the expiration date.

c. pH.

The pH of a radiopharmaceutical preparation is quite likely to vary from batch to batch. Since quick testing of this factor is feasible, it should be performed on a regular basis. The actual pH should be stated on the label of each preparation and should be within the physiologically acceptable range (5.5–8).

d. Isotonicity.

Isotonicity can usually be assured by appropriate setting up of the purification and formulation steps at the end of the preparation. In most cases it does not call for regular testing.

e. Stability.

The stability of most short-lived radiopharmaceuticals is limited by the physical half-life of the radionuclide. There are other limitations, however, which have to be considered, especially for oxidation- and radiation-sensitive compounds. While some radiopharmaceuticals, such as for example, 2-[^{18}F]fluoro-2-deoxy-D-glucose (2-^{18}FDG) (see Section 3.13.8.) and L-[*S-methyl*-^{11}C]methionine (see Section 3.5.7.), are very stable towards radio-decomposition up to radioactivity concentrations of 1 GBq/mL (27 mCi/mL), others such as *S*-[*N-methyl*-^{11}C]nomifensine are rather unstable (Pike *et al.*, 1990) and must be used immediately after final purification.

2.6. REFERENCES

Betriebsverordnung für pharmazeutische Unternehmer. (1988) Bundesgesetzblatt I, S. 546, 8th March 1985 bzw. Verordnung zur Änderung der Betriebsverordnung, Bundesgesetzblatt I, S. 480, 25th March 1988.

Bryant R. (1989) *The Pharmaceutical Quality Control Handbook*, Aster Publishing Corporation, Eugene, Org. USA,

Bundesministerium der Justiz. (1989) Allgemeine Verwaltungsvorschrift zur Anwendung der Arzeneimittelprüfrichtlinien. Bundesanzeiger 41, No. 243a, p. 5. (29th December).

Commission of the European Communities (1990) III/B/6. 'The rules governing medical products in the European Community, Vol. IV; Guide to good manufacturing practice for medicinal products.' (Draft supplementary guidelines for the manufacture of radiopharmaceuticals). No. III/3973/89-EN (April). Brussels, Belgium.

Commission of the European Communities. (1991) Annex to Council Directive 75/318/EEC. III 19062/90-EN (17th January). Brussels, Belgium.

Pike V.W., Kensett M.J., Turton, D.R., Waters S.L. and Silvester D.J. (1990) Labelled agents for PET studies of the dopaminergic system — some quality assurance methods, experience and issues. *Appl. Radiat. Isot.*, 41, 483–492.

Sharp J.R. (1983) Ed., *Guide to Good Pharmaceutical Manufacturing Practice*, HMSO London.

Vera Ruiz H., Marcus C.S., Pike V.W., Coenen H.H., Fowler J.S., Meyer G-J., Cox P.H., Vaalburg W., Cantineau R., Helus F. and Lambrecht R.M. (1990) Report of an International Atomic Energy Agency's Advisory Group Meeting on "Quality control of cyclotron-produced radiopharmaceuticals". *Nucl. Med. Biol.*, 17, 445–456.

Wolf A.P. (1981) Synthesis of organic compounds labeled with positron emitters and the carrier problem. *J. Label. Compd. Radiopharm.*, 18, 1–2. (Abstract).

3. QA and QC Recommendations for Frequently Used Short-lived Radiopharmaceuticals for PET

3.1. [1-^{11}C]ACETATE

3.1.1. *Introduction.* Although the heart can recruit its energy demands by a variety of metabolic processes, fatty acids constitute the main energy source for heart muscle under normal conditions. Whereas the availability of long-chain fatty acids is buffered by branching of the metabolic pathway into direct oxidation and storage in the triglyceride pool, acetate enters the tricarboxylic acid (Krebs) cycle at the last possible step by binding to coenzyme-A. At this stage its transition through myocardium reflects the activity of the Krebs cycle. Thus, [1-^{11}C]acetate can be used as a tracer for the measurement of myocardial oxygen utilisation (Buxton *et al.*, 1988, 1989; Walsh *et al.*, 1989; Kotzerke *et al.*, 1990).

3.1.2. *Radiochemistry.* [1-^{11}C]Acetate is most commonly produced via the reaction of the Grignard reagent, methylmagnesium bromide, with cyclotron-produced [^{11}C]carbon dioxide (Pike *et al.*, 1982, 1984; Brown *et al.*, 1987; Walsh *et al.*, 1989; Westera, 1991; Meyer *et al.*, 1993). Grignard reagent is available commercially and can be used from stock solutions. After a short reaction time the radioactive adduct is hydrolysed with water or aqueous acid. Most papers describe a purification by solvent extraction (Pike *et al.*, 1982, 1984; Brown *et al.*, 1987; Buxton *et al.*, 1989, Walsh, 1989; Westera, 1991). Modifications of this procedure have been mentioned by several authors, using simplified phase separation or distillation techniques (Brown *et al.*, 1987; Buxton *et al.*, 1989; Westera 1991; Norenberg *et al.*, 1992). Alternatively, and in order to avoid phase separation techniques, hydrolysis is carried out with a minimal amount of water, followed by evaporation of all solvents to dryness. Resolubilisation in a weakly acidic phosphate buffer and passage of this solution over a combined silver oxide-cation exchange cartridge and through a sterile 0.22 µm filter, yields an injectable solution of [1-^{11}C]acetate. Analysis is carried out by HPLC (Westera, 1991; Meyer *et al.*, 1993).

3.1.3. *Radionuclidic purity.* As with all organic ^{11}C-labelled compounds, radionuclidic purity is usually a negligible problem since all possible impurities are eliminated during the synthesis. As long as the production parameters are not changed, a thorough investigation of radionuclidic purity is only necessary during the set-up phase of the routine synthesis. In these tests the γ-ray spectrum must be identical to that of carbon-11, in that it exhibits a major photo peak at 0.511 MeV and possibly a sum peak at 1.02 MeV, depending on source geometry and detector efficiency. Since γ-ray spectroscopy cannot distinguish between the positron-emitters, it is mandatory to determine that the half-life of the product is 20.4 min, by a suitable detector system.

3.1.4. *Chemical purity.* All possible chemical impurities arise from the Grignard reagent, which is used in quantities of about 0.1–0.4 mmol per batch. Hydrolysis of excess methylmagnesium bromide yields methane, magnesium hydroxide and bromide. Organic by-products, like bromoethane, bromomethane, acetone or *t.*-butanol may arise from impurities in the Grignard reagent, its dimerisation or its decomposition. All organic impurities are separated from [1-^{11}C]acetate by solvent extraction or evaporation of the solvent to dryness after hydrolysis. In the former method the aqueous phase must be cleared of residual organic solvent by flushing it with inert gas. The conditions for complete removal must be elaborated using GC analysis and strictly adhered to in routine preparations.

Inorganic by-products, such as Mg^{2+} and Br^{-} ions, can be removed by silver oxide and cation exchange cartridges. However, taking into account the known toxicity levels of these ions, a separation does not seem necessary, provided the amount of Grignard reagent used in the reaction is limited to 0.1 mmol.

Analysis should be carried out by HPLC using an anion exchange column (*e.g.* Aminex™ 87H from BioRad, REZEX™ organic acid from Phenomenex or Nucleosil™-10-Anion from Macherey and Nagel) eluted with a weak aqueous mineral acid, such as 2.5mM-sulphuric acid (Buxton *et al.*, 1989; Meyer *et al.*, 1993). Acetate may be detected down to 0.1mM by detectors for absorbance at 210 nm. Salt concentrations of a few mM can be detected with a refractive index detector

3.1.5. *Radiochemical purity.* Incomplete reaction of [^{11}C]carbon dioxide with the Grignard reagent may leave [^{11}C]carbonate as a possible contaminant. This is most conveniently removed by purging the acid-reconstituted reaction mixture with nitrogen or any other inert gas. As a double safety measure, passage of the solution through a silver oxide column (*e.g.* OnGuard™-Ag by Dionex) removes any residual [^{11}C]carbonate. Reaction of excess Grignard reagent with the primary adduct between [^{11}C]carbon dioxide and the Grignard reagent may lead to by-products with a higher molecular weight, such as [2-^{11}C]acetone and *t.*-[2-^{11}C]butanol. These can be avoided by milder reaction conditions such as a reduced concentration of Grignard reagent and/or a shorter reaction time. Analysis can be carried out most conveniently by HPLC, preferably with an an ion exchange column as stated above. This should demonstrate the complete removal of any labelled carbonate.

3.1.6. *Specific radioactivity.* Since [^{11}C]carbon dioxide is usually produced no-carrier-added, the specific radioactivity may be as high as about 100–200 GBq/µmol (2.7–5.4 Ci/µmol) at the end of synthesis, even if no special precautions are taken. The specific radioactivity is reduced by any ingress of atmospheric carbon dioxide into the Grignard reagent. However, a lower specific radioactivity presents no problem in application, since acetate is quite abundant in blood under physiological conditions.

3.1.7. *Pharmaceutical quality.* Pharmaceutical quality is achieved by strict control of the determining parameters. For [1-^{11}C]acetate these consist of the following measures. The reaction system is set up from clean sterilised glassware and sterile medical tubing for each production batch. The [1-^{11}C]acetate is collected in a sterilised capped vial after passage through a sterile 0.22 µm filter. The pH of the product is adjusted to 7.0 ± 1.0 with a physiologically acceptable buffer. This is controlled in each individual batch. The isotonicity should be checked at regular intervals. The synthesis system must have been shown to produce apyrogenic and sterile products at least three times before products are prepared for administration to humans. Sterility and apyrogenicity of the product are checked frequently in routine production runs (every month) by taking samples and testing these by the standard procedures. In the Limulus test the product meets the requirements of the bacterial endotoxin tests, as stated under Section 2.5.5. Small samples of each batch should be withheld for retrospective testing of any relevant parameter if required.

[1-^{11}C]Acetate preparations containing up to 2 GBq (54 mCi) in 5 mL have been shown to be stable in aqueous solution at pH levels between 5.0 and 7.5 for two hours at room temperature (Meyer *et al.*, 1993).

3.1.8. *References.*

Brown M., Marshall D.R., Sobel B.E. and Bergmann S.R. (1987) Delineation of myocardial oxygen utilization with carbon-11-labeled acetate. *Circulation,* 76, 687–696.

Buxton D.B., Schwaiger M., Nguyen A., Phelps M.E. and Schelbert H.R. (1988) Radiolabeled acetate as a tracer of myocardial tricarboxylic acid cycle flux. *Circulation Res.,* 63, 628–634.

Buxton D.B., Nienaber C.A., Luxen A., Ratib O., Hansen H., Phelps M.E. and Schelbert H.R. (1989) Noninvasive quantitation of regional myocardial oxygen consumption in vivo with [1-^{11}C]acetate and dynamic positron emission tomography. *Circulation,* 79, 134–142.

Kotzerke J., Hicks R.J., Wolfe E., Herman W.H., Molina E., Kuhl D.E. and Schwaiger M. (1990) Three-dimensional assessment of myocardial oxidative metabolism: a new approach for regional determination of PET-derived carbon-11-acetate kinetics. *J. Nucl. Med.*, 31, 1876–1893.

Meyer G-J., Günther K., Matzke K-H., Harms Th. and Hundeshagen H. (1993) A modified preparation method for ^{11}C acetate, preventing liquid phase extraction steps. *J. Label. Compd. Radiopharm.,* 32, 182–183. (Abstract).

Norenberg J.P., Simpson N.R., Dunn B.B. and Kiesewetter D.O. (1992) Remote synthesis of [1-^{11}C]acetate. *Appl. Radiat. Isot.*, 43, 943–945.

Pike V.W,, Eakins M.N., Allan R.M. and Selwyn A.P. (1982) Preparation of [1-^{11}C]acetate — an agent for the study of myocardial metabolism by positron emission tomography. *Int. J. Appl. Radiat. Isot.,* 33, 505–512.

Pike V.W., Horlock P.L., Brown C. and Clark J.C. (1984) The remotely-controlled preparation of a ^{11}C-labelled radiopharmaceutical — [1-^{11}C]acetate. *Int. J. Appl. Radiat. Isot.,* 35, 623–627.

Walsh M.N., Geltman E.M., Brown M.A., Henes C.G., Weinheimer C.J., Sobel B.E. and Bergman S.R. (1989) Noninvasive estimation of regional myocardial oxygen consumption by positron emission tomography with carbon-11 acetate in patients with myocardial infarction. *J. Nucl. Med.*, 30, 1798–1808.

Westera G. (1991) Production and quality control of 11-C acetate. *Proc. 4th Eur. Symp. Radiopharmacy & Radiopharmaceuticals,* May 1st–4th, Baden, Switzerland. (Abstract).

3.2. *S*-[*CARBONYL*-^{11}C]CGP 12177

3.2.1. *Introduction.* Quantitation of β-adrenergic receptors in the heart offers new diagnostic information with direct therapeutic consequences for patients treated with β-blockers. For this purpose several antagonists such as propranolol, practolol, pindolol, carazolol and CGP 12177, have been labelled with carbon-11 or fluorine-18. Among these *S*-[*carbonyl*-^{11}C]CGP 12177 is the most promising and has been used for β-receptor characterisation *in vivo* (Delforge *et al.*, 1992).

3.2.2. *Radiochemistry*. Feasible routes to *S*-[*carbonyl*-^{11}C]CGP 12177 have been reported by several authors (Brady *et al.*, 1991; Hammadi and Crouzel, 1991) and involve addition of [^{11}C]phosgene to *S*-1-(2,3-diaminophenoxy)-3-(*t*.-butylamino)-2-propanol at room temperature [*cf.* the conditions for the preparation of racemic radioligand originally reported by Boullais *et al.* (1986)]. Synthesis of this cold precursor has been described from, for example, *S*-3-tosyloxy-1,2-propanediol acetonide (Hammadi and Crouzel, 1991) or *S*-glycidyl-3-nitrobenzenesulphonate (Aigbirhio *et al.*, 1992). [^{11}C]Phosgene can be prepared routinely from [^{11}C]methane (Landais and Crouzel, 1987).

3.2.3. *Radionuclidic purity*. As with all organic ^{11}C-labelled compounds, radionuclidic purity is usually a negligible problem since all possible impurities are eliminated during the synthesis. As long as the production parameters are not changed, a thorough investigation of radionuclidic purity is only necessary during the set-up phase of the routine synthesis. In these tests the γ-ray spectrum must be identical to that of carbon-11, in that it exhibits a major photo peak at 0.511 MeV and possibly a sum peak at 1.02 MeV, depending on source geometry and detector efficiency. Since γ-ray spectroscopy cannot distinguish between the positron-emitters, it is mandatory to determine that the half-life of the product is 20.4 min, by a suitable detector system.

3.2.4. *Chemical purity*. *S*-[*carbonyl*-^{11}C]CGP 12177 can be purified by HPLC using a reverse phase column (*e.g.* µ-Bondapak™ C-18, 30 cm x 7.8 mm i.d., 10 µm particle size) Waters Associates) eluted at 4 mL/min with physiological saline-ethanol (7:1 v/v) containing 2mM-phosphate buffer adjusted to pH 2.3. Precursor elutes at 2.5 min and the radioligand at 4.5 to 5.5 min. Ethanol is purged from the collected fraction of product by bubbling nitrogen through the solution for 2 min.

With respect to the pharmacodynamic effects of receptor ligands and their derivatives and their possible interference with PET measurements, control of the mass level of *S*-CGP 12177 itself (see specific radioactivity), the cold precursor and derived impurities is mandatory for each run. This must be checked routinely by HPLC analysis of the product. Each batch of *S*-precursor (or its chiral progenitor) should be checked for enantiomeric purity, for example by chiral HPLC (Aigbirhio *et al.*, 1992).

3.2.5. *Radiochemical purity*. The radiochemical purity of each batch of radioligand can be checked by the same HPLC system used to determine chemical purity, simply by adding a radioactivity detector. This should be performed routinely. Radiochemical purity should exceed 98%. Enantiomeric purity may be estimated by chiral HPLC on a sample of CGP 12177 produced from any given batch of the *S*-diamino-precursor (see Aigbirhio *et al.*, 1992). However, routine measurement is unnecessary as it has been demonstrated that the labelling reaction does not cause racemisation (Aigbirhio *et al.*, 1992).

3.2.6. *Specific radioactivity*. The specific radioactivity of *S*-[*carbonyl*-^{11}C]CGP 12177 mostly depends on the specific radioactivity of the [^{11}C]phosgene used for labelling. Higher specific radioactivity is obtained if the [^{11}C]phosgene is produced catalytically (Landais and Crouzel, 1987) rather than photochemically (Diksic *et al.*, 1982). The specific radioactivity is measured routinely by a radio-HPLC system, incorporating a highly sensitive UV spectrophotometer, and calibrated for mass with reference CGP 12177. The specific radioactivity should be in the range 20–60 GBq/µmol (*ca* 0.5–1.5 Ci/µmol) at the time of measurement. This value should be stated on the label of the radiopharmaceutical container together with the time of calibration.

3.2.7. *Pharmaceutical quality.* Pharmaceutical quality is achieved by strict control of the determining parameters. For *S*-[*carbonyl*-^{11}C]CGP 12177 these consist of the following measures. The reaction system is set up from clean sterilised glassware and sterile medical tubing for each production batch. The product eluted from the HPLC column is collected in a sterilised capped vial. After evaporation of most of the ethanol the residue is passed through a 0.22 μm sterile filter.

The isotonicity should be checked at regular intervals. The synthesis system must be shown to produce apyrogenic and sterile products at least three times before production for administration to humans. Sterility and apyrogenicity of the product should be checked frequently in routine production runs (every month) by taking samples and testing these by standard procedures. In the Limulus test the product meets the requirement of the bacterial endotoxin tests, as stated under Section 2.5.5. Small samples of each batch should be withheld for retrospective testing of any relevant parameter if required.

Formulated solutions of *S*-[*carbonyl*-^{11}C]CGP 12177 have not shown radiochemical instability over short periods (40 min) after preparation.

3.2.8. *References.*

Aigbirhio F., Pike V.W., Francotte E., Waters S.L., Banfield B., Jaeggi K.A. and Drake A. (1992) *S*-[1-(2,3,-Diaminophenoxy)]-3'-(*N*-*t*-butylamino)propan-2'-ol — simplified asymmetric synthesis with CD and chiral HPLC analysis. *Tetrahedron: Asymmetry*, 3, 539–554.

Boullais C., Crouzel C. and Syrota A. (1986) Synthesis of 4-(3-*t*.-butylamino-2-hydroxypropoxy)benzimidazol-2-[^{11}C]one (CGP 12177). *J. Label. Compd. Radiopharm.*, 23, 565–567.

Brady F., Luthra S.K., Tochon-Danguy H-J., Steel C.J., Waters S.L., Kensett M.J., Landais P., Shah F., Jaeggi K.A., Clark J.C. and Pike V.W. (1991) Asymmetric synthesis of a precursor for the automated radiosynthesis of *S*-(3'-*t*-butylamino-2'-hydroxypropoxy)-benzimidazol-2-[^{11}C]one (*S*-[^{11}C]CGP 12177) as a preferred radioligand for β-adrenergic receptors. *Appl. Radiat. Isot.*, 42, 621–628.

Delforge J., Syrota A., Lançon J-P., Nakajima K., Loc'h C., Janvier M., Vallois J.M., Cayla J. and Crouzel C. (1992) Cardiac beta-adrenergic receptor density measured in vivo using PET, CGP 12177 and a new graphic method. *J. Nucl. Med.*, 32, 739–748.

Diksic M., Jolly D. and Farrokhzad S. (1982) An on line synthesis of "no-carrier-added" [^{11}C]phosgene. *Int. J. Nucl. Med. Biol.*, 9, 283–285.

Hammadi A. and Crouzel C. (1991) Asymmetric synthesis of (2S)-and (2R)-4-(3-t-butylamino-2-hydroxypropoxy)-benzimidazol-2-[^{11}C]-one ((S)-and (R)-[^{11}C]-CGP 12177 from optically active precursors. *J. Label. Compd. Radiopharm.*, 29, 681–690.

Landais P. and Crouzel C. (1987) A new synthesis of carbon-11 labelled phosgene. *Appl. Radiat. Isot.*, 38, 297–300.

3.3. L-[*N-METHYL*-^{11}C]DEPRENYL

3.3.1. *Introduction.* The enzyme, monoamine oxidase type B (MAO-B), catalyses the oxidative deamination of endogenous and exogenous amines. L-[*N-methyl*-^{11}C]Deprenyl, a suicide inhibitor of the enzyme, has been used to map the presence of MAO-B both in living human and animal brain (MacGregor *et al.*, 1985; Arnett *et al.*, 1987; Axelsson *et al.*, 1987; Fowler *et al.*, 1987, 1988).

3.3.2. *Radiochemistry.* L-[*N-methyl*-^{11}C]Deprenyl has been prepared by methylation of the *nor*-precursor with [^{11}C]iodomethane (MacGregor *et al.*, 1988). Purification can be achieved by sample enrichment (C-18 reverse phase) followed by HPLC. Stereospecific synthesis of the *nor*-precursor has been described (MacGregor *et al.*, 1988).

3.3.3. *Radionuclidic purity.* As with all organic ^{11}C-labelled compounds, radionuclidic purity is usually a negligible problem since all possible impurities are eliminated during the synthesis. As long as the production parameters are not changed, a thorough investigation of radionuclidic purity is only necessary during the set-up phase of the routine synthesis. In these tests the γ-ray spectrum must be identical to that of carbon-11, in that it exhibits a major photo peak at 0.511 MeV and possibly a sum peak at 1.02 MeV, depending on source geometry and detector efficiency. Since γ-ray spectroscopy cannot distinguish between the positron-emitters, it is mandatory to determine that the half-life of the product is 20.4 min, by a suitable detector system.

3.3.4. *Chemical purity.* The product is purified by reverse phase HPLC on a C-18 column (*e.g.* μ-Bondapak™, 10 μm, 7.8 x 300 mm, Waters Associates) eluted with 10mM-ammonium formate-methanol (35:65 v/v). Under these conditions the product is well separated from starting materials. Since the amounts of reagents are necessarily large compared to the amount of product, peak tailing and the efficiency of the HPLC column should be regularly monitored. However, generally, the overall mass of reagents still allows adequate separation in one chromatographic cycle. Proof of chemical purity should be obtained by independent analytical methods, such as NMR spectroscopy and mass spectrometry on decayed products when setting up the production process. The purity of each batch of final product should be analyzed by reverse phase HPLC using a C-18 column (*e.g.* μ-Bondapak™, 10 μm, 4 x 250 mm, Waters Associates) eluted with 1mM-diammonium hydrogen orthophosphate-methanol (70:30 v/v). The preparative HPLC system, as well as the analytical, must be calibrated using appropriate standards.

3.3.5. *Radiochemical purity.* The radiochemical purity of each batch can be checked with the same HPLC system that is used for measuring chemical purity, simply by adding a suitable radioactivity detector. The separated L-[*N-methyl*-^{11}C]deprenyl should have a radiochemical purity of at least 98%. Enantiomeric purity should be estimated on at least one sample produced from any given batch of the *nor*-precursor.

3.3.6. *Specific radioactivity.* For quantitative PET studies there is a requirement to produce L-[*N-methyl*-^{11}C]deprenyl at high specific radioactivity. It may be determined accurately by HPLC methods equipped with both quantitative radioactivity and mass detection. As the UV extinction coefficient is particularly low, even at the λ_{max} of 260 nm, a highly sensitive spectrophotometer is required. The specific radioactivity should be in the range 30–65 GBq/μmol (0.5–1.8 Ci/μmol) at the end of synthesis.

3.3.7. *Pharmaceutical quality*. Pharmaceutical quality is achieved by strict control of the determining parameters. For L-[*N-methyl*-^{11}C]deprenyl these consist of the following measures. The reaction system is set up from clean sterilised glassware and sterile medical tubing for each production batch. The L-[*N-methyl*-^{11}C]deprenyl, eluted from the HPLC column, is collected in a sterilised capped vial. After evaporation of the mobile phase the residue is re-dissolved in sterile saline or phosphate buffer. Addition of ethanol during final formulation, for reasons of achieving solubility and stability, should not exceed 5% of volume for pharmacological safety. The final solution is passed through a 0.22 μm sterile filter.

The pH of the product is adjusted to 7.0 ± 1.0 with a physiologically acceptable buffer. This is controlled for each individual batch. The isotonicity should be checked at regular intervals. The synthesis system must be shown to produce apyrogenic and sterile products at least three times before production for administration to humans. Sterility and apyrogenicity of the product should be checked frequently in routine production runs (every month) by taking samples and testing these by standard procedures. In the Limulus test the product meets the requirement of the bacterial endotoxin tests, as stated under Section 2.5.5. Small samples of each batch should be withheld for retrospective testing of any relevant parameter if required.

High specific radioactivity L-[*N-methyl*-^{11}C]deprenyl preparations, containing up to 2 GBq in 10 mL, have been shown to be stable in aqueous solutions at a pH between 6.0 and 6.5 for up to two hours at room temperature.

3.3.8. *References*.

Arnett C.D., Fowler J.S., MacGregor R.R., Schlyer D.J., Wolf A.P., Långström B. and Halldin C. (1987) Turnover of brain monoamine oxidase measured *in vivo* by positron emission tomography using L-[^{11}C]deprenyl. *J. Neurochem.*, 49, 522–527.

Axelsson B.S., Långström B. and Matsson O. (1987) ^{11}C/^{14}C Kinetic isotope effects. *J. Am. Chem. Soc.*, 109, 7233–7235.

Fowler J.S., MacGregor R.R., Wolf A.P., Arnett C.D., Dewey S.L., Schlyer D., Christman D., Logan J., Smith M., Sachs H., Aquilonius S.M., Bjurling P., Halldin C., Hartvig P., Leenders K.L., Lundqvist H., Oreland L., Stålnacke C-G. and Långström B. (1987) Mapping human brain monoamine oxidase A and B with ^{11}C-labeled suicide inactivators and PET. *Science*, 235, 481–485.

Fowler J.S., Wolf A.P., MacGregor R.R., Dewey S.L., Logan J., Schlyer D.J. and Långström B. (1988) Mechanistic positron emission tomography studies: demonstration of a deuterium isotope effect in the monoamine oxidase-catalysed binding of [^{11}C]L-deprenyl in living baboon brain. *J. Neurochem.*, 51, 1524–1534.

MacGregor R.R., Halldin C., Fowler J.S., Wolf A.P., Arnett C.D., Långström B. and Alexoff D. (1985) Selective, irreversible in vivo binding of [^{11}C]clorgyline and [^{11}C]-L-deprenyl in mice: potential for measurement of functional monoamine oxidase activity in brain using positron emission tomography. *Biochem. Pharmacol.*, 34, 3207–3210.

MacGregor R.R., Fowler J.S., Wolf A.P., Halldin C. and Långström B. (1988) Synthesis of suicide inhibitors of monoamine oxidase: carbon-11 labelled clorgyline, L-deprenyl and D-deprenyl. *J. Label. Compd. Radiopharm.*, 25, 1–12.

3.4. [*N-METHYL*-^{11}C]FLUMAZENIL

3.4.1. *Introduction.* Since their introduction more than twenty years ago, benzodiazepines have been used in medical applications for the treatment of anxiety, insomnia and epilepsy. Several positron-emitting benzodiazepine receptor agonists (*e.g.* Comar *et al.*, 1979) have been prepared for use as radioligands in PET studies (for a review see Pike *et al.*, 1993). A search for central benzodiazepine receptor-selective radioligands led to the ^{11}C-labelling of the antagonist, flumazenil (Ro 15-1788).

[*N-methyl*-^{11}C]Flumazenil has been used for receptor characterisation in baboons *in vivo* (Mazière *et al.*, 1983; Hantraye *et al.*, 1984), brain regional distribution and saturation studies in humans (Samson *et al.*, 1985; Persson *et al.*, 1985, 1989; Shinotoh *et al.*, 1986) and for a demonstration of reduced benzodiazepine receptor binding in human epileptic foci (Savic *et al.*, 1988).

3.4.2. *Radiochemistry.* Flumazenil has been labelled with carbon-11 in the *N*-methyl and ethyl ester positions, either by *N*-methylation with [^{11}C]iodomethane (Mazière *et al.*, 1984; Suzuki *et al.*, 1985; Långström *et al.*, 1986; Halldin *et al.*, 1988) or by esterification with [1-^{11}C]iodoethane, respectively (Halldin *et al.*, 1988). Both [^{11}C]iodomethane and [1-^{11}C]iodoethane can be routinely prepared from [^{11}C]carbon dioxide using a one-pot apparatus (Långström *et al.*, 1986; Crouzel *et al.*, 1987). A shorter reaction time and a higher specific radioactivity generally result from using [^{11}C]iodomethane instead of the longer chain haloalkane, [1-^{11}C]iodoethane. Furthermore, the Grignard reagent used in the esterification approach, methylmagnesium bromide, must be freshly prepared to achieve a high and reproducible radiochemical yield and specific radioactivity. These factors make *N*-methylation more suitable for routine synthesis than esterification with [1-^{11}C]iodomethane. The precursor (Ro 15-5528) and flumazenil can be obtained on request (Hoffman-La Roche, Basel, Switzerland).

3.4.3. *Radionuclidic purity.* As with all organic ^{11}C-labelled compounds, radionuclidic purity is usually a negligible problem since all possible impurities are eliminated during the synthesis. As long as the production parameters are not changed, a thorough investigation of radionuclidic purity is only necessary during the set-up phase of the routine synthesis. In these tests the γ-ray spectrum must be identical to that of carbon-11, in that it exhibits a major photo peak at 0.511 MeV and possibly a sum peak at 1.02 MeV, depending on source geometry and detector efficiency. Since γ-ray spectroscopy cannot distinguish between the positron-emitters, it is mandatory to determine that the half-life of the product is 20.4 min, by a suitable detector system.

3.4.4. *Chemical purity.* [*N-methyl*-^{11}C]Flumazenil can be purified by HPLC using a μ-Bondapak™ C-18 column (300 x 7.8 mm, 10 μm, Waters Associates) eluted with 10mM-phosphoric acid-acetonitrile (75:25 v/v) at 4 mL/min, using absorbance at 254 nm for detection. The fraction collected between 15-17 min is evaporated and the residue is redissolved in a ternary mixture of propylene glycol-ethanol (7:3 v/v) plus sterile saline or phosphate buffer (3:5 v/v with a total volume of 8 mL). This is filtered through a sterile 0.22 µm filter yielding a solution which is sterile and apyrogenic. Routine HPLC analysis can be performed using a C-18 column eluted with 10mM-phosphoric acid-acetonitrile (75:25 v/v) at a flow rate of 2 mL/min or methanol-water (40:60 v/v) at 1 mL/min.

Small amounts (less than 5%, assuming an equal extinction coefficient) of an unidentified chemical impurity may be observed in crude [*N-methyl*-^{11}C]flumazenil. The chemical impurity elutes with a longer retention time than [*N-methyl*-^{11}C]flumazenil.

In view of the possible pharmacodynamic effect of receptor ligands and their derivatives, the control of the mass of flumazenil itself (see specific radioactivity) and of derived impurities is mandatory for each preparation. Derivatives especially may interfere with PET measurements.

The absence of organic solvents must be guaranteed by appropriate tests. To detect traces of organic solvents GC with FI-detection is most useful.

3.4.5. *Radiochemical purity*. Radiochemical purity can be controlled most effectively by adding a radioactivity detector to the HPLC system that is used for establishing chemical purity. Radioactive by-products may include fast-eluting compounds like iodomethane, methanol and methylamine (depending on reaction pathway). In the routine HPLC analysis of [*N-methyl*-^{11}C]flumazenil usually no radiochemical impurities can be detected. However, proof of radiochemical purity should be obtained by HPLC analysis of the purified end-product, using a system similar to that used for preparative purification.

3.4.6. *Specific radioactivity*. The specific radioactivity is especially critical for the efficacy of measuring receptor densities. The specific radioactivity will largely depend on that of [^{11}C]iodomethane, for which recommendations on production have been given previously (Crouzel *et al.*, 1987). Traces of compounds with affinity for the receptor, especially the starting material and its derivatives, will lower the binding of the radioligand. Therefore, carrier dilution and contamination with cold flumazenil and analogues (by-products), lower the apparent specific radioactivity. Therefore, this should be carefully controlled in each individual batch.

The specific radioactivity is analyzed routinely by HPLC with a highly sensitive UV absorbance spectrophotometer and the signal compared to standards. The specific radioactivity of [*N-methyl*-^{11}C]flumazenil should be in the range of 18.5–74 GBq/µmol (0.5–2 Ci/µmol) at calibration time and should be stated on the label of the radiopharmaceutical container together with the time of calibration.

3.4.7 *Pharmaceutical quality*. Pharmaceutical quality is achieved by strict control of the determining parameters. For [*N-methyl*-^{11}C]flumazenil these consist of the following measures. The reaction system is set up from clean sterilised glassware and sterile medical tubing for each production batch. The [*N-methyl*-^{11}C]flumazenil fraction eluting from the HPLC column is collected in a sterilised capped vial. After evaporation of the collected HPLC fraction the residue is redissolved in sterile saline or phosphate buffer and filtered through a 0.22 µm sterile filter. It may be necessary to add up to 5% ethanol to achieve solubility. The pH of the product is adjusted to 7.0 ± 1.0 with an appropriate buffer. This is controlled in each individual batch. The isotonicity should be checked at regular intervals. The system must have shown to produce apyrogenic and sterile products at least three times before production for administration to humans. Sterility and apyrogenicity of the product must be checked frequently in routine production runs (every month) by taking samples and testing these according to standard procedures. In the Limulus test the product meets the requirements of the bacterial endotoxin tests, as stated under Section 2.5.5. Small samples of each batch should be withheld for retrospective testing of any relevant parameter if required.

[*N-methyl*-^{11}C]Flumazenil has been found to be stable during storage. A propylene glycol-ethanol-saline solution of [*N-methyl*-^{11}C]flumazenil (8 mL) showed no deterioration in chemical or radiochemical purity with storage at room temperature for three hours.

3.4.8. *References.*

Crouzel C., Långström B., Pike V.W. and Coenen H.H. (1987) Recommendations for a practical production of ^{11}C-methyl iodide. *Appl. Radiat. Isot.*, 38, 601–604.

Comar D., Mazière M., Godot J.M., Berger G., Soussaline F., Menini Ch., Arfel G. and Naquet R. (1979) Visualisation of ^{11}C-flunitrazepam displacement in the brain of the live baboon. *Nature*, 280, 329–331.

Halldin C., Stone-Elander S., Thorell J-O., Persson A. and Sedvall G. (1988) ^{11}C-Labelling of Ro 15-1788 in two different positions and also ^{11}C-labelling of its main metabolite Ro 15-3890, for PET studies of benzodiazepine receptors. *Appl. Radiat. Isot.*, 39, 993–997.

Hantraye P., Kaijima M., Prenant C. Giubert B. Sastre J., Crouzel M., Naquet R., Comar D. and Mazière M. (1984) Central type benzodiazepine binding sites: a positron emission tomography study in the baboon brain. *Neurosci. Lett.*, 48, 115–120.

Långström B., Antoni G., Gullberg P., Halldin C., Någren K., Rimland A. and Svärd H. (1986) The synthesis of 1-^{11}C-labelled ethyl, propyl, butyl and isobutyl iodides and examples of alkylation reactions. *Appl. Radiat. Isot.*, 37, 1141–1145.

Mazière M., Prenant C., Sastre J., Crouzel M., Comar D. Hantraye P., Kaijima M., Guibert B. and Naquet R. (1983) ^{11}C-Ro 15-1788 et ^{11}C-flunitrazepam, deux coordinats pour l'étude par tomographie par positons des sites de liaision des benzodiazepines. *C. R. Acad. Sci. (Paris)*, 296, 871–876.

Mazière M., Hantraye P., Prenant C., Sastre J. and Comar D. (1984) Synthesis of ethyl 8-fluoro-5,6-dihydro-5-[^{11}C]methyl-6-oxo-4H-imidazo[1,5a][1,4]benzodiazepine-3-carboxylate (RO 15-1788-^{11}C): a specific radioligand for the in vivo study of central benzodiazepine receptors by positron emission tomography. *Appl. Radiat. Isot.*, 35, 973–976.

Persson A., Ehrin E., Eriksson L., Farde L., Hedström C-G., Litton J.E., Mindus P. and Sedvall G. (1985) Imaging of [^{11}C]-labelled RO 15-1788 binding to benzodiazepine receptors in the human brain by positron emission tomography. *J. Psychiat. Res.*, 19, 609–622.

Persson A., Pauli S., Halldin C., Stone-Elander S., Farde L., Sjögren I. and Sedvall G. (1989) Saturation analysis of specific ^{11}C-Ro 15-1788 binding to the human neocortex using positron emission tomography. *Human Psychopharmacology*, 4, 21–31.

Pike V.W., Halldin C., Crouzel C., Barré L., Nutt D.J., Osman S, Shah F., Turton D.R. and Waters S.L. (1993) Radioligands for PET studies of Bz receptors and PK (peripheral benzodiazepine) binding sites — current status. *Nucl. Med. Biol.*, In press.

Samson Y., Hantraye P., Baron J-C, Soussaline F., Comar D. and Mazière M. (1985) Kinetics and displacement of [^{11}C]RO 15-1788, a benzodiazepine antagonist, studied in human brain in vivo by positron emission tomography. *Eur. J. Pharmacol.*, 110, 247–251.

Savic I., Roland P., Sedvall G., Persson A., Pauli S. and Widén L. (1988) In-vivo demonstration of reduced benzodiazepine receptor binding in human epileptic foci. *Lancet,* ii, 863–866.
Shinotoh H., Yamasaki T., Inoue O., Itoh T., Suzuki K., Hashimoto K., Tateno Y. and Ikehira H. (1986) Visualization of specific binding sites of benzodiazepine in human brain. *J. Nucl. Med.,* 27, 1593–1599.
Suzuki K., Inoue O. Hashimoto K., Yamasaki T., Kuchiki M. and Tamate K. (1985) Computer-controlled large scale production of high specific activity [^{11}C]Ro 15-1788 for PET studies of benzodiazepine receptors. *Appl. Radiat. Isot.*, 36, 971–976.

3.5. ^{11}C-LABELLED L-METHIONINES

3.5.1. *Introduction.* L-[^{11}C]Methionine, labelled in its methyl position, has been used for brain and whole-body studies, mainly within the field of oncology (Bergström *et al.*, 1983, 1987a,b; Ericson *et al.*, 1985; Lilja *et al.*, 1985, 1989; Meyer *et al.*, 1985; Kubota *et al.*, 1985; Bustany *et al.*, 1986; Mosskin *et al.*, 1989; Meyer and Schober, 1990). Its accumulation in tissue reflects amino acid utilisation (transport, protein synthesis, transmethylation and other metabolic processes). The position of the ^{11}C-label with regard to data interpretation and the limitations for measuring protein synthesis rate have been discussed in a recent review (Vaalburg *et al.*, 1992). L-[1-^{11}C]Methionine has slight advantages over L-[*S-methyl*-^{11}C]methionine with respect to the interpretation of its accumulation data (Ishiwata *et al.*, 1988b) but would still be less suitable for quantitative protein synthesis rate determinations than other amino acids, such as L-[1-^{11}C]leucine. The main advantage of L-[*S-methyl*-^{11}C]methionine is its simple synthesis. This, in combination with the possibility to interpret the data in terms of a more complex utilisation, which is dominated by the transport component (Ericson *et al.*, 1985; Lilja *et al.*, 1985; Bergström *et al.*, 1987a; Meyer and Schober 1990), has led to its widespread use in clinical applications. L-[^{11}C]Methionine must be prepared as a sterile, isotonic aqueous solution, suitable for intravenous administration.

3.5.2. *Radiochemistry.* There are several reliable ways of preparing the radioisotope carbon-11. Production by the most frequently applied method, the ^{14}N(p,α)^{11}C reaction, implies that the radioactivity is obtained as [^{11}C]carbon dioxide or [^{11}C]methane, depending on whether pure nitrogen or a nitrogen-hydrogen mixture is used as a target gas. [^{11}C]Carbon dioxide or [^{11}C]methane are the starting materials for [^{11}C]iodomethane (*cf.* Crouzel *et al.*, 1987) and [^{11}C]cyanide (*cf.* Meyer *et al.*, 1990), respectively. These are the labelling agents in the main synthetic routes to L-[^{11}C]methionine. The labelled methionine can be produced either as L-[*S-methyl*-^{11}C]methionine (Comar *et al.*, 1976; Långström and Lundqvist, 1976; Långström *et al.*, 1987) or as racemic [1-^{11}C]methionine (Bolster *et al.*, 1986a,b). The latter may be resolved chromatographically to give the L-isomer.

*a. L-[*S-methyl-*^{11}C]Methionine.*

L-[*S*-methyl-^{11}C]Methionine is prepared by alkylation of the sulphide anion of L-homocysteine with [^{11}C]iodomethane. Two main approaches have been used to generate the anion:

i) By treating *S*-benzyl-L-homocysteine with liquid ammonia and sodium (Långström and Lundqvist, 1976; Långström *et al.*, 1987)

ii) By treating L-homocysteine thiolactone with sodium hydroxide in acetone (Comar *et al.*, 1976).

The two methods are reliable and give enantiomerically pure L-[^{11}C]methionine. However, some racemisation can occur in method ii if conditions are not well controlled (Lunqvist *et al.*, 1985; Ishiwata *et al.*, 1988a).

b. L-[1-^{11}C]Methionine.

Two main approaches to the synthesis of L-[1-^{11}C]methionine have been used:

i) The addition of [^{11}C]carbon dioxide to the carbanion generated by treating the corresponding isonitrile with a strong base, such as butyllithium in tetrahydrofuran, followed by acid hydrolysis (Bolster *et al.*, 1986a,b). This synthesis yields the labelled racemate.

ii) The Strecker-Bücherer synthesis can be applied by adding [^{11}C]hydrogen cyanide to 3-*S*-methyl-propylaldehyde in the presence of ammonium carbonate. The hydantoin obtained under heat and pressure is hydrolysed under basic conditions to yield the labelled racemate.

In both cases resolution of the labelled amino acid may be achieved by, for example, enantiomeric separation on a reversed phase column using a chiral eluent, such as copper-proline (D or L) (Bolster *et al.*, 1986a,b).

3.5.3. *Radionuclidic purity.* As with all organic ^{11}C-labelled compounds, radionuclidic purity is usually a negligible problem since all possible impurities are eliminated during the synthesis. As long as the production parameters are not changed, a thorough investigation of radionuclidic purity is only necessary during the set-up phase of the routine synthesis. In these tests the γ-ray spectrum must be identical to that of carbon-11, in that it exhibits a major photo peak at 0.511 MeV and possibly a sum peak at 1.02 MeV, depending on source geometry and detector efficiency. Since γ-ray spectroscopy cannot distinguish between the positron-emitters, it is mandatory to determine that the half-life of the product is 20.4 min, by a suitable detector system.

3.5.4. *Chemical purity.* Purified end-product is obtained by reverse phase HPLC of the reaction mixture on a C-18 column (4 x 250 mm) eluted with an aqueous phosphate buffer at about 2 mL/min. The retention time of the end-product is about 7–9 min. The precursor and all chemicals in the reaction mixture must be efficiently separated from the L-methionine. Since the amounts of reagents are large compared to the amount of end-product, chromatographic tailing must be carefully monitored. However, the overall mass of reagents is usually small enough to allow an efficient separation in one chromatographic cycle. Oxidative by-products, such as sulphoxide derivatives of methionine, have been identified. However, these have longer retention times than methionine and are separated efficiently by the standard HPLC procedure.

For syntheses that require a terminal chiral separation, analytical verification of enantiomeric purity should be demonstrated at regular intervals.

Proof of chemical purity should be obtained by HPLC analysis of the purified end-product, using a system similar to that used for preparative purification and by residue analysis. While analytical HPLC should be performed routinely, residue analysis is necessary only during the set-up phase of the synthesis.

3.5.5. *Radiochemical purity.* Radiochemical purity can be controlled most effectively by including radioactivity detection in the HPLC analysis used for establishing chemical purity. Radioactive side-products include fast-eluting compounds like iodomethane, methanol, and methylamine (depending on the reaction pathway), as well as some unidentified products with retention times longer than methionine. Possibly among these are oxidative by-products such as sulphoxide derivatives of methionine. The reaction mixture usually contains over 90% of the radioactivity as the desired end-product. It can be purified by preparative HPLC, leading to L-[^{11}C]methionine with a radiochemical purity > 98%. Proof of chemical purity should be obtained by analytical HPLC of the purified end-product, using a system similar to that used for preparative purification.

3.5.6. *Specific radioactivity.* The specific radioactivity of L-[^{11}C]methionine is usually sufficiently high, even without special precautions, as long as no carrier is added during the synthesis. The specific radioactivity should not be below 37 GBq/μmol (1 Ci/μmol) at the end of synthesis. It can be measured by quantitative photometric methods, using ninhydrin derivatisation and highly sensitive instrumentation as applied to amino acid analysis, or by HPLC and UV absorbance detection at 214 nm.

3.5.7. *Pharmaceutical quality.* Pharmaceutical quality is achieved by strict control of the determining parameters. These consist of the following measures. The reaction system is set up from clean sterilised glassware and sterile medical tubing for each production batch. The chromatographic column is autoclaved before installation and is eluted with sterilised buffer only. The eluate is collected in a sterilised capped vial after passage through a sterile 0.22 μm filter. The system must have been shown to produce apyrogenic and sterile products at least three times before production for administration to humans. Sterility and apyrogenicity of the product are checked frequently in routine production runs (every month) by keeping samples and testing these by the standard procedures. In the Limulus test the product meets the requirements of the bacterial endotoxin tests, as stated under Section 2.5.5. The pH of the product must be between 6.0 and 8.0, and the isotonicity should be checked at regular intervals. Small samples of each batch should be withheld for retrospective testing of any relevant parameter if required.

L-[^{11}C]Methionine preparations containing up to 4 GBq (108 mCi) in 5 mL have been shown to be stable in aqueous solutions at pH levels between 5.0 and 7.5 for two hours at room temperature.

3.5.8. *References.*

Bergström M., Collins V.P., Ehrin E., Ericson K., Eriksson L., Greitz T., Halldin C., von Holst H., Långström B., Lilja A., Lundqvist H. and Någren K. (1983) Discrepancies in brain tumor extent as shown by computed tomography and positron emission tomography using ^{68}Ga-EDTA, [^{11}C]glucose and [^{11}C]methionine. *J. Comput. Assist. Tomogr.*, 7, 1062–1066.

Bergström M., Lundqvist H., Ericson K., Lilja A., Johnström P., Långström B., von Holst H., Eriksson L. and Blomqvist G. (1987a) Comparison of the accumulation kinetics of L-(methyl-^{11}C)-methionine and D-(methyl-^{11}C)-methionine in brain tumors studied with positron emission tomography. *Acta Radiologica*, 28, 225–229.

Bergström M., Muhr C., Lundberg P.O., Bergström K., Lundqvist H., Antoni G., Fasth K-J. and Långström B. (1987b) Amino acid distribution and metabolism in pituitary adenomas using positron emission tomography with D-[^{11}C]methionine and L-[^{11}C]methionine. *J. Comput. Assist. Tomogr.*, 11, 384–389.

Bolster J.M., Vaalburg W., Elsinga Ph.H., Ishiwata K., Vissering H. and Woldring M.G. (1986a) The preparation of ^{11}C-carboxylic labelled L-methionine for measuring protein synthesis. *J. Label. Compd. Radiopharm.*, 23, 1081–1082. (Abstract).

Bolster J.M., Vaalburg W., Elsinga H., Wijnberg H. and Woldring M.G. (1986b) Synthesis of D/L [1-^{11}C]-methionine. *Appl. Radiat. Isot.*, 37, 1069–1070.

Bustany P., Chatel M., Derlon J.M., Darcel F., Sgouropuolos P., Soussaline F. and Syrota A. (1986) Brain tumor protein synthesis and histological grades: a study by positron emission tomography (PET) with C-11-L-Methionine. *J. Neurooncol.*, 3, 397–404.

Comar D., Cartron J.C., Mazière M. and Marazano C. (1976) Labelling and metabolism of methionine-methyl-^{11}C. *Eur. J. Nucl. Med.*, 1, 11–14.

Crouzel C., Långström B., Pike V.W. and Coenen H..H. (1987) Recommendations for a practical production of ^{11}C-methyl iodide. *Appl. Radiat. Isot.*, 38, 601–603.

Ericson K., Lilja A., Bergström M., Collins V.P., Eriksson L., Ehrin E., von Holst H., Lundqvist H., Långström B. and Mosskin M. (1985) Positron emission tomography with [^{11}C]methyl-L-methionine, [^{11}C]-D-glucose and [^{68}Ga]EDTA in supratentorial tumors. *J. Comput. Assist. Tomogr.*, 9, 683–689.

Ishiwata K., Ido T. and Vaalburg W. (1988a) Increased amounts of D-enantiomer dependent on alkaline concentration in the synthesis of L-[methyl-^{11}C]methionine. *Appl. Radiat. Isot.*, 39, 311–314.

Ishiwata K., Vaalburg W., Elsinga P.H., Paans A.M.J. and Woldring M.G. (1988b) Comparison of L-[1-^{11}C]methionine and L-methyl-[^{11}C]methionine for measuring in vivo protein synthesis rates with PET. *J. Nucl. Med.*, 29, 1419–1427.

Kubota K., Matzuzawa T., Ito M., Ito K., Fujiwara T., Abe Y., Yoshioka S., Fukuda H., Hatazawa J., Iwata R., Watanuki S. and Ido T. (1985) Lung tumor imaging by positron emission tomography using C-11 L-methionine. *J. Nucl. Med.*, 26, 37–42.

Långström B. and Lundqvist H. (1976) The preparation of ^{11}C-methyl iodide and its use in the synthesis of ^{11}C-methyl-L-methionine. *Int. J. Appl. Radiat. Isot.*, 27, 357–363.

Långström B., Halldin C., Antoni G., Gullberg P., Halldin C. Malmborg P., Någren K., Rimland A. and Svärd H. (1987) Synthesis of L- and D-methyl-^{11}C methionine. *J. Nucl. Med.*, 28, 1037–1040.

Lilja A., Bergström K., Hartvig P., Spannare B., Halldin C., Lundqvist H. and Långström B. (1985) Dynamic study of supratentorial gliomas with methyl-^{11}C-L-methionine and positron emission tomography. *A J N R* , 6, 505–514.

Lilja A., Lundqvist H., Olsson Y., Spännare B., Gullberg P. and Långström B. (1989) Positron emission tomography and computed tomography in differential diagnosis between recurrent or residual glioma and treatment-induced lesions. *Acta Radiol.*, 30, 121–128.

Lundqvist H., Långström B. and Malmqvist M. (1985) Determination of enantiomeric purity in biogenic ^{11}C-labelled amino acids by aminoacylation of t-RNA. *J. Radioanal. Nucl. Chem.*, 89, 79–87.

Meyer G-J. and Schober O. (1990) Evaluation of brain tumors by PET. In *Radiopharmaceuticals and Brain Pathology Studied with PET and SPECT*. Eds., Diksic M. and Reba R.C. Boca Raton Fl. CRC Press. pp 303–336.

Meyer G-J., Schober O. and Hundeshagen H. (1985) Uptake of ^{11}C-D- and ^{11}C-L-methionine in brain tumors. *Eur. J. Nucl. Med.*, 10, 373–376.
Meyer G-J., Osterholz A. and Harms T. (1990) A systematic investigation of [^{11}C]-HCN production. *Radiochim. Acta*, 50, 43–47.
Mosskin M., Ericson K., Hindmarsh T., von Holst H., Collins V.P., Bergström M., Eriksson L. and Johnström P. (1989) Positron emission tomography compared with magnetic resonance imaging and computed tomography in supratentorial gliomas using multiple stereotactic biopsies as reference. *Acta Radiol.*, 30, 225–232.
Vaalburg W., Coenen H.H., Crouzel C., Elsinga Ph.H., Långström B., Lemaire C. and Meyer G-J. (1992) Amino acids for the measurement of protein synthesis in vivo by PET. *Nucl. Med. Biol.*, 19, 227–237.

3.6. 3-*N*-[^{11}C]METHYLSPIPERONE

3.6.1. *Introduction.* Being one of the first receptor radioligands for PET, 3-*N*-[^{11}C]methylspiperone (^{11}C-MSP) (Wagner *et al.*, 1983) is still widely used to determine D_2 receptor density in neurological diseases and pharmacological states in patients (for a review see Mazière *et al.*, 1992). Andreason *et al.* (1988) have recently reviewed its usefulness compared to irreversible ligands for studies of psychiatric diseases, such as schizophrenia. ^{11}C-MSP has a high binding affinity to D_2 receptors and its pharmacokinetics and metabolic behaviour are very similar to those of 3-*N*-[^{18}F]methylspiperone (Arnett *et al.*, 1985; Fowler *et al.*, 1986).

3.6.2. *Radiochemistry.* ^{11}C-MSP is prepared by *N*-methylation of spiperone with [^{11}C]iodomethane. Mazière *et al.* (1992) have recently reviewed the various methods. They differ in use of solvent and base [CH_2Cl_2-*t.*-Bu_4NOH(*aq.*) (Burns *et al.*, 1984); acetone-NaOH(*aq.*) (Turton *et al.*, 1984); toluene-sodium salt, 18-crown-6 (Omokawa *et al.*, 1985); DMF-*t.*-Bu_4NOH(*aq.*) (Dannals *et al.*, 1986); DMF-NaH (Suzuki *et al.*, 1990)]. The radiochemical yields are very different and the highest specific radioactivities are reported by Burns *et al.* (1984), Dannals *et al.* (1986) and Suzuki *et al.* (1990). Spiperones are sensitive to treatment with base and to radiolysis at high dose. Suzuki *et al.* (1990) especially address how to avoid the decomposition of ^{11}C-MSP during work-up. Important for methylation is, of course, the effective production of [^{11}C]iodomethane for which recommendations have been given previously (Crouzel *et al.*, 1987).

3.6.3. *Radionuclidic purity.* As with all organic ^{11}C-labelled compounds, radionuclidic purity is usually a negligible problem since all possible impurities are eliminated during the synthesis. As long as the production parameters are not changed, a thorough investigation of radionuclidic purity is only necessary during the set-up phase of the routine synthesis. In these tests the γ-ray spectrum must be identical to that of carbon-11, in that it exhibits a major photo peak at 0.511 MeV and possibly a sum peak at 1.02 MeV, depending on source geometry and detector efficiency. Since γ-ray spectroscopy cannot distinguish between the positron-emitters, it is mandatory to determine that the half-life of the product is 20.4 min, by a suitable detector system.

3.6.4. *Chemical purity.* The starting material, spiperone, is commercially available. It should be checked for high purity to ensure labelling efficacy and to avoid by-products with possible D_2 receptor binding affinity. The method of choice is HPLC with a UV absorbance detector. This technique is also recommended for the final control of the chemical purity of the formulated end-product. Chromatographic conditions are given in the reports on synthesis (Burns *et al.*, 1984; Omokawa *et al.*, 1984; Turton *et al.*, 1984; Dannals *et al.*, 1986; Suzuki *et al.*, 1990). Several of the reports describing the separations of ^{18}F-labelled spiperone derivatives are also useful for comparison (see Section 3.15. on ^{18}F-labelled 3-*N*-alkylspiperones).

Spiperone and its derivatives may have pharmacodynamic effects and may interfere with PET measurement of D_2 receptors. Thus, the control of the mass level of spiperone (see specific radioactivity) and of any derived impurities is mandatory for each batch.

The absence of organic solvents and of phase transfer catalysts, if used, must be guaranteed by appropriate tests. GC with an FI-detector is most useful for the detection of trace organic solvents.

3.6.5. *Radiochemical purity.* By including a radioactivity detector in the HPLC apparatus used for establishing chemical purity, radiochemical purity can be measured simultaneously. Radioactive by-products may include fast-eluting compounds like iodomethane, methanol and methylamine, depending on synthetic method. Usually in the routine HPLC analysis of ^{11}C-MSP no radiochemical impurities are detected. However, radiochemical purity should be proved by further analysis of the end-product, using a HPLC system similar to that used for preparative purification. Since several HPLC conditions are described it is recommended to use different systems (based on RP-18 or silica gel) for preparation and purity analysis.

3.6.6. *Specific radioactivity.* The specific radioactivity is especially critical for the efficacy of measuring receptor densities. The specific radioactivity will largely depend on that of the [^{11}C]iodomethane, for which recommendations on optimisation were given previously (Crouzel *et al.*, 1987). Traces of compounds with affinity for D_2 receptors, especially the starting material, spiperone, will reduce the binding of the radioligand. Therefore, isotopic dilution and contamination with cold spiperone and analogues (by-products) lower the apparent specific radioactivity. Therefore, these should be carefully controlled in each individual batch.

The HPLC system used for establishing chemical and radiochemical purity can be used to measure specific radioactivity, since spiperone derivatives exhibit a high UV absorption. Specific radioactivities should be in the range of 10–50 GBq/µmol (270–1350 mCi/µmol) and the value should be stated on the label of the radiopharmaceutical container, together with the time of measurement.

3.6.7. *Pharmaceutical quality.* Pharmaceutical quality is achieved by strict control of the determining parameters. For ^{11}C-MSP these consist of the following measures. The reaction system is set up from clean sterilised glassware and sterile medical tubing for each production batch. The ^{11}C-MSP is collected from the HPLC column in a sterilised capped vial. After evaporation of the mobile phase the residue is redissolved in sterile saline or phosphate buffer. Addition of ethanol during final formulation, for reason of achieving solubility or stability, should not exceed 5% of volume for pharmacological safety. The final solution is passed through a 0.22 µm sterile filter.

The pH of the product is adjusted to 7.0 ± 1.0 with an appropriate physiologically acceptable buffer. This is controlled in each individual batch. The isotonicity should be checked at regular intervals. The system must be shown to produce apyrogenic and sterile products on at least three occasions before production for administration to humans. Sterility and apyrogenicity of the product are checked frequently in routine production runs (every month) by taking samples and testing these by the standard procedures. In the Limulus test the product meets the requirements of the bacterial endotoxin tests, as stated under Section 2.5.5. Small samples of each batch should be withheld for retrospective testing of any relevant parameter, if required.

High specific radioactivity ^{11}C-MSP was reported to be sensitive to radio-decomposition in saline at high dose (MacGregor *et al.*, 1987; Suzuki *et al.*, 1990). Autodecomposition, however, can be avoided by the presence of a hydroxyl radical scavenger (*e.g.* ethanol) during dispensing and storage (Suzuki *et al.*, 1990).

3.6.8. *References.*

Andreasen N.C., Carson R., Diksic M., Evans A., Farde L., Gjedde A., Hakim A., Lal S., Nair N., Sedvall G., Tune L. and Wong D. (1988) Workshop on schizophrenia, PET, and dopamine D2 receptors in the human neostriatum. *Schizophrenia Bull.*, 14, 471–484.

Arnett C.D., Fowler J.S., Wolf A.P., Shiue C-Y. and McPherson D.W. (1985) [^{18}F]*N*-Methylspiroperidol: the radioligand of choice for PETT studies of the dopamine receptor in human brain. *Life Sci.*, 36, 1359–1366.

Burns H.D., Dannals R.F., Långström B., Ravert H.T., Zemyan S.E., Duelfer T., Wong D.F., Frost J.J., Kuhar M.J. and Wagner H.N. (1984) (3-*N*-[^{11}C]methyl)Spiperone, a ligand binding to dopamine receptors: radiochemical synthesis and biodistribution studies in mice. *J. Nucl. Med.*, 25, 1222–1227.

Crouzel C, Långström B., Pike V.W. and Coenen H.H. (1987) Recommendations for a practical production of [^{11}C]methyl iodide. *Appl. Radiat. Isot.*, 38, 601–604.

Dannals R.F., Ravert H.T., Wilson A.A. and Wagner H.N. Jr. (1986) An improved synthesis of (3-*N*-[^{11}C]methyl)spiperone. *Appl. Radiat. Isot.*, 37, 433–434.

Fowler J.S., Arnett C.D., Wolf A.P., Shiue D-Y., MacGregor R.R., Halldin C., Långström B. and Wagner H.N. Jr. (1986) A direct comparison of the brain uptake and plasma clearance of *N*-[^{11}C]methylspiroperidol and [^{18}F]*N*-methylspiroperidol in baboon using PET. *Nucl. Med. Biol.*, 13, 281–284.

MacGregor R.R., Schlyer D.J., Fowler J.S., Wolf A.P. and Shiue C-Y. (1987) Fluorine-18-*N*-methylspiroperidol; radiolytic decomposition as a consequence of high specific activity and high dose levels. *J. Nucl. Med.*, 28, 60–67.

Mazière B, Coenen H.H., Halldin C., Någren K. and Pike V.W. (1992) PET radioligands for dopamine receptors and re-uptake sites: chemistry and biochemistry. *Nucl. Med. Biol.*, 19, 497–512.

Omokawa H., Tanaka A. Ito M., Nishihara Y., Inoue O. and Yamazaki T. (1985) Synthesis of *N*-methyl and *N*-^{11}C-methyl spiperone by phase transfer catalysis in anhydrous solvent. *Radioisotopes*, 34, 480–485.

Suzuki K., Inoue O., Tamate K. and Mikado F. (1990) Production of 3-*N*-[^{11}C]methylspiperone with high specific activity and high radiochemical purity for PET studies: suppression of its radiolysis. *Appl. Radiat. Isot.*, 41, 593–599.

Turton D.R., Pike V.W., Cartoon M., Widdowson D.A. and Matthews R.W. (1984) A method for the preparation of 2-(^{11}C)methyl-spiperone — an agent for studying dopamine receptor distribution *in vivo*. *J. Label. Compd. Radiopharm.*, 21, 1148–1149. (Abstract).

Wagner H.N. Jr., Burns H.D., Dannals R.F., Wong D.F., Långström B., Duelfer T., Frost J.J., Ravert H.T., Links J.M., Rosenbloom S.B., Lukas S., Kramer A.V. and Kuhar M.J. (1983) Imaging dopamine receptors in the human brain by positron tomography. *Science*, 221, 1264–1266.

3.7. [*O-METHYL*-^{11}C]RACLOPRIDE

3.7.1. *Introduction.* Raclopride has been shown to be a selective antagonist of dopamine D_2 receptors in animal experiments (Köhler *et al.*, 1985; Hall *et al.*, 1988). [^{11}C]Raclopride has been used in stereoselectivity studies (Farde *et al.*, 1988a) and in investigations of patients with various neurological and psychiatric disorders, including naive schizophrenics (Farde *et al.*, 1986, 1990), schizophrenics treated with antipsychotic drugs (Farde *et al.*, 1988b,) patients with pituitary adenomas (Muhr *et al.*, 1986) and patients with Parkinson's disease (Rinne *et al.*, 1990).

3.7.2. *Radiochemistry.* Raclopride can be labelled with carbon-11 either by *N*-ethylation with [1-^{11}C]iodoethane (Ehrin *et al.*, 1985) or by *O*-methylation with [^{11}C]iodomethane (Farde *et al.*, 1988a; Pike *et al.*, 1990; Mazière *et al.*, 1992). Both [^{11}C]iodomethane and [1-^{11}C]iodoethane can be routinely prepared from [^{11}C]carbon dioxide (Långström *et al.*, 1986; Crouzel *et al.*, 1987). [^{11}C]Iodomethane, requires a shorter reaction time and gives a higher specific radioactivity than [^{11}C]iodoethane. These factors make *O*-methylation more suitable for routine synthesis.

The enantiomerically pure precursor for *O*-methylation can be obtained by resolving 2-aminomethyl-1-ethylpyrrolidine by fractional recrystallisation of the di-tartrates. The enantiomeric excess should exceed 99.5% according to GC analysis of the diastereomeric *O*-methylmandelamides. Coupling of the resolved pyrrolidine amines with 3,5-dichloro-2,6-dimethoxybenzoyl chloride followed by *bis*-demethylation yields the pure *S*-precursor for [*O-methyl*-^{11}C]raclopride and the *R*-precursor for labelling its inactive enantiomer (Ehrin *et al.*, 1987). The *S*- and *R*-precursors (*O*-desmethylraclopride) and raclopride tartrate can be obtained on request (Astra Research Centre AB, S-151 85 Sodertälje, Sweden).

3.7.3. *Radionuclidic purity.* As with all organic ^{11}C-labelled compounds, radionuclidic purity is usually a negligible problem since all possible impurities are eliminated during the synthesis. As long as the production parameters are not changed, a thorough investigation of radionuclidic purity is only necessary during the set-up phase of the routine synthesis. In these tests the γ-ray spectrum must be identical to that of carbon-11, in that it exhibits a major photo peak at 0.511 MeV and possibly a sum peak at 1.02 MeV, depending on source geometry and detector efficiency. Since γ-ray spectroscopy cannot distinguish between the positron-emitters, it is mandatory to determine that the half-life of the product is 20.4 min, by a suitable detector system.

3.7.4. *Chemical purity.* Analysis of [*O-methyl*-^{11}C]raclopride is performed preferably by reverse phase HPLC using a C-18 column eluted with 10mM-phosphoric acid-acetonitrile (70:30 v/v) (Ehrin *et al.*, 1985; Pike *et al.*, 1990; Mazière *et al.*, 1992).

One possible chemical impurity has the same retention time as *O*-desmethylraclopride. The main source of *O*-desmethylraclopride is most probably breakthrough from the HPLC separation. The amounts are usually less than 2%. *O*-Desmethylraclopride has been found to be non-binding to dopamine receptors *in vitro* (Köhler *et al.*, 1985). The antipode of raclopride is 100-fold less active than raclopride in displacing [^{3}H]spiperone from dopamine D_2 receptors (de Paulis *et al.*, 1986). Thus, a small contamination with the antipode would not effect receptor binding. GC analysis shows *O*-desmethylraclopride to have over 99.8% enantiomeric excess.

Another chemical impurity that has been identified is *O*-ethyl-desmethylraclopride (Pike *et al.*, 1990). This most probably arises from *O*-ethylation of *O*-desmethylraclopride with iodoethane that is co-produced with [^{11}C]iodomethane through hydriodic acid cleavage when diethyl ether is used as solvent. This problem is solved by using THF instead of diethyl ether.

The absence of organic solvents must be guaranteed by appropriate tests. GC with an FI-detector is most useful for detecting traces of organic solvents.

3.7.5. *Radiochemical purity*. Radiochemical purity can be controlled most effectively by including a radioactivity detector in the HPLC apparatus used for establishing chemical purity. Radioactive by-products may include fast-eluting compounds like iodomethane, methanol and methylamine, depending on the synthetic method. An unidentified radiochemical impurity, that generally represents less than 2% of the total radioactivity, has been reported (Pike *et al.*, 1990). The reaction mixture usually contains over 90% of the radioactivity as the desired end-product. Preparative HPLC gives [*O-methyl*-^{11}C]raclopride with > 98% radiochemical purity. Radiochemical purity should be proved by analysis of the purified end-product by HPLC similar to that used in preparative purification.

3.7.6. *Specific radioactivity*. Specific radioactivity is especially critical for the efficacy of measuring receptor densities. The specific radioactivity will largely depend on that of [^{11}C]iodomethane, for which recommendations were given previously (Mazière *et al.*, 1992). Traces of compounds with affinity to D_2 receptors, especially the starting material and derivatives, will lower the binding of the radioligand. Therefore, isotopic dilution and contamination with cold raclopride and analogues (by-products), lower the apparent specific radioactivity. Therefore, these should be carefully controlled in each individual batch.

Analysis is routinely performed by HPLC with a highly sensitive UV absorbance detector and the signal is compared to standards. The specific radioactivity should be in the range of 18.5–74 GBq/μmol (0.5–2 Ci/μmol) at the time of calibration and the value should be stated on the label of the radiopharmaceutical container, together with the time of calibration.

3.7.7. *Pharmaceutical quality*. Pharmaceutical quality is achieved by strict control of the determining parameters. For [*O-methyl*-^{11}C]raclopride these consist of the following measures. The reaction system is set up from clean sterilised glassware and sterile medical tubing for each production batch. The [*O-methyl*-^{11}C]raclopride eluted from the HPLC column is collected in a sterilised capped vial. After evaporation of the mobile phase the residue is redissolved in sterile saline or phosphate buffer and filtered through a 0.22 μm sterile filter. The pH of the product is adjusted to 7.0 ± 1.0 with an appropriate buffer. This is controlled in each individual batch. The isotonicity should be checked at regular intervals.

The system must have shown to produce apyrogenic and sterile product at least three times before production for administration to humans. Sterility and apyrogenicity of the product are checked frequently in routine production runs (every month) by taking samples and testing these by standard procedures. In the Limulus test the product meets the requirements of the bacterial endotoxin tests, as stated under Section 2.5.5. Small samples of each batch should be withheld for retrospective testing of any relevant parameter if required.

[*O-methyl*-^{11}C]Raclopride has been found to be stable during storage. A formulated solution of [^{11}C]raclopride (450 MBq; 5 GBq/μmol; 7 mL) showed no deterioration in chemical or radiochemical purity during storage at room temperature for 74 min (Pike *et al.*, 1990).

3.7.8. *References*

Crouzel C., Långström B., Pike V.W. and Coenen H.H. (1987) Recommendations for a practical production of ^{11}C-methyl iodide. *Appl. Radiat. Isot.*, 38, 601–604.

de Paulis T., Kumar Y., Johansson L., Rämsby S., Hall H., Sällemark M., Ängeby-Möller K, Ögren S-O. (1986) Potential neuroleptic agents. 4. Chemistry, behavioral pharmacology, and inhibition of [^{3}H]spiperone binding of 3,5-disubstituted *N*-[(1-ethyl-2-pyrrolidinyl)methyl]-6-methoxysalicylamides. *J. Med. Chem.*, 29, 61–69.

Ehrin E., Farde L., de Paulis T., Eriksson L., Greitz T., Johnström P., Litton J-E., Nilsson J.L.G., Sedvall G., Stone-Elander S. and Ögren S-O. (1985) Preparation of ^{11}C-labelled raclopride, a new potent dopamine receptor antagonist: preliminary PET studies of cerebral dopamine receptors in the monkey. *Appl. Radiat. Isot.*, 36, 269–273.

Ehrin E., Gawell L., Högberg T., de Paulis T. and Ström P. (1987) Synthesis of [methoxy-^{3}H]- and [methoxy-^{11}C]-labelled raclopride, specific dopamine D_2 receptor ligands. *J. Label. Compd. Radiopharm.*, 24, 931–940.

Farde L., Hall H., Ehrin E. and Sedvall G. (1986) Quantitative analysis of dopamine D2 receptor binding in the living human brain by PET. *Science*, 231, 258-261.

Farde L., Pauli S., Hall H., Eriksson L., Halldin C., Högberg T., Nilsson L., Sjögren I. and Stone-Elander S. (1988a) Stereoselective binding of ^{11}C-raclopride in living human brain — a search for extrastriatal central D_2-dopamine receptors by PET. *Psychopharmacology*, 94, 471–478.

Farde L., Wiesel F-A., Halldin C. and Sedvall G. (1988b) Central D2-dopamine receptor occupancy in schizophrenic patients treated with antipsychotic drugs. *Arch. Gen. Psychiatry*, 45, 71–76.

Farde L., Wiesel F-A., Stone-Elander S., Halldin C., Nordström A-L., Hall H. and Sedvall G. (1990) D_2-dopamine receptors in neuroleptic-naive schizophrenic patients — a positron emission tomography study with [^{11}C]raclopride. *Arch. Gen. Psychiatry*, 47, 213–219.

Hall H., Köhler C., Gawell L., Farde L. and Sedvall G. (1988) Raclopride, a new selective ligand for the dopamine-D_2 receptors. *Prog. Neuro-Psychopharmacol. & Biol. Psychiat.*, 12, 559–568.

Köhler C., Hall H., Ogren S-O. and Gawell L. (1985) Specific in vitro and in vivo binding of [^{3}H]raclopride. A potent substituted benzamide drug with high affinity for D-2 dopamine receptors in the rat brain. *Biochem. Pharmacol.*, 34, 2251–2259.

Långström B., Antoni G., Gullberg P., Halldin C., Någren K., Rimland A. and Svärd H. (1986) The synthesis of 1-^{11}C-labelled ethyl, propyl, butyl and isobutyl iodides and examples of alkylation reactions. *Appl. Radiat. Isot.*, 37, 1141–1145.

Mazière B., Coenen H.H., Halldin C., Någren K. and Pike V.W. (1992) PET radioligands for dopamine receptors and re-uptake sites: chemistry and biochemistry. *Nucl. Med. Biol.*, 19, 497–512.

Muhr C., Bergström M., Lundberg P.O., Bergström K. and Långström B. (1986) In vivo measurement of dopamine receptors in pituitary adenomas using positron emission tomography. *Acta Radiol. Suppl.*, 369, 406–408.

Pike V.W., Kensett M.J., Turton D.R., Waters S.L. and Silvester D.J. (1990) Labelled agents for PET studies of the dopaminergic system — some quality assurance methods, experience and issues. *Appl. Radiat. Isot.*, 41, 483–494.

Rinne U.K., Laihinen J.O., Rinne J.O., Någren K., Bergman J. and Ruotsalainen U. (1990) Positron emission tomography demonstrates dopamine D_2 receptor supersensitivity in the striatum of patients with early Parkinson's disease. *Movement Disorders*, 5, 55–59.

3.8. [^{13}N]AMMONIA

3.8.1. *Introduction.* Besides its use as a precursor for the incorporation of nitrogen-13 into biomolecules, [^{13}N]ammonia is a highly diffusible tracer which, after intravenous injection, is efficiently extracted into tissue, where it remains for a considerable period due to various fast metabolic processes. Its application as a radiopharmaceutical for measuring regional blood flow in tissues such as heart and brain with PET is based on these properties.

Because of its short physical half-life, the control of the radionuclidic, radiochemical, chemical and pharmaceutical quality of [^{13}N]ammonia solutions for injection relies on good production practices, process control, rapid quality control procedures and on retrospective testing. Recently, a monograph on [^{13}N]ammonia for injection was proposed for the United States Pharmacopeia (United States Pharmacopeial Convention, 1989). That proposal is accompanied by a discussion stimulus (Gatley, 1989).

3.8.2. *Radiochemistry.* Nitrogen-13 ($t_{1/2}$ = 10 min) may be produced from carbon isotopes, using low energy protons in the ^{13}C(p,n)^{13}N reaction or deuterons in the ^{12}C(d,n)^{13}N reaction, or from oxygen, using higher energy protons in the ^{16}O(p, α)^{13}N reaction (see Qaim *et al.*, this volume).

The reaction on carbon-13 can be used with low energy proton cyclotrons. A disadvantage is the need for ^{13}C-enriched target material. The most common production process is the ^{16}O(p,α)^{13}N reaction. Though this reaction has the lowest cross section of the three, sufficient amounts of nitrogen-13 can be produced conveniently.

The most common method of [^{13}N]ammonia production is based on proton irradiation of water followed by reduction of the generated ^{13}N-labelled nitrates and nitrites. After irradiation of the target, the water is transferred to a reaction vessel that contains a reducing agent in alkaline medium. The ^{13}N-labelled nitrate and nitrite can be reduced by one of several agents, such as titanium(III) chloride or titanium(III) hydroxide in alkaline medium (Ido and Iwata, 1981; Tamaki *et al.*, 1985) or DeVarda's alloy in aqueous sodium hydroxide solution (Vaalburg *et al.*, 1975; Slegers *et al.*, 1980; Tilbury, 1981). The generated [^{13}N]ammonia is then distilled out of the reaction mixture by heating under a flow of gas and is finally trapped in a slightly acidic saline solution (*cf.* Tilbury, 1981; Vaalburg and Paans, 1989).

[^{13}N]Ammonia may be produced directly in the target in an adequate yield if the target water contains a small amount of ethanol as a scavenger for oxidising radicals (Wieland *et al.*, 1991). Feeding a slightly acidic solution to the target effluent facilitates the adsorption of [^{13}N]ammonium ion onto a small cation exchange cartridge, from which an injectable [^{13}N]ammonia solution can be eluted with saline.

With low energy cyclotrons [^{13}N]ammonia can be produced directly in a porous carbon target flushed with water (Bida *et al.*, 1986). Here too [^{13}N]ammonia is formed by radical-induced reactions between nucleogenic nitrogen-13 atoms generated by the ^{13}C(d,n)^{13}N or ^{13}C(p,n)^{13}N reaction and water. The ratio of oxidative products to reduced products depends on the flow of water through the porous carbon.

3.8.3. *Radionuclidic purity.* Besides some non-volatile cationic radionuclidic impurities in the unprocessed target-water, which arise from the target window foil, small amounts of ^{15}O- and ^{18}F-labelled impurities are produced by the ^{16}O(p,pn)^{15}O and ^{18}O(p,n)^{18}F reactions. The amounts depend on the incoming particle energy. The removal of radionuclidic impurities can be achieved by various methods, depending on the production parameters and the production pathway.

Production pathways based on the reduction of oxyanions of nitrogen-13, which require a distillation step, are likely to remove [^{18}F]fluoride and cationic radionuclidic impurities very effectively. In this process only oxygen-15, possibly in the form of water, is detected as a radionuclidic contaminant in the [^{13}N]ammonia solution. A 10–20 min period between nitrogen-13 production and application may be introduced to allow the oxygen-15 to decay. This radionuclidic contaminant is also eliminated by evaporation of the target water before the reduction step or adsorption of the final [^{13}N]ammonia as [^{13}N]ammonium ion on a cation exchange cartridge and subsequent elution.

All direct production pathways for [^{13}N]ammonia (*e.g.* in water targets containing ethanol) are likely to produce raw products that contain cationic radionuclidic impurities arising from the target foils. Their composition and amount depends on the target-foil material, the beam intensity and the beam energy. In most cases it will be necessary to remove the cationic radionuclidic impurities by adsorption of the [^{13}N]ammonia on a cation exchange column followed by fractional desorption. This also eliminates possible oxygen-15 contamination. Since contamination of [^{13}N]ammonium ion with other radionuclides is more likely than with many other short-lived radiopharmaceuticals, checks on radionuclidic purity are recommended not only during the set-up phase of the synthesis, but at regular intervals.

In these tests the γ-ray spectrum must be identical to that of nitrogen-13 in that it exhibits a major photo peak at 0.511 MeV and possibly a sum peak at 1.02 MeV, depending on source geometry and detector efficiency. Since γ-ray spectroscopy cannot distinguish between the positron-emitters it is mandatory to determine that the half-life of the product is 10 min, by a suitable detector system.

3.8.4. *Chemical purity.* Tests have to be carried out to demonstrate the absence of any unlabelled reagent in the final product. Possible chemical impurities may arise from reducing agents like DeVarda's alloy or titanium (III) chloride. Traces of these compounds or their components can possibly be carried over during the distillation process. For aluminum detection in the end-product, simple and sensitive photometric methods are commercially available (*e.g.* Spectroquant™, Merck). The absence of titanium can be analyzed qualitatively with spot tests (Feigl and Oesper, 1972) or quantitatively by highly sensitive colorimetric assays, for example that based on the use of salicylic acid (Müller, 1967). The chemical identity of no-carrier-added quantities of [^{13}N]ammonia can be established by radio-HPLC on a cation exchange column.

3.8.5. *Radiochemical purity.* Radio-HPLC is advisable for the determination of radiochemical purity. Cation exchange is preferable to partition chromatography since the former leads to a higher retention and a better separation of possible impurities, such as [^{13}N]hydrazine and [^{13}N]methylamine.

3.8.6. *Specific radioactivity.* Although no carrier is added in production, the product is not carrier-free. Carrier dilution arises mainly from small amounts of ammonium salts or traces of nitrogen compounds that are also reduced to ammonia. As a control for undesired carrier a negative colour test with Nessler's reagent has been suggested (United States Pharmacopeial Convention, 1989). Quantitative determination of the carrier content with highly sensitive photometric methods (*e.g.* Spectroquant™, Merck) is feasible down to a level of 0.01 mg/L. This allows the determination of carrier dilution up to specific radioactivity values of nearly 2 TBq/µmol (50 Ci/µmol).

3.8.7. *Pharmaceutical quality.* Pharmaceutical quality is achieved by strict control of the determining parameters. These consist of the following measures. The reaction system is set up from clean sterilised glassware and sterile medical tubing for each production batch. The anion exchange column is autoclaved before installation and is eluted with sterile mobile phase only. The eluate is collected in a sterilised capped vial after passage through a sterile 0.22 µm filter. The system must be shown to produce apyrogenic and sterile product on at least three occasions before production for human administration. Sterility and apyrogenicity of the product are checked frequently in routine production runs (every month) by using samples and testing these by the standard procedures. In the Limulus test the product meets the requirements of the bacterial endotoxin tests, as stated under Section 2.5.5. The pH of the product, must be 7.0 ± 1.0, and the isotonicity should be checked at regular intervals. Small samples of each batch should be withheld for retrospective testing of any relevant parameter if required.

3.8.8. *References.*

Bida G., Wieland B.W., Ruth T.J., Schmidt D.G., Hendry G.O. and Keen K.E. (1986) An economical target for nitrogen-13 production by proton bombardment of a slurry of carbon-13 powder on O-16 water. *J. Label. Compd. Radiopharm.*, 23, 1217-1219. (Abstract).

Feigl F. and Oesper R. (1972) Spot tests in inorganic analysis. Amsterdam, Elsevier.

Gatley J. (1989) USP Standards for nitrogen-13 ammonia injection. *U.S. Pharmacopeial Forum*, 5400–5401.

Ido T. and Iwata R. (1981) Fully automated synthesis of $^{13}NH_3$. *J. Label. Compd. Radiopharm.*, 18, 244–245. (Abstract).

Müller G.O. (1967) Praktikum der quantitativen chemischen Analyse. Leipzig. S. Hitzel Verlag, pp 254–256.

Slegers G., Vandecasteele C. and Sambre J. (1980) Cyclotron production of ^{13}N-labelled ammonia for medical use. *J. Radioanal. Chem.*, 59, 585–587.

Tamaki N., Yonekura Y., Senda M., Kureshi S.A., Saji H., Kodama S., Konishi Y., Ban T., Kambara H., Kawai C. and Torizuka K. (1985) Myocardial positron computed tomography with ^{13}N-ammonia at rest and during exercise. *Eur. J. Nucl. Med.*, 11, 246–251.

Tilbury R.S. (1981) The chemical forms of ^{13}N produced in various nuclear reactions and chemical environments. In *Short-Lived Radionuclides in Chemistry and Biology*. ACS Advances in Chemistry Series Monograph. Eds. Root J. and Krohn K. Washington DC, American Chemical Society, pp. 261–267.

United States Pharmacopeial Convention (1989) 'Nitrogen-13 ammonia injection'. *U.S. Pharmacopeial Forum*, 5331–5333.

Vaalburg W. and Paans A.M.J. (1989) Short-lived positron emitting radionuclides. In *Radionuclides Production II*. Ed., Helus F. Boca Raton Fl. CRC Press Inc. pp. 47–99.

Vaalburg W., Kamphuis J.A.A,. Beerling van der Molen H.D., Reiffers S., Rijskamp A. and Woldring M.G. (1975) An improved method for the cyclotron production of ^{13}N-labelled ammonia. *Int. J. Appl. Radiat. Isot.*, 26, 316–318.

Wieland B., Bida G., Padgett H., Hendry G., Zippi E., Kabalka G., Morelle J-L., Verbruggen R. and Ghyoot M. (1991) In-target production of nitrogen-13 ammonia via proton irradiation of dilute aqueous ethanol and acetic acid mixtures. *Appl. Radiat. Isot.*, 42, 1095–1098.

3.9. ^{15}O-LABELLED GASES

3.9.1. *Introduction.* The production of the short-lived radioisotope, oxygen-15 ($t_{1/2}$ = 2.04 min) and its conversion into labelled oxygen, carbon dioxide, carbon monoxide, water and *n*-butanol has been the subject of much research at centres using positron emission tomography (PET) (Clark and Buckingham, 1975). In these various chemical forms, oxygen-15 is being used clinically to study oxygen metabolism, blood flow and blood volume (Ter Pogossian *et al.*, 1975; Frackowiak *et al.*, 1980). Since these radiopharmaceuticals are now routinely prepared at many PET centres, their production, especially with respect to quality assurance and quality control, was previously reviewed by an EEC Task Group (Clark *et al.*, 1987).

Specific quality control methods for ^{15}O-labelled gases were described by the EEC Task Group and included acceptable limits for impurities (radionuclidic, chemical and radiochemical) plus levels of detection. This monograph fully endorses those recommendations. Discussion of *n*-[^{15}O]butanol and [^{15}O]water production, which also appeared in the earlier report, are here the subject of separate entries (Sections 3.10. and 3.11., respectively).

Compliance with the general guidelines for quality assurance and quality control of short-lived radiopharmaceuticals are also fully supported here and should be regarded as a prerequisite for any group wishing to produce clinical materials labelled with oxygen-15. Given that the half-life of oxygen-15 is only 2 min, it is a challenge to incorporate quality control methods into on-line or batch production procedures, such as decay curve analysis to determine radionuclidic impurities and pharmacopoeial tests for pyrogen content and sterility. Therefore, in the production of oxygen-15 labelled gases, it is imperative that GMP rules are strictly adhered to as these are the only real means of assuring the quality of the final product.

3.9.2. *Radiochemistry.* Typically oxygen-15 is produced via the $^{14}N(d,n)^{15}O$ nuclear reaction. Others that can be used include the $^{16}O(p,d)^{15}O$ reaction, which requires protons of greater than 14 MeV (Beaver *et al.*, 1976; Ruth 1985; Krohn *et al.*, 1986), the $^{15}N(p,n)^{15}O$ reaction, which can use 5 MeV protons (Sajjad *et al.*, 1984; Wieland *et al.*, 1986) and the $^{16}O(p,pn)^{15}O$ reaction (Beaver *et al.*, 1976; Fernandez-Rubio *et al.*, 1981; Ruth 1985). For further details see Qaim *et al.* (in this volume).

The nuclear reactions starting with nitrogen as target material require molecular oxygen carrier (at concentrations ranging from 0.2–4%) in order to recover the oxygen-15 as molecular oxygen. Conversion of [^{15}O]oxygen into [^{15}O]carbon dioxide using activated charcoal at 400°C is feasible but not very effective. Therefore, direct production by irradiation of a carbon dioxide (2%) in nitrogen is more commonly employed. Conversion of [^{15}O]oxygen into [^{15}O]carbon monoxide can be achieved with activated charcoal at 1000°C. Conversion of [^{15}O]carbon dioxide into [^{15}O]carbon monoxide or [^{15}O]oxygen has also been reported (Iwata *et al.*, 1988).

3.9.3. *Radionuclidic purity.* The $^{14}N(d,n)^{15}O$ reaction in a nitrogen gas target yields oxygen-15 with only small amounts of other contaminating radionuclides, provided that the deuteron energy is kept at the lower end of the excitation function (*i.e.* 7 MeV) and the target gas mixture does not contain any significant impurities.

Unavoidable contaminants are of the order of 0.1% nitrogen-13 ($t_{1/2}$ = 10 min) and of the order of 0.05% carbon-11 ($t_{1/2}$ = 20 min), arising from the $^{14}N(d,t)^{13}N$, $^{16}O(d,\alpha n)^{13}N$, and $^{14}N(d,\alpha n)^{11}C$ reactions, respectively. The limits of these impurities should be verified by decay analysis. The absence of any other radionuclidic impurities should be checked by γ-ray spectroscopy after the decay of oxygen-15. In these tests the γ-ray spectrum must be identical to that of oxygen-15, in that it exhibits a major photo peak at 0.511 MeV and possibly a sum peak at 1.02 MeV, their ratio depending on the detector geometry. Since γ-ray spectroscopy cannot distinguish between the positron-emitters, it is mandatory to determine that the half-life of the product is 2.06 min, as determined by a suitable detector system,.

In the case of direct [^{15}O]carbon dioxide production in a nitrogen target with 2% carbon dioxide carrier, up to 1% nitrogen-13 can arise from the $^{12}C(d,n)^{13}N$ reaction. The $^{16}O(p,d)^{15}O$ reaction is likely to produce higher levels of nitrogen-13 contamination by the $^{16}O(p,\alpha)^{13}N$ reaction.

Since the levels of radionuclidic impurities are unlikely to change in a standardised production scheme, the levels of contamination need to be measured during the set-up of production or after changes of beam-particle energy or of target gas starting material.

3.9.4. *Chemical purity.* Since carrier is added in most procedures producing ^{15}O-labelled gases, nearly all the gaseous chemical impurities are labelled and are thus present as radiochemical impurities as well. The essential instrument for any analysis of these materials is the radio-gaschromatograph, though it is not suitable for all the necessary quality assurance and quality control measurements of atmospheric gas impurities (Clark *et al.*, 1987). In particular, for [^{15}O]carbon monoxide the actual concentration of carbon monoxide that is administered to patients has to be strictly controlled by careful consideration of the target volume (for single breath inhalation) and the target gas flow (for continuous inhalation). At a carrier gas concentration of 0.5% oxygen, the carbon monoxide level becomes 1%, which cannot be tolerated in procedures involving continuous inhalation. Using 0.25% oxygen carrier, and a twenty-fold dilution with air, a carbon monoxide concentration of 0.025% is obtained and this has been reported to be safe in a continuous inhalation protocol limited to 15 min (Clark *et al.*, 1987) However, the actual carboxyhaemoglobin concentration in the subject is the crucial factor so even these levels of carbon monoxide have to be subjected to scrutiny when particularly susceptible patients are being studied. The radio-gaschromatograph and a small volume I.R. photometer, which is particularly suitable for the estimation of carbon monoxide concentration, can be plumbed 'in-line' with the production process to enable the most efficient analysis (Strijckmans *et al.*, 1989).

It is important to use more appropriate methods than GC when analyzing for certain other contaminants (Clark *et al.*, 1987) such as ozone and the oxides of nitrogen. Proof of the absence of these noxious gases, following purification of the desired ^{15}O-labelled product, is essential.

3.9.5. *Radiochemical purity.* Possible radiochemical contaminants of the ^{15}O-labelled gases ($^{15}O_2$, $C^{15}O_2$, $C^{15}O$) are the ^{15}O-labelled oxides of nitrogen ($N_2{}^{15}O$, $N^{15}O_x$, and $^{13}N_2O$) and possibly ozone. These can be effectively removed by the use of soda lime and charcoal adsorbers. [^{15}O]Carbon monoxide and [^{15}O]carbon dioxide can be contaminated by each other and by [^{15}O]oxygen. [^{15}O]Carbon monoxide can be purified from traces of [^{15}O]carbon dioxide by soda lime, but the purification of [^{15}O]carbon dioxide from traces of [^{15}O]carbon monoxide is more difficult to achieve. Mixed iron oxide can be used for this purpose but becomes less effective with time so that strict monitoring of the product by radio-GC is required.

The calibration of the radio-gaschromatograph should be well documented and ideally all batches of ^{15}O-labelled materials should be analyzed prior to dispensing. Most systems described in the literature have used two columns (Porapak™ Q and molecular sieve 5A). However, the fully microprocessor-controlled automatic on-line production of ^{15}O-labelled oxygen, carbon monoxide and carbon dioxide, using a concentric dual column (CTRI; Alltech Associates) that contains both packing materials, has distinct advantages (Strijckmans *et al.*, 1989). A facility for feeding back the quality control results via the microprocessor to adjust the production parameters can be of considerable assistance.

3.9.6. *Specific radioactivity.* Due to the necessary addition of carrier to all target gases for the production of ^{15}O-labelled products (except for [^{15}O]carbon monoxide) their specific radioactivity is low, but this is of no consequence for their clinical application.

3.9.7. *Pharmaceutical quality.* While gas applications do not necessarily require sterilisation or special precautions to prevent contamination by pyrogens, they nevertheless should pass through micro-filters before entering the patient to ensure that the gas is 'particulate-free'. However, very special consideration has to be given to the quality assurance and quality control procedures of materials prepared for injection or infusion (see Sections 3.10. and 3.11. for *n*-[^{15}O]butanol and [^{15}O]water, respectively).

3.9.8. *References.*

Beaver J.E., Finn R.D. and Hupf H.B. (1976) A new method for the production of high concentration oxygen-15 labelled carbon dioxide with protons. *Appl. Radiat. Isot.,* 27, 195–197.

Clark J.C. and Buckingham P.D. (1975) *Short-Lived Radioactive Gases for Clinical Use.* Butterworths, London.

Clark J.C., Crouzel C., Meyer G-J. and Strijckmans K. (1987) Current methodology for oxygen-15 production for clinical use. *Appl. Radiat. Isot.,* 38, 597–600.

Fernandez-Rubio F., Finn R. and Gilson A.J. (1981) Alchemy with short-lived radionuclides. *IEEE Trans. Nucl. Sci.,* NS-28, 1921–1923.

Frackowiak R.S.J,. Lenzi G.L., Jones T. and Heather J.D. (1980) Quantitative measurement of regional cerebral blood flow and oxygen metabolism in man using ^{15}O and positron emission tomography: theory, procedure and normal values. *J. Comput. Assist. Tomogr.,* 4, 727–736.

Iwata R., Ido T., Fujisawa Y. and Yamazaki S. (1988) On-line interconversion of $[^{15}O]O_2$ and $[^{15}O]CO_2$ via metal oxide by isotopic exchange. *Appl. Radiat. Isot.,* 39, 1207–1211.

Krohn K.A., Link J.M., Lewellen T.K., Risler R., Eenmaa J. and Maier M. (1986) The use of 50 MeV protons to produce C-11 and O-15. *J. Label. Compd. Radiopharm.,* 23, 1190–1192.

Ruth T.J. (1985) The production of ^{18}F-F_2 and ^{15}O-O_2 sequentially from the same target chamber. *Appl. Radiat. Isot.,* 36, 107–110.

Sajjad M., Lambrecht R.M. and Wolf A.P. (1984) Excitation function for the $^{15}N(p,n)^{15}O$ reaction. *Radiochim. Acta,* 36, 159–162.

Strijckmans K., Sambre J. and De Guchteneire F. (1989) Automated production and quality control of $^{15}O_2$ and $C^{15}O_2$. *J. Label. Compd. Radiopharm.,* 26, 458–459. (Abstract).

Ter Pogossian M.M., Phelps M.E., Hoffman E.J. and Mullani N.A. (1975) A positron-emission transaxial tomograph for nuclear imaging (PETT). *Radiology,* 114, 89–98.

Wieland B.W., Schmidt D.G., Bida G., Ruth T.J. and Hendry G.O. (1986) Efficient, economical production of oxygen-15 labeled tracers with low energy protons. *J. Label. Compd. Radiopharm.,* 23, 1214–1216. (Abstract).

3.10. *n*-[^{15}O]BUTANOL

3.10.1. *Introduction.* *n*-[^{15}O]Butanol is being used to study blood flow in the brain and potentially in other organs. Its advantage over [^{15}O]water is based on its better partition coefficient, which is nearly 1.0, compared to 0.9 for water (Herscovitch *et al.,* 1987; Herholz *et al.,* 1989). Since *n*-[^{15}O]butanol is most commonly prepared from [^{15}O]oxygen, it is mandatory to consider the quality assurance and quality control criteria for ^{15}O-labelled gases, as proposed in Section 3.9.

3.10.2. *Radiochemistry.* *n*-[^{15}O]Butanol is most often prepared by the reaction of [^{15}O]oxygen with tri-*n*-butyl borane, loaded onto an alumina SepPak™ cartridge (Kabalka *et al.,* 1985; Berridge *et al.,* 1986, 1990; Takahashi *et al.,* 1986; Bauer and Wagner, 1991). In order to recover oxygen-15 in the form of molecular oxygen, carrier oxygen is included in the nitrogen gas target at concentrations ranging from 0.2-0.5%. After the gas-solid reaction, labelled *n*-butanol can be eluted from the cartridge with water. Purification is achieved by adsorption of the product on a C-18 SepPak™ cartridge and subsequent elution with an ethanol-water mixture. An automated system is described by Crouzel *et al.* (this volume).

3.10.3. *Radionuclidic purity.* The commonly used nuclear reactions for oxygen-15 production in gas targets, namely the $^{14}N(d,n)^{15}O$ reaction or, where suitable deuterons are lacking, the $^{15}N(p,n)^{15}O$ reaction, yield a product with only small amounts of other radionuclides, provided the target gas mixture does not contain any significant impurities and the particle energy is kept at the lower side of the excitation function (*e.g.* 7 MeV for the $^{14}N(d,n)^{15}O$ reaction). Unavoidable contaminants from the $^{14}N(d,n)^{15}O$ process are nitrogen-13 (up to 0.1%) and carbon-11 (up to 0.05%), arising from the $^{14}N(d,t)^{13}N$, $^{16}O(d,\alpha n)^{13}N$ and $^{14}N(d,\alpha n)^{11}C$ processes. In tests for radionuclidic purity the γ-ray spectrum must be identical to that of oxygen-15, in that it exhibits a major photo peak at 0.511 MeV and possibly a sum peak at 1.02 MeV, depending on source geometry and detector efficiency. The absence of any other impurities should be checked by γ-ray spectroscopy after the decay of oxygen-15. Since γ-ray spectroscopy cannot distinguish between the positron-emitters, it is mandatory to determine that the half-life of the product is 2.06 min, by a suitable detector system. The limits for contaminants should be verified by decay analysis.

The $^{16}O(p,d)^{15}O$ process, which requires protons of greater than 14 MeV, is likely to produce higher levels of nitrogen-13 contamination by the $^{16}O(p,\alpha)^{13}N$ reaction.

Levels of radionuclidic impurities need to be measured not only during the set-up of production and after changes of beam-particle energies and target-gas cylinders, but also on a regular basis during production.

3.10.4. *Chemical purity.* Inactive chemical impurities in *n*-[^{15}O]butanol, may consist of low levels of boric acid and its derivatives (< 1 μg). These should be be removed by passing the products of hydrolysis over an anion exchange column. The purity of the end-product can be checked quickly with HPLC, using an 4 x 250 mm RP-18 column, eluted with acetonitrile-water (1:9 v/v) at 2.5 mL/min. On this system water, *n*-butanol and the boron compound elute with retention times of 0.25 min, 1.0 min and 1.5 min, respectively (Bauer and Wagner, 1991). For further details see Crouzel *et al.* (this volume).

3.10.5. *Radiochemical purity.* Possible contaminants of all ^{15}O-labelled gases are oxides of nitrogen and ozone. These are effectively removed by soda lime and charcoal absorbers. Their absence should be monitored by measures indicated for the quality assurance and quality control of ^{15}O-labelled gases (Section 3.9) and [^{15}O]water (Section 3.11). If these impurities breakthrough they may interact with tri-*n*-butyl-borane. The purity of the end-product can be checked quickly by HPLC, as stated above, with radioactivity detection (Bauer and Wagner, 1991). For further details see Crouzel *et al.* (this volume).

3.10.6. *Specific radioactivity.* Due to the necessary presence of carrier in all targets for the production of oxygen-15, specific radioactivity is low. A specific radioactivity in the range of 3–10 GBq/mmol (81–270 mCi/mmol) has been reported for *n*-[^{15}O]butanol, corresponding to 25 ± 10 mg of *n*-butanol per injection of *ca* 1.5 GBq (40.5 mCi). In order to keep the maximal concentration to this level, the concentration of oxygen in the target gas must be limited to 0.5% (Berridge *et al.*, 1989; Bauer and Wagner, 1991). The actual concentration can be checked by HPLC or GC.

3.10.7. *Pharmaceutical quality.* Special consideration has to be given to the quality control of materials prepared for injection or infusion. Good manufacturing procedures are required to check and assure that the materials are safe for administration with respect to non-toxicity, sterility and apyrogenicity. This can be achieved by the use of disposable sterile components and/or the efficient cleaning of components from bacteriological contamination. It is absolutely mandatory that the solution containing the *n*-[^{15}O]butanol is passed over a sterile 0.22 µm filter before entering the patient.

The pH of the product should be checked during the set-up of the production and thereafter at regular intervals.

The isotonicity is unlikely to be influenced by the synthetic set up and needs no special attention except during the set up phase.

The system must have shown to produce apyrogenic and sterile products on at least three occasions before production for administration to humans. Sterility and apyrogenicity of the product are checked frequently in routine production runs (every month) by taking samples and testing these by standard procedures. In the Limulus test the product meets the requirements of the bacterial endotoxin tests, as stated under Section 2.5.5. A small sample of at least one batch per week should be withheld for retrospective testing of any relevant parameter if required.

Descriptions of the preparation of *n*-[^{15}O]butanol, that have incorporated these procedures, have appeared in the recent literature (Berridge *et al.*, 1989; Takahashi *et al.*, 1986; Bauer and Wagner *et al.*, 1991)

3.10.8. *References.*

Bauer B. and Wagner R. (1991) Improved synthesis of (^{15}O)butanol for clinical use. *J. Label. Compd. Radiopharm.*, 30, 69–71. (Abstract).

Berridge M.S., Franceschini M.P., Tewson T.J. and Gould K.L. (1986) Preparation of oxygen-15 butanol for positron tomography. *J. Nucl. Med.*, 27, 834–837.

Berridge M.S., Cassidy E.H. and Terris A.H. (1990) A routine, automated synthesis of oxygen-15-labelled butanol for positron tomography. *J. Nucl. Med.*, 31, 1727–1731.

Herholz K., Pietrzyk U., Wienhard K., Hebold I., Pawlik G., Wagner R., Holthoff V., Klinkhammer P. and Heiss W.D. (1989) Regional cerebral blood flow measurement with intravenous ^{15}O-water bolus and ^{18}F-fluoro-methane inhalation. *Stroke*, 20, 1174–1181.

Herscovitch P., Raichle M.E., Kilbourn M.R. and Welch M.J. (1987) Positron emission tomography measurement of cerebral blood flow and permeability-surface area product of water using ^{15}O-water and ^{11}C-butanol. *J. Cerebr. Blood Flow.*, 7, 527–542.

Kabalka G.W., Lambrecht R.M., Sajjad M., Fowler J.S., Kunda S.A., McCollum G.W. and MacGregor R. (1985) Synthesis of ^{15}O-labelled butanol via organoborane chemistry. *Appl. Radiat. Isot.*, 36, 853–855.

Takahashi K., Murakami M., Hagami E., Sasaki H., Kondo Y., Mizusawa S., Nakamichi H., Iida H., Miura S., Kanno I., Uemura K. and Ido T. (1986) Radiosynthesis of

^{15}O-labelled butanol available for clinical use. *J. Label. Compd. Radiopharm.*, 23, 1111–1113. (Abstract).

3.11. [^{15}O]WATER

3.11.1. *Introduction.* [^{15}O]Water is being used to study blood flow in various organs, mainly the brain (Frackowiak *et al.*, 1980; Lammertsma *et al.*, 1990) and the heart (Bergman *et al.*, 1989; Lammertsma and Mazoyer, 1990). It has also been applied to measure the perfusion status of tumours (Strauss and Conti, 1991) and the amount of extravascular water in the lungs (Schober *et al.*, 1985; Schuster *et al.*, 1986). In many older studies [^{15}O]water has been administered by inhalation of [^{15}O]carbon dioxide, which is transformed instantaneously to labelled water in the lungs. Advanced PET-study protocols, for the quantitative analysis of flow, demand reproducible and strictly defined input functions. These can be achieved more adequately by infusion techniques than by inhalation. This has led to an increasing request for [^{15}O]water for bolus, ramp, or steady-state infusion.

Since [^{15}O]water is most commonly prepared from [^{15}O]oxygen, it is mandatory to consider the quality assurance and quality control criteria for ^{15}O-labelled gases, as proposed in Section 3.9. A monograph on [^{15}O]water has recently been proposed for the United States Pharmacopeia (United States Pharmacopeial Convention, 1992).

3.11.2. *Radiochemistry.* [^{15}O]Water is most commonly prepared from [^{15}O]oxygen by reaction with hydrogen using a palladium catalyst. In order to recover oxygen-15 as [^{15}O]oxygen, carrier oxygen, at concentrations ranging from 0.2–4%, is added to the target gas nitrogen (Clark *et al.*, 1987).

Alternatively, [^{15}O]water can be produced 'in-target', if hydrogen is added to the target gas at a concentration of about 2% (Hagami *et al.*, 1986). Production is usually carried out 'on-line'. In the most common process the irradiated target-gas is mixed with hydrogen and is then passed over the catalyst at about 180°C. The gas-stream containing the labelled water vapour is then either bubbled through a saline reservoir (Meyer *et al.*, 1986; Matzke *et al.*, 1993), or is exchanged with saline in a small dialytic membrane filter (Clark and Tochon-Danguy, 1991) from where it can be pumped precisely into the patient (see Crouzel *et al.*, this volume).

3.11.3. *Radionuclidic purity.* The commonly used reactions, namely the $^{14}N(d,n)^{15}O$ reaction, or where suitable deuterons are lacking, the $^{15}N(p,n)^{15}O$ reaction, yield oxygen-15 with only small amounts of other radionuclides, provided that the target gas mixture does not contain any significant impurities and the particle energy is kept on the lower side of the excitation function (*e.g.* 7 MeV for the $^{14}N(d,n)^{15}O$ reaction). Unavoidable contaminants from the $^{14}N(d,n)^{15}O$ process are up to 0.1% nitrogen-13 and up to 0.05% carbon-11, which arise from the $^{14}N(d,t)^{13}N$, $^{16}O(d,\alpha n)^{13}N$, and $^{14}N(d,\alpha n)^{11}C$ reactions. In tests of radionuclidic purity the γ-ray spectrum must be identical to that of oxygen-15, in that it exhibits a major photo peak at 0.511 MeV and possibly a sum peak at 1.02 MeV, depending on source geometry and detector efficiency. The absence of any other impurities should be checked by γ-ray spectroscopy after the decay of oxygen-15. Since γ-ray spectroscopy cannot distinguish between the positron-emitters, it is mandatory to determine that the half-life of the product is 2.06 min, by a suitable detector system. The limits for contaminants should be verified by decay analysis.

The $^{16}O(p,d)^{15}O$ process, which requires protons of greater than 14 MeV, is likely to produce higher levels of nitrogen-13 contamination by the $^{16}O(p,\alpha)^{13}N$ reaction.

Since the levels of radionuclidic impurities are unlikely to change in a certain production scheme, the contamination levels need to be measured only during the set-up of the production and after changes of beam-particle energies and target-gas cylinders.

3.11.4. *Chemical purity.* Ammonia is a possible chemical impurity in [^{15}O]water. This may arise either from catalytic conversion of hydrogen and nitrogen on the palladium catalyst or by radiolysis if in-target production is used. The amount of ammonia in the water to be injected can be analyzed by titrimetric and/or photometric (Spectroquant™; Merck) methods. It should not increase the pH of the injection solution above 7.5.

3.11.5. *Radiochemical purity.* The identity and purity of [^{15}O]water should be checked by radio-GC (Clark *et al.*, 1987). Possible contaminants of all ^{15}O-labelled gases are ^{15}O-labelled oxides of nitrogen and ozone. These are effectively removed by soda lime and charcoal adsorbers. Their absence should be monitored by measures indicated in the quality assurance and quality control of ^{15}O-labelled gases (Section 3.9.). Oxides of nitrogen impurities these may that breakthrough may accumulate in the saline reservoir for injection, from where they can be removed only by adsorption on an anion exchange resin.

3.11.6. *Specific radioactivity.* Due to the necessary addition of carrier to all target gases for the production of ^{15}O-labelled products, their specific radioactivity is low. For [^{15}O]water this is of no consequence for its clinical application.

3.11.7. *Pharmaceutical quality.* Special consideration has to be given to the quality control of materials prepared for injection or infusion. Good manufacturing procedures are required to check and assure that the materials are safe for administration *i.e.* non-toxic, sterile and apyrogenic. This can be achieved by the use of disposable sterile components and/or the efficient cleaning of components from bacteriological contamination. It is absolutely mandatory that the solution containing the [^{15}O]water is passed through a sterile 0.22 μm filter before entering the patient.

The pH of the product should be checked during the set-up of the production and thereafter at regular intervals.

The isotonicity is unlikely to be influenced by the synthetic set up and needs no special attention except during the set up phase. Before administration to humans the system must have shown to produce apyrogenic and sterile products on at least three occasions. Sterility and apyrogenicity of the product are checked frequently in routine production runs (every month) by using samples and testing these by the standard procedures. In the Limulus test the product meets the requirements of the bacterial endotoxin tests, as stated under Section 2.5.5. A small sample of at least one batch per week should be withheld for retrospective testing of any relevant parameter if required.

Descriptions of the preparation of [^{15}O]water which have incorporated these procedures have appeared in the recent literature (Hagami *et al.*, 1986; Meyer *et al.*, 1986; Clark and Tochon-Danguy, 1991; Matzke *et al.*, 1993).

3.11.8. *References.*

Bergman S.R., Herrero P., Markham J., Weinheimer C.J. and Walsh M.N. (1989) Noninvasive quantitation of myocardial blood flow in human subjects with oxygen 15-labeled water and positron emission tomography. *J. Am. Coll. Cardiol.*, 14, 639–652.

Clark J.C. and Tochon-Danguy H. (1991) R2D2, — a bedside [oxygen-15]water infuser. *PSI Proceedings 92-01*, pp 234–235. ISSN 1019-6447. Proc. IV. Int. Workshop on Targetry and Target Chemistry; Sept 9–12th; Villigen, Switzerland, 1991. (Abstract).

Clark J.C., Crouzel C., Meyer G-J. and Strijckmans K. (1987) Current methodology for oxygen-15 production for clinical use. *Appl. Radiat. Isot.*, 38, 597–600.

Frackowiak R.S.J., Lenzi G.L., Jones T, and Heather J.D. (1980) Quantitative measurement of regional cerebral blood flow and oxygen metabolism in man using ^{15}O and positron emission tomography: theory, procedure and normal values. *J. Comput. Assist. Tomogr.*, 4, 727–736.

Hagami E., Murakami M., Takahashi K., Kanno I., Aizawa Y., Hachiya T., Shoji Y., Shishido F. and Uemura K. (1986) Studies on the direct synthesis of [O-15]H_2O. *Kakuigaku (Nuclear Medicine, Japan)* 23, 351–358. (In Japanese with English abstract.)

Lammertsma A.A. and Mazoyer B. (1990) EEC concerted action on cellular degeneration and regeneration studied with PET. Modelling expert meeting blood flow measurement with PET. *Eur. J. Nucl. Med.*, 16, 807–812.

Lammertsma A.A., Cunningham V.J., Deiber M.P., Heather J.D., Bloomfield P.M,. Nutt J., Frackowiak R.S.J. and Jones T. (1990) Combination of dynamic and integral methods for generating reproducible functional CBF images. *J. Cerebr. Blood Flow Metab.*, 10, 675–686.

Matzke K-H., Meyer G-J. and Hundeshagen H. (1993) An advanced system for the administration of ^{15}O-water. *J. Label. Compd. Radiopharm.*, 32, 459–460. (Abstract).

Meyer G-J., Osterholz A. and Hundeshagen H. (1986) ^{15}O-Water constant infusion system for clinical routine application. *J. Label. Compd. Radiopharm.*, 23, 1209–1210. (Abstract).

Schober O., Meyer G-J., Bossaller C., Creutzig H., Lichtlen P.R. and Hundeshagen H. (1985) Quantitative determination of regional extravascular lung water and regional blood volume in congestive heart failure. *Eur. J. Nucl. Med.*, 10, 17–24.

Schuster D.P., Marklin G.F. and Mintun M.A. (1986) Regional changes in extravascular lung water detected by positron emission tomography. *J. Appl. Physiol.*, 60, 1170–1178.

Strauss L.G. and Conti P.S. (1991) The application of PET in clinical oncology. *J. Nucl. Med.*, 32, 623–648.

United States Pharmacopeial Convention (1992). *U.S. Pharmacopeial Forum*, p. 4305.

3.12. [^{18}F]FLUORIDE

3.12.1. *Introduction.* The affinity of [^{18}F]fluoride for bone was recognised as early as 1940 (Volker *et al.*, 1940). Its usefulness as a bone-scanning agent for the detection of skeletal lesions had been demonstrated long before the development of positron emission tomography (PET) (Bernstein and Katz, 1953). Although its use for routine bone-scanning has been taken over completely by ^{99m}Tc-phosphonate complexes, the development of PET has led to new strategies for the clinical use and application of [^{18}F]fluoride (Cochavi *et al.*, 1979). In combination with PET it allows for the quantitation of bone metabolism (Charkes *et al.*, 1978, 1979; Hawkins *et al.*, 1990), which offers itself as a sophisticated tool for therapy control in bone transplantation and reconstitution. Furthermore, the high sensitivity and resolution of PET has been claimed to be advantageous for 3-D whole-body bone-scanning for the early diagnosis of metastases (Yeh *et al.*, 1980; Hoh *et al.*, 1991). A monograph on [^{18}F]fluoride proposed for the United States Pharmacopeia is now under revision (Gatley and Finn, 1992).

3.12.2. *Radiochemistry.* [^{18}F]Fluoride is readily prepared simply by passing [^{18}F]fluorine, as produced by the ^{20}Ne(d,α)^{18}F nuclear reaction in neon gas with 0.1%–0.5% fluorine, through water [for recent reviews of fluorine-18 production see Guillaume *et al.* (1991) and Qaim *et al.* (this volume)]. Alternatively, [^{18}F]fluoride is produced directly in target via the ^{18}O(p,n)^{18}F process in [^{18}O]water or via the ^{16}O(^{3}He,p)^{18}F in regular water. In these cases [^{18}F]fluoride should be adsorbed on an anion exchange column (*cf.* Schlyer *et al.*, 1990) followed by washing with water and elution with saline. This procedure also enables a simple recovery of ^{18}O-enriched target water. Reactor-produced [^{18}F]fluoride can be purified via conversion into [^{18}F]fluorotrimethylsilane and subsequent decomposition (Rosenthal *et al.*, 1985; Gatley, 1989; Gatley and Finn, 1992).

3.12.3. *Radionuclidic purity.* The quality of [^{18}F]fluorine produced by the ^{20}Ne(d,α)^{18}F nuclear reaction is high. Possible radionuclidic impurities, such as very short-lived isotopes ($t_{1/2} < 30$ s) of sodium and neon, decay during the work-up.

The radionuclidic purity of [^{18}F]fluoride produced via the ^{18}O(p,n)^{18}F process in [^{18}O]water is more crucial and demands for control. Fixation of [^{18}F]fluoride on an anion exchange column followed by washing with water and elution with saline is recommended. It allows a separation of cationic radionuclidic impurities, that arise from the target window foil and vary according to the foil material (Rosenthal *et al.*, 1985; Kilbourn, 1990). Although this procedure enables recycling of the ^{18}O-enriched target water, it must be mentioned that with decreasing ^{18}O-enrichment of the target water the amount of nitrogen-13 increases via the (p,α) reaction on oxygen-16. Since nitrogen-13 may be adsorbed on the anion exchange column in the form of oxyanions of nitrogen-13, either fractional desorption from such a column or a sufficient decay-time for nitrogen-13 is recommended.

Less frequently applied methods of [^{18}F]fluoride production include the ^{16}O(^{3}He,p)^{18}F process or the use of a reactor. The former method may possibly lead to contamination by beryllium-7 via a fragmentation channel (Knust and Machulla, 1983) while reactor [^{18}F]fluoride production is accompanied by tritium formation (see Vera Ruiz, 1988). In both cases purification of [^{18}F]fluoride on an anion exchange column as stated above is recommended.

Radionuclidic purity and identity should be tested by γ-ray spectroscopy and half-life measurement. As long as the production parameters are not changed, a thorough investigation of radionuclidic purity is only necessary during the set-up phase of the routine synthesis. In these tests the γ-ray spectrum must exhibit a major photo peak at 0.511 MeV and possibly a sum peak at 1.02 MeV depending on source geometry and detector efficiency. Since γ-ray spectroscopy cannot distinguish between positron-emitters, it is mandatory to demonstrate that the half-life of the product is 110 min, by a suitable detector system.

3.12.4. *Chemical purity.* It is rather unlikely that significant chemical impurities are introduced during the production of [^{18}F]fluoride by the common methods, except that using a reactor. In the case of production from a water target, fixation of [^{18}F]fluoride on an anion exchange column followed by washing with water and elution with saline is recommended. This process will remove low level cationic contaminants. Anionic contaminants have been discussed by Solin *et al.* (1988). Where [^{18}F]fluoride is produced from carrier-added [^{18}F]fluorine target gas, the trap for collection must not contain any saline or buffer but pure water, which only after degassing from residual molecular fluorine should be made isotonic.

3.12.5. *Radiochemical purity.* The definite chemical composition of [^{18}F]fluoride has been discussed in some detail (Noto and Nicolini, 1975; Nickles *et al.*, 1986), considering the possibilities for complex formation and reaction with impurities. Since [^{18}F]fluoride prepared by the aforementioned methods undergoes nucleophilic substitution reactions, it does not seem to be necessary to confirm its chemical identity further. In cases of doubt, HPLC on an anion exchange column should be performed, using an electrochemical or ion-sensitive detector.

3.12.6. *Specific radioactivity.* The specific radioactivity is determined by the amount of fluoride introduced into the system during the synthesis. For no-carrier-added [^{18}F]fluoride the specific radioactivity may reach values of about 1 TBq/µmol (27 Ci/µmol). Verification of high specific radioactivity necessitates HPLC on an anion exchange column with an electrochemical or ion-sensitive detector.

For production via [^{18}F]fluorine the amount of carrier fluorine in the target gas determines the specific radioactivity. The amount of fluorine is a function of the concentration of fluorine in the target gas, the target volume and the target gas pressure. The amount of carrier may vary from 0.01 to 0.2 mmol, depending on target design parameters. The specific radioactivities obtainable under such conditions vary accordingly from 20 to 400 GBq/mmol (0.504–10.8 Ci/mmol) (See Guillaume *et al.*, 1992).

3.12.7. *Pharmaceutical quality.* This is achieved by strict control of the determining parameters. These consist of the following measures. The [^{18}F]fluoride collection system is set up from clean sterilised glassware and sterile medical tubing for each production batch. The ion exchange resin is stored under *iso*-propanol and washed with sterile water. The end-product is collected in a sterilised capped vial after passage through a sterile 0.22 µm filter. The system must have shown to produce apyrogenic and sterile [^{18}F]fluoride solutions on at least three occasions before production for administration to humans. Sterility and apyrogenicity of the product are checked frequently in routine production runs (every month) by taking samples and testing these by the standard procedures. In the Limulus test the product meets the requirements of the bacterial endotoxin tests as stated under Section 2.5.5. The pH of the product must be between 6.0 and 8.0 and the isotonicity should be checked at regular intervals. Small samples of each batch should be withheld for retrospective testing of any relevant parameter if required.

3.12.8. *References.*

Bernstein R.B. and Katz J.J. (1953) Fluorine-18: preparation, properties and uses. *Nucleonics*, 11, 46–51.

Charkes N.D., Makler P.T. and Philips C. (1978) Studies of skeletal tracer kinetics. I. Digital-computer solution of a five compartment model of [^{18}F]fluoride kinetics in humans. *J. Nucl. Med.,* 19, 1301–1309.

Charkes N.D., Brookes M. and Makler P.T. Jr (1979) Studies of skeletal tracer kinetics: II. Evaluation of a five-compartment model of [^{18}F]fluoride kinetics in rats. *J. Nucl. Med.,* 20, 1150–1157.

Cochavi S., Pohost G.M., Elmaleh D.R. and Strauss H.W. (1979) Traverse-sectional imaging with Na^{18}F in myocardial infarction. *J. Nucl. Med.,* 20, 1013–1017.

Gatley S.J. (1989) Rapid production and trapping of [^{18}F]fluorotrimethylsilane, and its use in nucleophilic fluorine-18 labeling without an aqueous evaporation step. *Appl. Radiat. Isot.,* 40, 541–544.

Gatley J.S and Finn R.D. (1992) USP standards for sodium fluoride F 18 Injection, a rediscovered radiopharmaceutical. *Pharmacopeial Forum,* 18, 2961–2963.

Guillaume M. Luxen A., Nebeling B., Argentini M., Clark J.C. and Pike V.W. (1991) Recommendations for fluorine-18 production. *Appl. Radiat. Isot.,* 42, 749–762.

Hawkins R.A., Choi Y., Hoh C., Huang S.C., Shiepers, Dahlbom M., Hoffman E.J., Barrio J.R., Satyamurthy N. and Phelps M.E. (1990) A method for determining bone metabolic rates with F-18 fluoride ion and PET. *J. Nucl. Med.,* 31, 778–779. (Abstract).

Hoh C.K., Hawkins R.A., Choi Y., Dahlbom M., Huang S.C., Satyamurthy N., Barrio J., Seeger L., Schiepers C.W., Phelps M.E. and Maddahi J. (1991) Total body skeletal imaging with F-18 ion and PET. *J. Nucl. Med.,* 32, 1025. (Abstract)

Kilbourn M.R. (1990) Fluorine-18 labeling of radiopharmaceuticals. *National Sciences Series NAS-NS3203.* Washington, DC, National Academy Press.

Knust E.J. and Machulla H-J. (1983) High yield production of ^{18}F in a water target via the ^{16}O(^{3}He,p)^{18}F reaction. *Int. J. Appl. Radiat. Isot.,* 34, 1627–1628.

Nickles R.J., Gatley S.J., Votaw J. and Kornguth M.L. (1986) Production of reactive fluorine-18. *Appl. Radiat. Isot.,* 37, 649–661.

Noto M.G and Nicolini J.O. (1975) The radiochemical purity determination of ^{18}F preparations. *J. Radioanal. Chem.,* 24, 85–87.

Rosenthal M.S., Bosch A.L., Nickles R.J. and Gatley S.J. (1985) Synthesis and some characteristics of no-carrier added [^{18}F]fluorotrimethylsilane. *Appl. Radiat. Isot.,* 36, 318–319.

Schlyer D.J., Bastos M.A.V., Alexoff D. and Wolf A.P. (1990) Separation of [^{18}F]fluoride from [^{18}O]water using anion exchange resin. *Appl. Radiat. Isot.,* 41, 531–533.

Solin O., Bergman J., Haaparanta M. and Reissell A. (1988) Production of ^{18}F from water targets. Specific radioactivity and anionic contaminants. *Appl. Radiat. Isot.,* 39, 1065–1072.

Vera Ruiz H. (1988) Report of an International Atomic Energy Agency's consultants meeting on fluorine-18: reactor production and utilization. *Appl. Radiat. Isot.,* 39, 31–39.

Volker J.F., Carpenter-Hodge H., Wilson H.J. and Van-Vooris S.N. (1940) The adsorption of fluorides by enamel, dentin and hydroxyapatite as shown by the radioactive isotope. *J. Biol. Chem.,* 134, 543–548.

Yeh S. D. J., Benua R.S., Grando R. and Graham M.C. (1980) Fluorine-18 positron emission tomography of bone lesions. *J. Nucl. Med.,* 21, 56. (Abstract).

3.13. 2-[^{18}F]FLUORO-2-DEOXY-D-GLUCOSE

3.13.1. *Introduction.* 2-[^{18}F]Fluoro-2-deoxy-D-glucose (2-^{18}FDG) is certainly the most frequently used organic radiopharmaceutical in studies with positron emission tomography (PET). It is used to measure glucose metabolism in tumours, heart and especially brain in various disease states. Corresponding to its importance and wide application, numerous reports have dealt with the efficient preparation of 2-^{18}FDG since the first reports from Gallagher *et al.* (1977) and Ido *et al.* (1978). Some papers review the wealth of literature on the production of 2-^{18}FDG and also enclose aspects of product quality control (Bida *et al.*, 1984; Fowler and Wolf 1986). A previous report from an EEC task group focused on recommendations for optimal labelling procedures (Coenen *et al.*, 1987) and a recent review discussed in detail points of concern and possible pitfalls for most known syntheses, including precursor and [^{18}F]fluoride preparation (Tewson, 1989). The study of this literature is recommended. 2-^{18}FDG was the first PET radiopharmaceutical to be included in the United States Pharmacopeia (United States Pharmacopeial Convention, 1989). Specific purity criteria for the purity of 2-^{18}FDG preparations are laid down in the USP monograph.

3.13.2. *Radiochemistry.* The method of choice and the most widely applied is that of nucleophilic substitution in 1,3,4,6-*tetra-O*-acetyl-2-*O*-trifluoromethane-sulphonyl-β-D-manno-pyranose with [^{18}F]fluoride, promoted by Kryptofix™ 2.2.2. (aminopolyether 2.2.2.) (Hamacher *et al.*, 1986). [^{18}F]Fluoride is most commonly produced by the ^{18}O(p,n)^{18}F nuclear reaction in [^{18}O]water, using protons at energies from 16–8 MeV (for reviews see Guillaume *et al.*, 1991; Qaim *et al.*, this volume). The aqueous [^{18}F]fluoride from the production target is adsorbed on an anion exchange resin, eluted with aqueous potassium carbonate solution and dried by evaporation (see Schlyer 1990). Addition of dry acetonitrile and Kryptofix™ 2.2.2. enhance the nucleophilicity of the [^{18}F]fluoride so that it reacts easily with *tetra*-acetylated mannosyltriflate in acetonitrile at elevated temperature. Removal of Kryptofix™ 2.2.2. can be achieved by different methods, all using separation cartridges, either in polar (Padgett *et al.*, 1989) or non-polar (Hamacher *et al.*, 1990) form. Final acid hydrolysis of the protected radiofluorinated sugar and subsequent flash-chromatography on a series of materials (ion retardation resin, Al_2O_3, Si 60-RP18) yields an injectable solution of 2-^{18}FDG. Variations of the method substitute Kryptofix™ 2.2.2. with *t.*-alkyl ammonium salts (Brodack *et al.*, 1988; Knust *et al.*, 1989; Johnson *et al.*, 1993).

An alternative method, which makes use of a solid-phase catalysed nucleophilic substitution, has been reported recently (Toorongian *et al.*, 1990). This method also avoids Kryptofix™ 2.2.2. The end-product has to be checked for the absence of the derivatisation agent.

Only a few groups still use an electrophilic pathway. Here the preferred route is the reaction of [^{18}F]acetyl hypofluorite with *tri-O*-acetyl-D-glucal (Bida *et al.*, 1984). Quality control considerations therefore relate mainly to the favoured nucleophilic method but general standards of product quality, as recommended, have to be met by any procedure of preparation. For pharmaceutical quality and production reliability, remotely controlled or automated closed synthesis systems with in-process feedback control (Hamacher *et al.*, 1990) are preferred to open systems with time control only (*e.g.* Padgett *et al.*, 1989).

3.13.3. *Radionuclidic purity.* The quality of [^{18}F]fluorine for electrophilic radiofluorination as produced by the ^{20}Ne(d,α)^{18}F nuclear reaction is high. Possible impurities, such as very short-lived isotopes of sodium and neon, decay during work-up and are eliminated during the synthesis.

The radionuclidic purity of [^{18}F]fluoride, produced via the ^{18}O(p,n)^{18}F process in [^{18}O]water, is more crucial and calls for control, since the quality of [^{18}F]fluoride will not only determine the radionuclidic purity of the final product but also its reactivity in the nucleophilic substitution. With decreasing concentration of [^{18}O]water the amount of nitrogen-13 increases via the (p,α) reaction on oxygen-16. Fixation of [^{18}F]fluoride on an anion exchange column is recommended. It allows the removal of cationic radionuclidic impurities, which arise from the target window foil and vary according to the foil material (Hamacher *et al.*, 1990; Schlyer *et al.*, 1990). Furthermore, this procedure enables simple recycling of the ^{18}O-enriched target water.

Radionuclidic purity and identity should be tested by γ-ray spectroscopy and half-life measurement. As long as the production parameters are not changed, a thorough investigation of radionuclidic purity is necessary only during the set-up phase of the routine synthesis. In these tests the γ-ray spectrum must exhibit a major photo peak at 0.511 MeV and possibly a sum peak at 1.02 MeV depending on source geometry and detector efficiency. Since γ-ray spectroscopy cannot distinguish between positron-emitters, it is mandatory that the half-life of the product is determined to be 110 min, by a suitable detector system.

3.13.4. *Chemical purity.* The precursors, 1,3,4,6-*tetra-O*-acetyl-2-*O*-trifluoromethane-sulphonyl-β-D-manno-pyranose or *tri-O*-acetyl-D-glucal, have to be checked for purity, even if obtained commercially. The method of choice is TLC.

For quality control of the final formulated product, the necessary tests and their frequency depend to some extend on the labelling method and technical procedure used.

The absence of organic solvents and of Kryptofix™ 2.2.2. must be guaranteed by appropriate tests. Partially hydrolysed precursor should pose no problems if the conditions for hydrolysis are strictly controlled (see below). Nevertheless, analytical verification of complete hydrolysis by HPLC should be carried out at defined intervals. Further, the amount of D-glucose depending on the labelling procedure, should be determined and given on the label of the ampoule of the radiopharmaceutical.

Special considerations apply to testing for Kryptofix™ 2.2.2, although a twofold extraction with 0.1M-hydrochloric acid will completely remove it (Hamacher *et al.*, 1990; Moerlein *et al.*, 1989). However, its poor detectability, on the one hand, and its toxicity with LD_{50} values of 32 mg/kg (*i.v.*) in mouse and 35 mg/kg (*i.v.*) in rat (Baudot *et al.*, 1977)], on the other hand, cause some concern. The frequency of testing may be reduced after gaining confidence in the applied synthetic procedure. Elemental analysis, mass spectrometry and chromatography have been used to determine minimal levels of Kryptofix™ 2.2.2. TLC, using silica gel layers and methanol-aqueous ammonia (9:1 v/v) (Chaly and Dahl, 1989) or methanol with 0.1% triethylamine (Vora *et al.*, 1985) as mobile phase, appear presently to be the most practical methods. The detection limit of this method is 0.025 mg/mL if 2 μL are spotted onto the TLC plate. This corresponds to 0.25 mg per batch in a 10 mL preparation, which is 10^4 times less than the LD_{50} value in rats.

GC with an FI-detector is certainly most appropriate to detect traces of organic solvents. Where production is from cyclotron-produced [^{18}F]fluorine (or an electrophilic derivative) determination of the ratio of 2-^{18}FDG to its epimer, 2-[^{18}F]fluoro-2-deoxy-D-mannose is important. For this purpose, GC after silylation (Shiue *et al.*, 1985) is not recommended as a technique for routine use.

For the determination of the mass of sugars by HPLC the best system appears to be a reverse phase amino column with acetonitrile-water as eluent (Tewson 1983; Vora *et al.*, 1985). Besides RI detectors the use of electrochemical detectors has been reported (Santos and Baldwin. 1987). These extremely sensitive devices have led to the detection of small amounts of 2-chloro-2-deoxy-D-glucose, formed under certain conditions of hydrolysis with hydrochloric acid during the synthesis of 2-^{18}FDG (Alexoff *et al.*, 1992). It is not clear yet if such a system can also be used for the simultaneous detection of Kryptofix™ 2.2.2. which would make it suitable for routine use.

3.13.5. *Radiochemical purity.* Besides the level of 2-^{18}FDG the absence of unreacted [^{18}F]fluoride, of partially acetylated [^{18}F]fluoro-deoxy-glucose derivatives, of [^{18}F]fluoro-deoxy-mannose, or other ^{18}F-labelled sugars can be ensured by radioanalytical methods. From these the actual content of 2-^{18}FDG, of partially acetylated 2-^{18}FDG and of free [^{18}F]fluoride should be determined in each batch.

The purification of 2-^{18}FDG from partially acetylated 2-^{18}FDG by means of HPLC, as performed by some groups, is usually unnecessary. Experience shows that appropriate synthesis conditions (concentrations, volumes) and devices (volume, reaction vessel) will ensure reliable hydrolysis. The presence of 2-^{18}FDM, or other radiofluorinated sugars, will largely depend on the labelling method and techniques used. Their lower limits or absence in the final preparation have to be standardised during the establishment of the routine labelling procedure. It is recommended to retest for these contaminants less frequently (*i.e.* after each 10th batch and after any changes in the procedure or to the synthesis device, including repairs).

TLC also allows easy detection of [^{18}F]fluoride but is less suitable for quantifying other ^{18}F-labelled fluoro sugars. Various analytical procedures have been described (Barrio *et al.*, 1981; Fowler *et al.*,.1981; Ehrenkaufer *et al.*, 1984; Hamacher *et al.*, 1986; Chaly and Dahl, 1989). TLC is certainly the most practical method for separating 2-^{18}FDG from 2-^{18}FDM (Van Rijn *et al.*, 1985). HPLC methods are preferable, however, as the quantitative determination of radiochemical impurities is easier. 2-^{18}FDG is easily separated from ^{18}F-labelled sugar derivatives by various methods, but separation from [^{18}F]fluoride can be a problem due to tailing effects. Reverse phase columns are not suitable, but exclusion chromatography on so called 'sugar columns' can be used with water as eluent. A reverse phase amino column eluted with acetonitrile-water is often used (Tewson 1983; Vora *et al.*, 1985). However, [^{18}F]fluoride can only be eluted from this column by injection of at least 1 mg of cold fluoride for displacement. The best chromatographic system so far appears to be anion exchange on a Dionex PA 100 column with 0.1M-sodium hydroxide as eluent. This allows isocratic separation of [^{18}F]fluoride, glucose, 2-^{18}FDG and partially hydrolysed sugars.

3.13.6. *Specific radioactivity.* The specific radioactivity is determined by the amount of fluoride introduced into the system during the synthesis. For synthesis by nucleophilic substitution with no-carrier-added [^{18}F]fluoride, the specific radioactivity may reach values of about 1 TBq/μmol (27 Ci/μmol). However, it should be considered that the radiopharmaceutical is quasi-diluted by amounts of D-glucose in the 40 μmol range. In the case of synthesis by electrophilic substitution, the carrier fluorine in the target gas determines the specific radioactivity. The former is a function of the concentration of fluorine in the target gas, the target volume, and the target gas pressure. The amount of carrier may vary from 0.01 to 0.2 mmol, depending on target design parameters. The specific radioactivities obtainable under such conditions vary accordingly from 20 to 400 GBq/mmol (0.54–8 Ci/mmol). The 2-^{18}FDG in these productions contains glucose amounts in the range of 100 to 300 µmol. Although the specific radioactivity is not crucial in any of the known applications of 2-^{18}FDG, it should be measured during the production set-up. The order of magnitude of the specific radioactivity or the minimal specific radioactivity at time of calibration should be stated on the label, as well as the maximal amount of D-glucose.

3.13.7. *Pharmaceutical quality*. This is achieved by strict control of the determining parameters. These consist of the following measures. The synthesis apparatus is set up from clean sterilised glassware and sterile medical tubing for each production batch. The chromatography column is autoclaved before installation and is washed with sterilised water only. The eluate is collected in sterilised capped vials after passage through a sterile 0.22 µm filter. The system must have shown to produce apyrogenic and sterile products on at least three occasions before production for administration to humans. Sterility and apyrogenicity of the product are checked frequently in routine production runs (every month) by using samples and testing these by the standard procedures. In the Limulus test the product meets the requirements of the bacterial endotoxin tests as stated under Section 2.5.5. The pH of the product must stay between 6.0 and 8.0, and the isotonicity should be checked at regular intervals. Small samples of each batch should be withheld for retrospective testing of any relevant parameter if required.

2-^{18}FDG, stored in saline solution, proved to be stable to hydrolysis and radiolysis for several hours as tested by various groups (KFA Jülich; BNL Brookhaven) with batches of > 10 GBq (> 300 mCi). It is also stable to standard autoclaving procedures (*e.g.* 130°C for 8 min). Stability should be tested after the new implementation of a production method or any change thereto.

3.13.8. *Comparison with the US pharmacopeia (USP)*. On three points our recommendations differ from the USP (United States Pharmacopeial Convention, 1989). First, we withstand from recommending GC as an analytical method for testing the epimeric purity of 2-^{18}FDG, since this method seems to be too complicated for routine application. Furthermore the USP does not require, methods for Kryptofix™ 2.2.2. determination, which we suggest should be included in the quality assurance tests. Finally it is not mentioned in the USP that the specific radioactivity should be stated on the label of the individual preparation. All other quality criteria and methods which are given in the USP entry are generally agreed upon.

3.13.9. *References*.

Alexoff D.L., Casati R., Fowler J.S,. Wolf A.P., Shea C., Schlyer D.R. and Shiue C-Y. (1992) Ion chromatographic analysis of high specific activity ^{18}FDG preparations and detection of the chemical impurity 2-chloro-2-deoxy-D-glucose. *Appl. Radiat. Isot.*, 43, 1313–1322.

Barrio J.R., MacDonald N.S., Robinson G.D., Najafi A., Cook J.S. and Kuhl D.E. (1981) Remote, semiautomated production of F-18 labeled 2-deoxy-2-fluoro-D-glucose. *J. Nucl. Med.*, 22, 372–375.

Baudot P, Jacque M. and Robin M. (1977) Effect of diaza-polyoxa-macrobicyclic complexing agent on the urinary elimination of lead in lead-poisoned rats. *Toxicol. Appl. Pharmacol.*, 41, 113–118.

Bida G.T., Satyamurthy N. and Barrio J.R. (1984) The synthesis of 2-[F-18]fluoro-2-deoxy-D-glucose using glycals: a reexamination. *J. Nucl. Med.*, 25, 1327–1334.

Brodack J.W., Dence C.S., Kilbourn M.R. and Welch M.J. (1988) Robotic production of 2-deoxy-2-[^{18}F]fluoro-D-glucose: a routine method of synthesis using tetrabutylammonium [^{18}F]fluoride. *Appl. Radiat. Isot.*, 39, 699–703.

Chaly T. and Dahl J.R. (1989) Thin layer chromatographic detection of Kryptofix 2.2.2 in the routine synthesis of [^{18}F]2-fluoro-2-deoxy-D-glucose. *Nucl. Med. Biol.*, 16, 385–387.

Coenen H.H., Pike V.W., Stöcklin G. and Wagner R. (1987) Recommendation for a practical production of 2-[^{18}F]fluoro-2-deoxy-D-glucose. *Appl. Radiat. Isot.*, 38, 605–610.

Ehrenkaufer R.E., Potocki J.F. and Jewett D.M. (1984) Simple synthesis of F-18 labeled 2-fluoro-2-deoxy-D-glucose: concise communication. *J. Nucl. Med.*, 25, 333–337.

Fowler J.S. and Wolf A.P. (1986) 2-Deoxy-2-[^{18}F]-fluoro-D-glucose for metabolic studies: current status. *Appl. Radiat. Isot.*, 37, 663–668.

Fowler J.S., MacGregor R.R., Wolf A.P., Farrell A.A., Karlstrom K.I. and Ruth T.J. (1981) A shielded synthesis system for production of 2-deoxy-2-[^{18}F]fluoro-D-glucose. *J. Nucl. Med.*, 22, 376–380.

Gallagher B.M., Ansari A., Atkins H., Casella V., Christman D.R., Fowler J.S., Ido T, MacGregor R.R., Som P., Wam C.N., Wolf A.P., Kuhl D.E. and Reivich M. (1977) Radiopharmaceuticals XXVII. ^{18}F-Labeled 2-deoxy-2-fluoro-D-glucose as a radiopharmaceutical for measuring regional myocardial glucose metabolism in vivo: tissue distribution and imaging studies in animals. *J. Nucl. Med.*, 18, 990–996.

Guillaume M., Luxen A., Nebeling B., Argentini M., Clark J.C. and Pike V.W. (1991) Recommendations for fluorine-18 production. *Appl. Radiat. Isot.*, 42, 749–762.

Hamacher K., Coenen H.H. and Stöcklin G. (1986) Efficient stereospecific synthesis of no-carrier-added 2-[^{18}F]-fluoro-2-deoxy-D-glucose using aminopolyether supported nucleophilic substitution. *J. Nucl. Med.*, 27, 235–238.

Hamacher K., Blessing G. and Nebeling B. (1990) Computer aided synthesis (CAS) of no-carrier-added 2-[^{18}F]fluoro-2-deoxy-D-glucose: an efficient automated system for the aminopolyether-supported nucleophilic fluorination. *Appl. Radiat. Isot.*, 41, 49–55.

Ido T., Wan C-N., Casella V., Fowler J.S.,Wolf A.P. Reivich M and Kuhl D.E. (1978) Labeled 2-deoxy-D-glucose analogs. ^{18}F-Labeled 2-deoxy-2-fluoro-D-glucose, 2-deoxy-2-fluoro-D-mannose, and ^{14}C-2-deoxy-2-fluoro-D-glucose. *J. Label. Compd. Radiopharm.*, 14, 175–183.

Johnson B.F,. Maylotte D.H., Sabourin C.L., Finn R. and Kothari P. (1993) Synthesis of 2-[^{18}F]FDG using tetraalkylammonium bicarbonate. *J. Label Compd. Radiopharm.*, 32, 562–564. (Abstract).

Knust E.J., Wortmann R. and Machulla H-J. (1989) Synthesis of ^{18}F-2-deoxy-2-fluoro-D-glucose and ^{18}F-3-deoxy-3-fluoro-D-glucose with no carrier added ^{18}F-fluoride. *J. Radioanal. Nucl. Chem.*, 132, 85–91

Moerlein S.M., Brodack J.W., Siegel B.A. and Welch M.J. (1989) Elimination of contaminant Kryptofix 2.2.2 in the routine production of 2-[^{18}F]fluoro-2-deoxy-D-glucose. *Appl. Radiat. Isot.*, 40, 741–743.

Padgett H.C., Schmidt D.G., Luxen A., Bida G.T., Satyamurthy N. and Barrio J.R. (1989) Computer-controlled radiochemical synthesis: a chemistry process control unit for the automated production of radiochemicals. *Appl. Radiat. Isot.*, 40, 433–445.

Santos L.M. and Baldwin R.P. (1987) Liquid chromatography/electrochemical detection of carbohydrates at a cobalt pthalocyanine containing chemically modified electrode. *Anal. Chem.*, 59, 1766-1770.

Schlyer D.J., Bastos M., Alexoff A.V. and Wolf A.P. (1990) Separation of [^{18}F]fluoride from ^{18}O water using anion exchange resin. *Appl. Radiat. Isot.*, 41, 531–533.

Shiue C-Y., Fowler J.S., Wolf A.P., Alexoff D. and MacGregor R.R. (1985) Gas-liquid chromatographic determination of relative amounts of 2-deoxy-2-fluoro-D-glucose and 2-deoxy-2-fluoro-D-mannose synthesized from various methods. *J. Label. Compd. Radiopharm.*, 22, 503–508.

Tewson T.J. (1983) Synthesis of no-carrier added fluorine-18 2-deoxy-2-fluoro-D-glucose. *J. Nucl. Med.*, 24, 718–721.

Tewson T.J. (1989) Procedures, pitfalls and solutions in the production of [^{18}F]2-deoxy-2-fluoro-D-glucose: a paradigm in the routine synthesis of fluorine-18 radiopharmaceuticals. *Nucl. Med. Biol.*, 16, 533–551.

Toorongian S.A., Mulholland G.K., Jewett D.M., Bachelor M.A. and Kilbourn M.R. (1990) Routine production of 2-deoxy-2-[^{18}F]fluoro-D-glucose by direct nucleophilic exchange on a quaternary 4-aminopyridinium resin. *Nucl. Med. Biol.*, 17, 273–279.

United States Pharmacopoeial Convention. (1989) Fluorodeoxyglucose F-18 Injection Monograph. *United States Pharmacopoeia National Formulary* XXI: Suppl. 9, 3190.

Van Rijn C.J.S, Herscheid J.D.M., Visser G.W.M. and Hoekstra A. (1985) On the stereoselectivity of the reaction of [^{18}F]acetylhypofluorite with glucals. *Appl. Radiat. Isot.*, 36, 111–115.

Vora M.M., Boothe T.E., Finn R.D., Kothari P.J., Emran A.M., Carroll S.T. and Gilson A.J. (1985) Multimillicurie preparation of 2-[^{18}F]-fluoro-2-deoxy-D-glucose via nucleophilic displacement with fluorine-18 labelled fluoride. I. Purification and quality control procedures. *J. Label. Compd. Radiopharm.*, 22, 953–960.

3.14. L-6-[^{18}F]FLUORO-DOPA

3.14.1. *Introduction.* L-6-[^{18}F]Fluoro-3,4-dihydroxyphenylalanine, (6-[^{18}F]fluoro-L-DOPA, 6-^{18}FDOPA), an analogue of L-DOPA, is used to assess presynaptic dopaminergic function *in vivo* (Garnett *et al.*, 1983a,b; Leenders *et al.*, 1986) and provides opportunities to examine changes in dopamine neurotransmission in clinically dysfunctional patients (Martin *et al.*, 1989; Lindvall *et al.*, 1990). The production of 6-^{18}FDOPA and its metabolism *in vivo* have been the subject of a recent critical review (Luxen *et al.*, 1992) and the radiopharmaceutical has been considered for the United States Pharmacopeia (United States Pharmacopeial Convention, 1991). Stimuli to the revision process have been published (Barrio, 1990)

3.14.2. *Radiochemistry.* The production of radiofluorination agents such as [^{18}F]fluorine, [^{18}F]acetyl hypofluorite and [^{18}F]fluoride, and the subsequent production of 6-^{18}FDOPA from these agents has been critically reviewed elsewhere (Coenen *et al.*, 1988; Luxen *et al.*, 1992).

Direct electrophilic radiofluorination of L-DOPA provides a mixture of regioisomers (Chirakal *et al.*, 1986; Adam *et al.*, 1986; Coenen *et al.*, 1988), which can be separated by HPLC. This is best achieved on a large diameter reverse phase column of high efficiency, using 70mM-potassium dihydrogen orthophosphate as eluent (Pike *et al.*, 1990). The collected product, after quality control and sterile filtration, is then suitable for clinical use.

To overcome the problem of non-regioselective fluorination, several radiofluorodemetalation reactions have been developed which produce 6-^{18}FDOPA in about 11% radiochemical yield (Luxen *et al.*, 1990; for a review see Luxen *et al.*, 1992). However, the mercurated precursors should be checked for chiral purity before use.

After radiofluorination of the mercurated precursor, purification and hydrolysis, the reaction mixture is brought to a defined volume (4–5 mL) by adding HPLC solvent, filtered through a 0.22 μm membrane filter and injected onto the HPLC column (C-18, 5–10 μm particle size, 8–16 mm i.d., 250–300 mm long). It seems advisable, however, to purify the sample before HPLC by passing it over a C-18 cartridge (*e.g.* Chromabond™ C-18 or SepPak™ C-18) and to wash it with 1 mL of water, to decolorise the solution. Elution with 5mM-sodium acetate solution, containing 1mM-EDTA, acetic acid (0.1%) and ascorbic acid (0.01%), at a flow rate of 7 mL/min, yields the 6-^{18}FDOPA with a retention time between 12 and 15 min, depending on the exact conditions used. EDTA has a protective effect against auto-oxidation of 6-FDOPA, which also occurs in acidic solutions (Chen *et al.*, 1989). Normally, the collected peak does not exceed 10 mL in volume and after adjustment to isotonicity, sterile filtration and quality control, the product is ready for clinical use.

6-^{18}FDOPA has recently been made via nucleophilic substitution with nca [^{18}F]fluoride, seeking advantages of high levels of radioactivity and high specific radioactivity (Lemaire *et al.*, 1990).

3.14.3. *Radionuclidic purity.* The quality of [^{18}F]fluorine for electrophilic radiofluorination, as produced by the ^{20}Ne(d,α)^{18}F nuclear reaction, is high. Possible impurities, such as very short-lived isotopes of sodium and neon, decay during the work-up and are eliminated during the synthesis.

The radionuclidic purity of [^{18}F]fluoride produced via the ^{18}O(p,n)^{18}F process on [^{18}O]water is more crucial and demands control, since the quality of [^{18}F]fluoride will not only determine the radionuclidic purity of the final product but also its reactivity in nucleophilic substitution. With decreasing concentration of [^{18}O]water the amount of nitrogen-13 increases via the ^{16}O(p,α)^{13}N reaction. Fixation of [^{18}F]fluoride on an anion exchange column is recommended. It allows the separation of cationic radionuclidic impurities which arise from the target window foil and vary according to the foil material (Adam *et al.*, 1986; Pike *et al.*, 1990). Furthermore this procedure enables simple recycling of the target water.

Radionuclidic purity and identity should be tested by γ-ray spectroscopy and half-life measurements. As long as the production parameters are not changed, a thorough investigation of radionuclidic purity is necessary only during the set-up phase of the routine synthesis. In these tests the γ-ray spectrum must exhibit a major photo peak at 0.511 MeV and possibly a sum peak at 1.02 MeV depending on source geometry and detector efficiency. Since γ-ray spectroscopy cannot distinguish between positron-emitters, it is mandatory to determine that the half-life of the product is 110 min, by a suitable detector system.

3.14.4. *Chemical purity.* Routine quality control is performed based on HPLC using a mass detector such as a detector for absorbance at 220 nm (Dunn *et al.*, 1991) or 280 nm (Pike *et al.*, 1990; Luxen *et al.*, 1990), or an electrochemical detector (Chen *et al.*, 1989). The response of the mass detector should be calibrated to allow identified impurities to be assayed.

L-DOPA and L-6-hydroxy-DOPA are the main possible contaminants, depending on the synthesis employed. L-6-Hydroxy-DOPA is converted into the potent neurotoxin, L-6-hydroxydopamine *in vivo* (Sachs and Jonsson, 1972) and 50 µg has been suggested as the upper acceptable limit for L-6-hydroxy-DOPA in any single injected dose (Pike *et al.*, 1990).

Many techniques may be used to analyze 6-^{18}FDOPA that has been prepared by carrier-added electrophilic methods. Especially useful is proton-decoupled ^{19}F-NMR spectroscopy which can, when applied with other techniques, confirm product identity and accurately quantify contamination by positional isomers (Chirakal *et al.*, 1984). Accepted values for the chemical shift and coupling constants for each isomer have been tabulated (Firnau *et al.*, 1986). Mass spectrometry can also be used to identify chemical impurities (Pike *et al.*, 1990). Reference L-DOPA and D,L-6-hydroxy-DOPA are available commercially, though it should be noted that the latter is unstable in solution.

Radiofluorodemercuration procedures may give rise to mercury breakthrough and careful control of a possible mercury contamination of the injectable preparation is mandatory. Atomic absorption spectrometry is the method of choice for trace analysis of mercury (Clarkson *et al.*, 1968) and should therefore be performed regularly during the set up and standardisation phase. By following the recommendations for synthesis given in a recent review (Luxen *et al.*, 1990), levels of mercury below 20 ppb can be expected. Such a concentration in a typical injection volume of 10 mL would lead to a dose of 3 ng/kg in a 70 kg subject, a value which is far below the smallest toxic dose of 5 mg/kg appearing in estimations of the toxicology of mercury (Henschler and Lehnert, 1989; Seiler and Sigel, 1988). The United States Pharmacopeial Convention (1991) has proposed that mercury content should be less than 0.5 µg/mL in L-6-[^{18}F]fluoro-DOPA preparations.

Although a fast and reliable method for routine control of every batch is called for, the colorimetric tests using chelating agents are not sensitive enough to detect these low concentrations (detection limit > 5 ppm). However, ionic mercury levels can be measured using an HPLC method based on reverse phase ion-pair chromatography which is reported to detect ionic mercury down to 10 ppb (Luxen and Barrio, 1988). Alternatively, a simple purification method based on Chelex™-S resin for demercuration has been reported (Wagner, 1993).

Methods have been reported for the preparation of multi-milligrammes of the standards D,L-6-fluoro-DOPA, L-6-fluoro-DOPA (Grierson and Adam, 1985), D-6-fluoro-DOPA (Luxen and Barrio, 1988), D,L-2-fluoro-DOPA and D,L-5-fluoro-DOPA (Creveling and Kirk, 1985). Analytical procedures should be calibrated regularly using such reference compounds. As yet they are unavailable commercially.

3.14.5. *Radiochemical purity.* Different methods of production may give rise to different types and levels of radiochemical impurities. Quality control for radiochemical purity should be performed routinely by reverse phase HPLC (Chen *et al.*, 1989; Dunn *et al.*, 1991; Pike *et al.*, 1990) or ion pair chromatography (Coenen *et al.*, 1988; Luxen *et al.*, 1990) equipped with radioactivity detection. Both methods are able to detect [^{18}F]fluoride and any ^{18}F-containing compounds present as regioisomers or as partially hydrolysed intermediates. Enantiomeric purity should be estimated on at least one sample produced from any given batch of precursor. This can be achieved by chiral TLC (Coenen *et al.*, 1988; Pike *et al.*, 1990; Wagner, 1992) or more accurately by ligand exchange HPLC (Chen *et al.*, 1989; Luxen *et al.*, 1990).

The USP (United States Pharmacopeial Convention, 1990) recommends that 6-^{18}FDOPA should represent not less than 95% of the total radioactivity and that not less than 95% of the total radioactivity measured should be present as the L-isomer.

3.14.6. *Specific radioactivity.* To date there is no requirement to produce 6-^{18}FDOPA at high specific radioactivity. It may be determined accurately from HPLC methods equipped with both quantitative radioactivity and mass detection (Chen *et al.*, 1989; Pike *et al.*, 1990). However, large variations of the specific radioactivity may affect the quality of clinical data. The USP recommends that specific radioactivity should not be less than 3.7 GBq/mmol (100 mCi/2.2 mg).

3.14.7. *Pharmaceutical quality.* Pharmaceutical quality is achieved by strict control of the determining parameters. For 6-^{18}FDOPA these consist of the following measures. The reaction system is set up from clean sterilised glassware and sterile medical tubing for each production batch. The 6-^{18}FDOPA fraction eluting from the HPLC column is collected in a sterilised capped vial.

EDTA and ascorbic acid, added during final formulation, for the purpose of achieving stability, should not exceed 0.1% of weight for pharmacological safety. The final solution is passed through a sterile 0.22 μm filter.

The pH of the product is adjusted to 7.0 ± 1.0 with an appropriate buffer. This is controlled in each individual batch. The isotonicity should be checked at regular intervals. The synthesis apparatus must have shown to produce apyrogenic and sterile products on at least three occasions before production for human administration. Sterility and apyrogenicity of the product are checked frequently in routine production runs (every month) by using samples and testing these by the standard procedures. In the Limulus test the product meets the requirements of the bacterial endotoxin tests, as stated under Section 2.5.5. Small samples of each batch should be withheld for retrospective testing if required.

The stability of formulated 6-^{18}FDOPA may depend on local production conditions. Significant radiochemical instability has been reported in the absence of EDTA (Chen *et al.*, 1989). Such instability may relate to the degree of metal contamination, oxygen concentration and also pH, well known factors in the oxidation of L-DOPA (Jameson, 1968) However, others have observed no such instability (Pike *et al.*, 1990). It is recommended that the shelf-life be checked occasionally by HPLC on typical preparations, and product stabilisation considered if necessary.

3.14.8. *References.*

Adam M.J., Ruth T.J., Grierson J.R., Abeysekera B. and Pate B.D. (1986) Routine synthesis of L-[^{18}F]6-fluorodopa with fluorine-18 acetyl hypofluorite. *J. Nucl. Med.*, 27, 1462–1466.

Barrio J.R. (1990) USP Standards for fluorine-18 labeled 6-fluoro-L-Dopa injection. *Pharmacopeial Forum*, 16, 320–321.

Chen J-J., Huang S-J., Finn R.D., Kirk K.L. Francis B.E., Adams H.R., Cohen R.M., Chiueh C.C. (1989) Quality control procedure for 6-[^{18}F]fluoro-L-DOPA: a presynaptic PET imaging ligand for brain dopamine neurons. *J. Nucl. Med.*, 30, 1249–1256.

Chirakal R., Firnau G., Couse J. and Garnett E.S. (1984) Radiofluorination with ^{18}F-labelled acetyl hypofluorite: [^{18}F]L-6-fluorodopa. *Int. J. Appl. Radiat. Isot.*, 35, 651–653.

Chirakal R., Firnau G. and Garnett E.S. (1986) High yield synthesis of 6-[^{18}F]fluoro-L-DOPA. *J. Nucl. Med.*, 27, 417–421.

Clarkson T.W., Greenwood M.R. and Magos L. (1968) Atomic adsorption determination of total, inorganic and organic mercury in biological fluids. In *Clinical Chemistry and Chemical Toxicology of Metals*. Ed. Brown S.S. New York. Elsevier/North Holland, p. 201.

Coenen H.H., Franken K., Kling P. and Stöcklin G. (1988) Direct electrophilic radiofluorination of phenylalanine, tyrosine and dopa. *Appl. Radiat. Isot.*, 39, 1243–1250.

Creveling C.R. and Kirk K.L. (1985) The effect of ring-fluorination on the rate of O-methylation of dihydroxyphenylalanine (DOPA) by catechol-O-methyltransferase: significance in the development of ^{18}F-PETT scanning agents. *Biochem. Biophys. Res. Commun.*, 130, 1123–1131.

Dunn B.B., Channing M.A., Adams H.R., Goldstein D.S., Kirk K.L., Kiesewetter D.O. (1991) A single column, rapid quality control procedure for 6-[^{18}F]fluoro-L-DOPA and 6-[^{18}F]fluorodopamine PET imaging agents. *Nucl. Med. Biol.*, 18, 209–213.

Firnau G., Garnett E.S., Chirakal R., Sood S., Nahmias C. and Schrobilgen G. (1986) [^{18}F]Fluoro-L-DOPA for the in vivo study of intracerebral dopamine. *Appl. Radiat. Isot.*, 37, 669–675.

Garnett E.S., Firnau G. and Nahmias C. (1983a) Dopamine visualized in the basal ganglia of living man. *Nature*, 305, 137–138.

Garnett E.S., Firnau G., Nahmias C. and Chirakal R. (1983b) Striatal dopamine metabolism in living monkeys examined by positron emission tomography. *Brain Res.*, 280, 169–171.

Grierson J.R. and Adam M.J. (1985) *In-situ* preparation of a chemically bonded chiral stationary phase for the separation of aromatic α-amino acid enantiomers. *J. Chromatogr.*, 325, 103–109.

Henschler D. and Lehnert G. (Eds) (1989) *DFG: Biologische Arbeitsstoff-Toleranz-Werte (Bat-Werte) und Expositionsequivalente für krebserzeugende Arbeitsstoffe.* Weinheim. VCH-Verlag.

Jameson R.F. (1968) The oxidation of L-β-(3:4-dihydroxyphenyl)alanine (DOPA) by molecular oxygen in the presence of Fe^{III} as catalyst. In *Progress in Coordination Chemistry*. Ed. Cais M. *Proc. 11th Internat. Conf. Coordination Chem.*, 1968 Amsterdam. Elsevier. pp. 23–25.

Leenders K.L. Palmer A.J., Quinn N., Clark J.C., Firnau G., Garnett E.S., Nahmias C., Jones T. and Marsden C.D. (1986) Brain dopamine metabolism in patients with Parkinson's disease measured with positron emission tomography. *J. Neurol. Neurosurg. Psychiat.*, 49, 853–860.

Lemaire C., Guillaume M., Cantineau R. and Christiaens L. (1990) No-carrier-added regioselective preparation of 6-[^{18}F]fluoro-L-DOPA. *J. Nucl. Med.*, 31, 1247–1251.

Lindvall O., Brundin P., Widner H., Rehncrona S., Gustavii B. Frackowiak R., Leenders K.L., Sawle G., Rothwell J.C., Marsden C.D. and Bjorklund A. (1990) Grafts of fetal dopamine neurons survive and improve motor function in Parkinson's disease. *Science*, 247, 574.

Luxen A. and Barrio J.R. (1988) Fluorination of substituted veratroles via regioselective mercuration. *Tetrahedron Lett.*, 29, 1501–1504.

Luxen A., Perlmutter M., Bida G.T., Van Moffaert G., Cook J.S. Satyamurthy N., Phelps M.E. and Barrio J.R. (1990) Remote, semiautomated production of 6-[^{18}F]fluoro-L-dopa for human studies with PET. *Appl. Radiat. Isot.*, 41, 275–281.

Luxen A., Guillaume M., Melega W.P., Pike V.W., Solin O. and Wagner R. (1992) Production of 6-[^{18}F]fluoro-L-DOPA and its metabolism *in vivo* — a critical review. *Nucl. Med. Biol.*, 19, 149–158.

Martin W.R.W., Palmer M.R., Patlak C.S. and Calne D.B. (1989) Nigrostriatal function in humans studied with positron emission tomography. *Ann. Neurol.*, 26, 535.

Pike V.W., Kensett M.J., Turton D.R., Waters S.L. and Silvester D.J. (1990) Labelled agents for PET studies of the dopaminergic system — some quality assurance methods, experience and issues. *Appl. Radiat. Isot.*, 41, 483-492.

Sachs C. and Jonsson G. (1972) Selective 6-hydroxy-DOPA induced degeneration of central and peripheral noradrenalin neurons. *Brain Res.*, 40, 563.

Seiler H.G. and Sigel H. (1988) *Handbook on toxicity of inorganic compounds.* New York, Basel. Marcel Dekker.

United States Pharmacopeial Convention. (1991) Fluorodopa F-18 injection. *Pharmacopeial Forum*, 17, 1582–1584.

Wagner R. (1993) Removal of mercury contamination from 6-F-DOPA preparations. *J. Label. Compd. Radiopharm.*, 32, 250. (Abstract).

3.15. ^{18}F-LABELLED 3-*N*-ALKYLSPIPERONES

3.15.1. *Introduction.* Due to the advantageous half-life of fluorine-18 ($t_{1/2}$ = 110 min), 3-*N*-[^{18}F]methylspiperone (^{18}FMSP) and 3-*N*-[^{18}F]fluoroethylspiperone (^{18}FESP) are the most widely used 'irreversible' ligands for the determination of cerebral D2-receptor densities with positron emission tomography (PET) (for recent reviews see Stöcklin, 1991 and Mazière *et al.*, 1992). The radiofluorinated butyrophenones have a high binding affinity like 3-*N*-[^{11}C]methylspiperone (Section 3.6.) and have proved useful for quantitation of D_2 receptor density in monkey and human PET studies in various disease states, and especially to measure D_2 receptor occupancy by neuroleptic drugs (Arnett *et al.*, 1985; Coenen *et al.*, 1987; Barrio *et al.*, 1989). ^{18}FMSP and ^{18}FESP exhibit an almost identical pharmacokinetic and metabolic behaviour (Arnett *et al.*, 1985).

3.15.2. *Radiochemistry.* With respect to the high specific radioactivity needed with receptor ligands only nucleophilic radiofluorination with no-carrier-added [^{18}F]fluoride is appropriate for labelling FMSP and FESP. There are several ways for preparing both ^{18}F-labelled butyrophenones (for reviews see Kilbourn and Welch, 1986; Mazière *et al.*, 1992). ^{18}FESP can be produced by substitution on functional 3-*N*-ethylene derivatives of spiperone (Kiesewetter *et al.*, 1986; Satyamurthy *et al.*, 1990). The most practical and reliable method appears to be via [^{18}F]fluoroethylation of spiperone after Kryptofix™ 2.2.2. (aminopolyether 2.2.2.)-activated nucleophilic substitution on disubstituted ethanes in acetonitrile (Kiesewetter *et al.*, 1986; Coenen *et al.*, 1987; Plenevaux *et al.*, 1991). ^{18}FMSP is either prepared by a multistep synthesis starting with nucleophilic substitution on for example *p*-nitrobenzaldehyde (Shiue *et al.*, 1986) or by direct [^{18}F]fluoro for nitro exchange on *p*-nitro-desfluoro-*N*-methylspiperone using an aminopolyether (2.2.2.)-potassium oxalate-carbonate buffer system in dimethyl sulphoxide (Hamacher *et al.*, 1991). By all four methods the final product is obtained directly and finally is purified by means of reverse or normal phase HPLC (Coenen *et al.*, 1987; Adam *et al.*, 1989; Barrio *et al.*, 1989; Hamacher *et al.*, 1991). The preparation via direct substitution on the nitro- or functional 3-*N*-ethylene compounds demands synthesis of the precursors. For the *N*-fluoroalkylation method and for the four step radiosynthesis the precursors, spiperone and *p*-nitrobenzaldehyde, are commercially available.

3.15.3. *Radionuclidic purity*. The quality of [^{18}F]fluoride obtained from an appropriate nuclear reaction and target will not only determine the radionuclidic purity of the final product but also its reactivity in the nucleophilic substitution process. Most common and efficient is the $^{18}O(p,n)^{18}F$ process on ^{18}O-enriched water. With decreasing concentration of [^{18}O]water the amount of nitrogen-13 increases via the (p,α) reaction on oxygen-16. Fixation of [^{18}F]fluoride on an anion exchange column is recommended. It allows a separation of cationic radionuclidic impurities which arise from the target window foil and vary according to the foil material (Shiue *et al.*, 1986; Hamacher *et al.*, 1991). Furthermore, this procedure enables simple recycling of the ^{18}O-enriched target water.

Radionuclidic purity and identity should be tested by γ-ray spectroscopy and half-life measurements. As long as the production parameters are not changed, a thorough investigation of radionuclidic purity is necessary only during the set-up phase of the routine synthesis. In these tests the γ-ray spectrum must exhibit a major photo peak at 0.511 MeV and possibly a sum peak at 1.02 MeV depending on source geometry and detector efficiency. Since γ-ray spectroscopy cannot distinguish between positron-emitters, it is mandatory to determine that the half-life of the product is 110 min as determined by a suitable detector system.

3.15.4. *Chemical purity*. If commercially purchased or synthesised, the precursors, such as the *N*-methylspirodecanone moiety, spiperone, or functionalised spiperones, have to be checked for high purity. This is to ensure labelling efficacy but moreover to prevent formation of spiperone derivatives which could lower the apparent specific activity. The method of choice is HPLC.

Semi-preparative and analytical HPLC is also recommended to assure and control the chemical purity of the formulated product. With respect to the potential pharmacodynamic effect of spiperone derivatives and also to their interference with the PET measurement this is mandatory for each run. Analysis can be performed by one of the HPLC methods mentioned above in conjunction with a UV absorbance detector. The method has to be appropriate to the used labelling method and correspondingly to the type of by-products likely to be encountered. For example, although the separation from precursor is uncritical, the elevated temperatures applied in [^{18}F]fluoro for nitro exchange on

3-*N*-methyl-nitro-desfluorospiperone required the use of a twofold HPLC system, using a RP-18 and a special end-capped RP-8 column, in order to separate the desired end-product from traces of unknown by-products (Hamacher *et al.*, 1991)

The absence of solvents and of Kryptofix™ 2.2.2, if used, must be guaranteed by appropriate tests. To detect traces of solvents, GC with an FI-detector is recommended. Testing for Kryptofix™ 2.2.2. should be done regularly as described for the quality control of 2-^{18}FDG (Section 3.13.). (N.B. spiperone and Kryptofix™ both form ammonium salts.)

3.15.5. *Radiochemical purity.* Radiochemical purity can be assessed by the HPLC procedures used for establishing chemical purity, simply by incorporating a radioactivity detector. Radioactive by-products will depend on the labelling method used. Proof of radiochemical purity should be obtained by additional analytical HPLC of the purified end-product, using an HPLC system similar to that used for preparative purification. Since several HPLC conditions are described it is recommended to use different systems (RP-18 or silica gel) for preparation and purity analysis. A TLC method has been used especially for the detection of [^{18}F]fluoride in the case of ^{18}FESP synthesis (Barrio *et al.*, 1989; Satyamurthy *et al.*, 1990) but this appears insufficient for detecting products of similar lipophilicity to the desired radiotracer.

3.15.6. *Specific radioactivity.* The specific radioactivity is especially critical for the efficacy of quantitation of D_2 receptor densities. Traces of compounds with affinity to the receptor will compete with binding of the radioligand. Therefore, isotopic dilution and contamination with cold spiperone analogues (by-products) will reduce the apparent specific radioactivity. These must be carefully controlled in each individual batch. It must be noted that spiperones are sensitive to treatment with base and fluoride is a good leaving group from aromatic rings. Thus, liberation of fluoride has been found in radiofluoroalkylation reactions leading to isotopic dilution. It is recommended to separate the intermediate radiofluoroalkylation agent from the disubstituted ethane (Plenevaux *et al.*, 1991). In direct substitution reactions on spiperone derivatives (Kiesewetter *et al.*, 1986; Satyamurthy *et al.*, 1990) cleavage of fluoride has to be controlled depending on the reaction conditions. The same HPLC systems can be used as for establishing the chemical and radiochemical purity since spiperones exhibit a high UV absorption. Specific radioactivities should be in the range of 10 to 50 GBq/µmol (0.27–1.35 Ci/µmol) at EOS and should be stated on the label of the radiopharmaceutical container together with the time of calibration.

3.15.7. *Pharmaceutical quality.* Pharmaceutical quality is achieved by strict control of the determining parameters. For ^{18}F-alkylated spiperones these consist of the following measures. The reaction system is set up from clean sterilised glassware and sterile medical tubing for each production batch. The ^{18}F-alkylated spiperone fraction eluting from the HPLC column is collected in a sterilised capped vial. After evaporation of the collected HPLC fraction the residue is redissolved in sterile saline or phosphate buffer. Addition of ethanol during final formulation, for the purpose of achieving solubility or stability, should not exceed 5% of volume for pharmacological safety. The final solution is passed through a 0.22 µm sterile filter.

The pH of the product, is adjusted to 7.0 ± 1.0 with an appropriate buffer. This is controlled in each individual batch. The isotonicity should be checked at regular intervals. The synthesis apparatus must have shown to produce apyrogenic and sterile products on at least three occasions before production for human administration. Sterility and apyrogenicity of the product are checked frequently in routine production runs (every month) by using samples and testing these by the standard procedures. In the Limulus test the product meets the requirements of the bacterial endotoxin tests, as stated under Section 2.5.5. Small samples of each batch should be withheld for retrospective testing of any relevant parameter if required.

^{18}FMSP of high specific radioactivity was reported to be sensitive to radiolytic decomposition when stored in pure saline solution at high dose (MacGregor *et al.*, 1987). Self-decomposition, however, can be avoided in presence of hydroxyl radical scavenger during dispensing and storage (Suzuki *et al.*, 1990). ^{18}FESP (0.5 GBq ;13.5 mCi) stored in saline solution with 5% ethanol proved to be stable for > 4 hours at room temperature. Stability has to be ensured for the given ^{18}F-labelled spiperone derivative depending on production, dispensing and delivery conditions.

3.15.8. *References.*

Adam M.J., Grierson J.R. and Jivan S. (1989) An improved HPLC system for the analysis and purification of organic amine radiopharmaceuticals. *Appl. Radiat. Isot.*, 40, 91–92.

Arnett C.D., Fowler J.S., Wolf A.P., Shiue C-Y. and McPherson D.W. (1985) [^{18}F]N-Methylspiroperidol: the radioligand of choice for PETT studies of the dopamine receptor in human brain. *Life Sci.*, 36, 1359–1366.

Barrio J.R., Satyamurthy N., Huang S.C., Keen R.E., Nissenson C.H.K., Hoffman J.M., Ackermann R.F., Bahn M.M., Mazziotta J.C. and Phelps M.E. (1989) 3-(2'-[^{18}F]-Fluoroethyl)-spiperone: *in vivo* biochemical and kinetic characterization in rodents, non human primates, and humans. *J. Cerebr. Blood Flow Metab.*, 9, 830–839.

Chi D.Y., Kilbourn M.R., Katzenellenbogen J.A. Brodack J.W. and Welch M.J. (1986) Synthesis of no-carrier-added N-([^{18}F]fluoroalkyl)spiperone derivatives. *Appl. Radiat. Isot.*, 37, 1173–1180.

Coenen H.H., Laufer P., Stöcklin G., Wienhard K., Pawlik G., Böcher-Schwarz H.G. and Heiss W-D. (1987) 3-N-(2-[^{18}F]-Fluoroethyl)-spiperone: a novel ligand for cerebral dopamine receptor studies with PET. *Life Sci.*, 40, 81– 88.

Hamacher K., Nebeling B., Coenen H.H. and Stöcklin G. (1991) [^{18}F]N-Methylspiperone: direct n.c.a. nucleophilic [^{18}F]fluorination of *N*-methyl-4-nitrospiperone for remote controlled routine production of n.c.a. [^{18}F]MSP. *J. Label Compd. Radiopharm.*, 30, 353–354. (Abstract).

Kiesewetter D.O., Eckelman W.C., Cohen R.M., Finn R.D. and Larson S.M. (1986) Syntheses and D_2 receptor affinities of derivatives of spiperone containing aliphatic halogens. *Appl. Radiat. Isot.*, 37, 1181–1188.

Kilbourn M.R. and Welch M.J. (1986) Fluorine-18 labeled receptor based radiopharmaceuticals. *Appl. Radiat. Isot.*, 37, 677–683.

MacGregor R.R. Schlyer D.J., Fowler J.S., Wolf A.P. and Shiue C-Y. (1987) Fluorine-18-*N*-methylspiroperidol: radiolytic decomposition as a consequence of high specific activity and high dose levels. *J. Nucl. Med.*, 28, 60–67.

Mazière B., Coenen H.H., Halldin C., Någren K. and Pike V.W. (1992) PET radioligands for dopamine receptors and re-uptake sites: chemistry and biochemistry. *Nucl. Med. Biol.*, 19, 497–512.

Plenevaux A., Cantineau R., Labar D., Lemaire C. and Guillaume M. (1991) Routine production and improvement in the purification of 3-N-(2'-[^{18}F]fluoroethyl)spiperone for clinical use. *J. Label. Compd. Radiopharm.*, 30, 382–384. (Abstract).

Satyamurthy N., Barrio J.R., Bida G.T., Huang S-C., Mazziotta J.C. and Phelps M.E. (1990) 3-(2'-[^{18}F]Fluoroethyl)-spiperone, a potent dopamine antagonist: synthesis, structural analysis and in-vivo utilization in humans. *Appl. Radiat Isot.*, 41, 113–129.

Shiue C-Y., Fowler J.S., Wolf A.P., McPherson D.W., Arnett C.D. and Zecca L. (1986) No-carrier-added fluorine-18-labeled *N*-methylspiroperidol: synthesis and biodistribution in mice. *J. Nucl. Med.*, 27, 226–234.

Stöcklin G. (1991) Radioligands for PET studies of D_2-receptors: butyrophenone and ergot derivatives. In *Brain Dopaminergic Systems: Imaging with Positron Emission Tomography.* Baron J.C., Comar D., Farde L., Martinot J.L. and Mazoyer B., Eds. Dordrecht, Kluwer Academic Publishers. pp 5–22.

Suzuki K., Inoue O., Tamate K. and Mikado F. (1990) Production of 3-N-[^{11}C]methylspiperone with high specific activity and high radiochemical purity for PET studies: suppression of its radiolysis. *Appl. Radiat. Isot.*, 41, 593–599.

4. Appendix 1. Sources of Precursors and Standards for QA/QC

4.1. NON-COMMERIAL PRECURSORS AND STANDARDS—SOURCES/INFORMATION

4.1.1. *Precursors.*

S-[*carbonyl*-^{11}C]CGP 12177 precursor	MRC Cyclotron Unit, London
N-Desmethyl-L-deprenyl	Britannia Pharmaceuticals Chinoin
N-Desmethyl-flumazenil	Hoffman-La Roche
N-Desmethyl-raclopride	Astra Research Centre
[*O-methyl*-^{11}C]Diprenorphine precursor	MRC Cyclotron Unit, London
D-Homocysteine thiolactone	MHH Hannover
R,S-[*N-methyl*-^{11}C]PK 11195 precursor	MRC Cyclotron Unit, London Rhône-Poulenc Rorer
R/S-[*N-methyl*-^{11}C]PK 11195 precursor	MRC Cyclotron Unit, London
3-*N*-Methyl-4'-desfluoro-4'-nitrospiperone	Institut für Nuklearchemie, KFA, Jülich
[1-^{11}C]Tyrosine precursor	PET Centre, Groningen
[^{18}F]Altanserin precursor	Centre de Recherches du Cyclotron, Liège Erasme Hospital, Brussels

4.1.2. *Standards.*

L-6-Fluoro-DOPA	Erasme Hospital, Brussels,
L-6-Fluoro-Dopamine	Erasme Hospital, Brsussels
L-6-Fluoro-DOPA metabolites	Erasme Hospital, Brussels
Flumazenil	Hoffman-La Roche
R,S-PK 11195	Rhône-Poulenc Rorer
Raclopride	Astra Research Centre
Setoperone	Janssen Pharmaceutica

4.2. COMMERCIAL SOURCES

4.2.1. *Precursors.*

N-Desmethyl SCH 23390	Research Biochemicals Inc.
6-^{18}F-DOPA precursor (Hg precursor)	Bis Chem Inc. Research Biochemicals Inc.
6-^{18}F-DOPA precursor (L-3-MeO-Tyr)	Sigma Chem Co. Ltd.
2-^{18}FDG precursor	Aldrich Chem Co. Ltd. Research Biochemicals Inc.
D-Homocysteine thiolactone	Sigma Chem Co. Ltd.
L-Homocysteine thiolactone	Sigma Chem Co. Ltd.
Metaraminol	Sigma Chem Co. Ltd.
Spiperone	Research Biochemicals Inc., Sigma Chem. Co. Ltd.
QNB	Research Biochemicals Inc.

4.2.2. *Standards.*

R,S-CGP 12177	Research Biochemicals Inc.
L-Deprenyl	Research Biochemicals Inc.
Diprenorphine	MacFarlan Smith Ltd.
3-*N*-Methylspiperone	Research Biochemicals Inc.
L-*m*-tyrosine	CIDtech Research Inc
MQNB	Research Biochemicals Inc.
2-Fluoro-2-deoxy-D-glucose	Research Biochemicals Inc.
R,S-PK 11195	Research Biochemicals Inc.
Scopolamine	Research Biochemicals Inc.
	Sigma Chem Co. Ltd.
SCH 23390	Research Biochemicals Inc.

4.3. ADDRESSES

Addresses for PET centres mentioned in Section 4.1. may be found under the list of contributors at the beginning of this book. Addresses for pharmaceutical companies and commercial suppliers mentioned in Sections 4.1. and 4.2. are as follows.

Aldrich Chemical Co Ltd.
The Old Brickyard,
New Road,
Gilingham,
DORSET SP8 4BR
U.K.
Tel. 0800 71 71 81
FAX 0800 37 85 38

Astra Research Centre
S-15185 SODERTALJE
Sweden
Tel. (46) 755 329 80
FAX (46) 755 665 53

Bis Chem. Inc.
2245 Ch St Francois,
Dorval,
QUEBEC
Canada

Britannia Pharmaceuticals Ltd.
Forum House,
Brighton Road,
Redhill,
SURREY RH16YS
U.K.
Tel. 0737 773741
FAX 0737 773116

Chinoin
Pharmaceutical and Chemical Works Ltd.,
Research Centre,
PO Box 110,
H-1325 BUDAPEST
Hungary
Tel. 690 900

CIDtech Research Inc.
268 Lakeshore Road E.,
Suite 530,
Mississauga,
ONTARIO L5G 1H1
Canada
Tel. (416) 891 2411
FAX (416) 271 4522

Hoffman-La Roche Co.
CH-4002 BASLE
Switzerland
Tel. 061 688 11 11
FAX 061 691 9391

Janssen Pharmaceutica
Turnhoutsweg,
30-B-2340 BEERSE
Belgium
Tel. 014 60 21 11.

Macfarlan Smith Ltd.
Wheatfield Road,
EDINBURGH EH11 2QA
U.K.
Tel. 031-337 2434
FAX 031 337 9813

Research Biochemicals Inc.
One Strathmore Road,
NATICK MA 01760-2418
USA
Tel. 508 651 8151
FAX 508 655 1359.

Rhône-Poulenc Rorer
Centre de Recherche de vitry-Alfortville,
13 Quai Jules Guesde - BP 14,
94403 VITRY SUR SEINE, Cedex
France
Tel. (1) 45 73 85 11
FAX (1) 45 73 81 29

Sigma Chemical Company Ltd.
Fancy Road,
Poole,
DORSET BH17 7NH
U.K.
Tel. 0202 733114
FAX Group 2/3 0202 715460

PET RADIOPHARMACEUTICAL METABOLISM — PLASMA METABOLITE ANALYSIS

Bernard Mazière, Robert Cantineau, Heinz H. Coenen, Marcel Guillaume, Christer Halldin, André Luxen, Christian Loc'h and Sajinder K. Luthra

ABSTRACT. PET radiopharmaceutical metabolism is discussed in general. Methodology for determining the proportion of unchanged radiopharmaceutical in plasma is discussed with regard to preparation of sample, current analytical techniques, sources of errors and pitfalls. The literature on metabolite analysis in plasma is discussed for several popular radiopharmaceuticals, including labelled amino acids, flow tracers and radioligands for acetylcholine, adrenergic, benzodiazepine, dopamine and serotonin receptors.

1. Introduction

Radiopharmaceuticals, like any other drugs or chemicals, may be liable to rapid chemical transformation after their administration *in vivo* to humans. For drugs and compounds in general the analytical chemist is able to identify the various products of biotransformation in terms of concentrations and kinetics, but only, for example, by the extensive use of chromatography and other techniques. For radiopharmaceuticals the situation is simpler as radiochemists are concerned only with the parent radiopharmaceutical and its radioactive metabolites; the radiolabel itself facilitates detection.

Positron emission tomography (PET) is a technique used to quantitatively image functional parameters *in vivo*, including tissue metabolism, neurotransmission and receptor occupancy; PET is not only a quantitative *in vivo* methodology in terms of radioactivity measurement but also in terms of functional imaging. The image of the distribution of the radioactivity has to be expressed in terms of the concentration distribution of the injected radiopharmaceutical. Ultimately, these radiopharmaceutical concentrations will be transformed into data with physiological, pathological or pharmacological significance (*e.g.* consumption or incorporation rate, receptor density or affinity) by the use of various bio-mathematical models.

All the data that are used in these models have to be expressed in terms of the concentration of the ligand or tracer. This requires that radioactivity concentration must be transformed into mass concentration. This transformation is performed by dividing the radioactivity of the unchanged radiopharmaceutical by the specific radioactivity of the injected radiopharmaceutical, assuming that the metabolism of the radiopharmaceutical is identical to that of the corresponding unlabelled compound. However, PET cannot

G. Stöcklin and V. W. Pike (eds.), Radiopharmaceuticals for Positron Emission Tomography, 151–178.

distinguish between different chemical species, it only measures radioactivity concentration. In other words, to be able to calculate the concentration of unchanged radiopharmaceutical accurately it is necessary to determine the fraction of unchanged radiopharmaceutical in serial plasma samples after injection. Methodology for determining the fraction of unchanged radiopharmaceutical is the main focus of this chapter. It is generally assumed that the tissue uptake of radioactivity *in vivo* in PET regions of interest (ROI's) is the unchanged radiopharmaceutical. This can only be verified by analyzing tissue samples. Since generally this type of study can only be performed using animals, caution should be exercised when extrapolating data to human studies.

2. Radiopharmaceutical Metabolism

Radiopharmaceutical metabolism or drug metabolism in general has been described as a 'detoxification mechanism'. The latter however is a misleading term because the resulting products or metabolites can also be toxic. Therefore the term 'detoxification' when one means 'metabolism' is certainly to be avoided. In fact most of these transformations result in compounds that are more water-soluble and hence more readily excreted (La Dù *et al.*, 1971; Testa and Jenner, 1976; Jenner and Testa, 1980).

Most drugs are metabolized in the liver but drug metabolism may also take place in the kidneys, intestines and lungs. Generally, the involvement of brain in metabolism is very low. Metabolising enzymes can occur in mitochondrial and microsomal fractions. The microsomal drug metabolising system consists of a multi-enzymatic complex including cytochrome P-450 and two flavoproteins: the NADPH-cytochrome c reductase and the NADH-cytochrome b5 reductase. The mechanism requires NADP, molecular oxygen and Mg^{2+} (Cooper *et al.*, 1979; Lu and West 1980; Siler Master and Okita, 1980; Strobel *et al.*, 1980; Schenkman *et al.*, 1981; Taylor and Francis, 1984).

Like drug metabolism in general (Williams 1960; Chamberlain, 1987), radiopharmaceutical metabolism can be classified into two phases. In the first phase the radiopharmaceutical is attacked by a single enzyme to effect a simple change in its chemical structure. Such reactions are usually oxidations, reductions or hydrolyses and usually result in a structure with a new functional group or 'handle' that is conveniently utilised in the second phase. Phase II involves the addition of a hydrophilic moiety to a functional group already existing in the radiopharmaceutical, or a functional group in a derivative resulting from phase I, so forming a water-soluble conjugate that can be readily excreted via the urine. More than one derivative from phase I may be transformed through phase II.

2.1. PHASE I METABOLISM

2.1.1. *Oxidation.* Aromatic compounds are generally metabolized by direct hydroxylation while aliphatic compounds are metabolised by ω-hydroxylation to the primary alcohol. Alcohols are then further oxidised to aldehydes and ketones and finally aldehydes are subsequently oxidised to acids. Aromatic ethers are converted into phenols by *O*-dealkylation, the alkyl group being lost as the corresponding aldehyde. Aromatic amines are hydroxylated to the corresponding hydroxyamino compounds. Tertiary amines may be oxidised to the *N*-oxide, notably the main route of metabolism of some benzodiazepines. Secondary amines are dealkylated to primary amines and the corresponding aldehydes.

2.1.2. *Reduction.* The metabolism of ketones may be expected to result, to some degree, in the formation of alcohols. Carbon-carbon double bonds are in some instances reduced to their saturated equivalents. Nitro groups are reduced to the primary amines (as, for example, in the metabolism of the benzodiazepine, nitrazepam).

2.1.3. *Hydrolysis.* All types of esters are readily hydrolysed by a variety of specific or nonspecific esterases. However, these esterases may be specific to certain species and tissues and the importance of hydrolysis in the metabolism of a particular compound is not easy to predict. Amides are also hydrolysed but not as readily as esters.

2.2. PHASE II METABOLISM

2.2.1. *Glucuronidation.* This is the most common and extensively studied mode of phase II metabolism and involves the conjugation of the radiopharmaceutical, or one of its phase I metabolites, with glucuronic acid. The conjugation may take place through an ether type linkage with alcohols and phenols, the highly water-soluble derivative being rapidly excreted in the urine. The conjugation may alternatively take place through an ester linkage with carboxylic acids.

2.2.2. *Sulphonation.* Conjugation with sulphuric acid can be the second most important method of conjugation for radiopharmaceuticals and for their metabolites, particularly for phenols and alcohols.

2.2.3. *Acetylation.* Acetylation is another common metabolic step, usually classed as phase II type metabolism. Aromatic amides are most susceptible.

2.3. METABOLIC PATHWAYS

The above reactions are not mutually exclusive. One reaction could provide a substrate suitable for another perhaps to give a metabolic sequence incorporating many steps of different type. On the other hand, the radiopharmaceutical may be subject to several different concurrent conversions. For example, chlorpromazine is metabolized by 7-hydroxylation, *S*-oxidation and *N*-demethylation, with these three conversions leading to 8 possible metabolites. A radiopharmaceutical may be susceptible to all these reactions. However, the extent of any particular reaction or chain of reactions will, of course, depend on the ability of the radiopharmaceutical or of its metabolites to act as substrates for particular enzymes.

Numerous factors may influence the most likely metabolic pathways of a radiopharmaceutical:

- Dose (and frequency) of administration
- Species, strain, age, sex and weight of animal used (Breimer, 1983; Wilson, 1984)
- Diet and nutritional status
- Route and time of administration
- Interaction with other drugs
- Physiological abnormalities

Hence, it is practically impossible to forecast the stability of a drug *in vivo*.

The above summary is intended to recall the range of reactions that can take place for radiopharmaceuticals and also to show how difficult, if not impossible, it is to predict the metabolism of any particular radiopharmaceutical. Consequently, each radiopharmaceutical has to be studied individually to ascertain the metabolites which are likely to appear in biological fluids and/or tissues and which will affect PET data interpretation.

3. Preparation of the Sample

For modelling purposes, the biological samples which are commonly analyzed for radiopharmaceutical metabolites are blood, plasma or tissues. Since only a few analytical techniques are adequately specific to assay the radiopharmaceutical in the biological sample directly, often the first problem is to separate the radiopharmaceutical (and its metabolites) from the endogenous material.

3.1. DISRUPTION OF SOLID BIOLOGICAL SAMPLES

It is a general rule in biochemical analysis that the ease with which a sample can be analyzed increases with its degree of fluidity. For this obvious reason, tissue samples have to be subjected to mechanical procedures before being analyzed. Among the procedures which can be used to disrupt biological samples before analysis, we can distinguish 'mortar and pestle' techniques with the all-glass or glass-Teflon™ Potter systems, blades techniques with such commercial devices as the Waring Blender, the Virtis-Sorvall or the Polytron apparatus and sonication techniques. When using these procedures one must be aware that they may affect the sample in several undesirable ways. Some may lead to real chemical changes in the radiopharmaceutical (by, for example, temperature effects, metal chelation or conjugate hydrolysis) and some may make subsequent handling more difficult by forming foams or emulsions. This mechanical cell or tissue disruption can be performed in various buffers or directly in an organic solvent. The nature of the solvent which will be used as the medium for such procedures is critical.

3.2. PROTEIN ELIMINATION

One of the main features of aqueous solutions or homogenates from disrupted biological samples is the presence of a large amount of protein which often has a strong affinity for the radiopharmaceutical of interest. Hence, direct removal of protein could also remove the 'protein-bound' fraction of the radiopharmaceutical. In order to measure all unchanged radiopharmaceutical, it is necessary to eliminate the binding of the radiopharmaceutical to the protein.

As the rapidity of action of proteolytic enzymes is not compatible with the short half-lives of the usual radioactive labels (20, 10 and 110 min for ^{11}C, ^{13}N, ^{18}F respectively), the protein has to be filtered off or precipitated to obtain a protein-free aqueous solution suitable for a subsequent extraction with an organic solvent.

For protein filtration, classical dialysis techniques, which are too slow for the short half-life of the radionuclide, are replaced by ultrafiltration techniques using molecular weight cutting membranes. Great care must be taken to minimise the adsorption of the radiolabelled compounds onto the protein or onto the filtration membrane. Ultrafiltration is the classical way to determine the proportions of bound and free radiolabelled compound. During the precipitation process the protein is denatured and usually any previously bound radiopharmaceutical remains in solution. Saturation with various salts (ammonium sulphate, zinc sulphate-sodium hydroxide, aluminium chloride) often confers excellent efficiency, but a high salt concentration in the supernatant liquid can be a drawback for subsequent analysis.

Another popular technical solution for protein precipitation is to use acidic reagents such as metaphosphoric, trichloroacetic or perchloric acids. However, such strong acids may have detrimental effects on the radiopharmaceutical that is to be extracted. Thus, such procedures should be carefully tested on reference compounds for absence of destructive effect.

Any problem of instability of a radiopharmaceutical at low pH can be circumvented by using a single organic solvent to denature and precipitate the protein and to extract the radiolabelled compound. Methanol or ethanol are often used for this purpose, two volumes of alcohol being required for complete denaturation of a plasma sample. Acetonitrile is a very popular solvent because it is often compatible with subsequent HPLC analysis. Only one and a half volumes are required for complete protein denaturation.

Protein can also be eliminated by chromatography. The use of an internal-surface reverse phase (ISRP) chromatography column (Westerlund, 1987) permits simultaneous one-step elimination of protein and also separation of the unchanged radiopharmaceutical from its metabolites. ISRP particles have two surfaces, outer and inner. Each one is functional with regard to the two types of solute molecules of interest in serum analysis. The outer surfaces of the particles separate protein from the radiopharmaceutical and metabolites while the inner surfaces separate the radiopharmaceutical and metabolites from each other. Proteins are too large to reach the inner surfaces of the particles. Therefore, unretained proteins pass right through an ISRP column which, in this respect, acts like an exclusion chromatography column. However, the radiopharmaceutical and any metabolites can penetrate to the inner surfaces where they are retained and separated according to the principles of adsorption chromatography.

4. Current Analytical Techniques

Usually the radiopharmaceutical and its metabolites have to be extracted into an organic solvent before analysis. Ease of extraction from the aqueous fluid (biological fluid and/or added buffers) into an organic solvent will depend on the solvent used. The aim of such a treatment is to extract all the radioactivity and to leave behind the undesired interfering material. This is commonly achieved by a combination of steps where the polarity of the extracting solvent and/or the pH of the aqueous phase are adjusted.

'Plasma tracer analysis', because it is focused on one compound, the unchanged radiopharmaceutical, is easier than procedures requiring identification of unknown metabolites. A wealth of methods for biochemical or pharmacological analysis are in principle available to use in combination with appropriate radiodetection devices for the examination of the metabolism of radiopharmaceuticals. Restrictions arise from the short half-lives of positron-emitters and the often no-carrier-added (n.c.a.) amounts of radiopharmaceutical present. Some recent books provide much detailed information on radiochromatographic techniques (Van Rijk, 1986; Wieland *et al.*, 1986; Theobald 1989).

Requirements for analytical methods are:

— Capacity to separate radiopharmaceutical completely from all metabolites

— Simplicity and high speed because of the need for kinetic data from high sample numbers and because of the short half-lives of the radionuclides

— Cheapness for routine use in a clinical setting.

The most basic method is radio-HPLC since it combines high speed with high resolution. Also, radio-HPLC conditions are usually known from the (routine) preparation and analysis of the radiopharmaceutical. Therefore, radio-HPLC recommends itself as a standard method, at least for the evaluation of technically simpler chromatographic methods. The possibility of on-line radioactivity detection in combination with a computer-based data acquisition system facilitates data calculation and documentation. Depending on the device used, detection limits can be as low as 1 Bq/μL (27 pCi/μL). However, collection of the eluate in fractions for discontinuous radioactivity measurement is recommended for samples with low radioactivity. The disadvantages of radio-HPLC are the relatively high cost of hardware and finite sample throughput.

If plasma samples are manipulated before radio-HPLC analysis by extraction and/or concentration procedures, possible losses of the radiopharmaceutical, especially in the case of highly lipophilic no-carrier-added compounds may occur. It is necessary to check for such losses. Direct injection of plasma onto a HPLC column will give the most reliable results but risks clogging the column. A pre-column (guard column) is necessary to help avoid this problem. Two recent developments in column packings allow the direct application of biological matrices (plasma), namely i) internal-surface-reverse-phase (ISRP) materials (Westerlund; 1987) and ii) shielded hydrophobic phases (Gisch *et al.*, 1988).

Problems of sample treatment and preparation also occur with TLC since application volumes must be very small and pre-concentration steps are necessary. Many analyses can be processed simultaneously using TLC scanner that is highly sensitive for radioactivity. In most cases resolution with simple classical TLC is insufficient. However, newer developments like high pressure-TLC (HPLTC) and overpressure-TLC (OPTLC) combine high resolution with short analysis times. OPTLC comes especially close to HPLC in efficiency. The whole TLC plate is in a pressurised chamber and the compounds to be separated are carried with a forced flow. The theoretical plate height does not change with length of development (Chatain, 1986; Newman 1986).

Small gel-exclusion columns and membrane filter techniques are only useful for sample preparation for subsequent chromatographic analyses. However, small derivatised adsorption columns can often be used directly to determine the radiopharmaceutical in plasma samples via 'solid phase extraction' (SPE). In this method the elutropic properties of the radiopharmaceutical have to be sufficiently different from those of the metabolites to allow it to be fixed selectively on the matrix while metabolites are eluted, or vice versa. The selection of the column material, as in HPLC, depends on the chemical and physicochemical properties of the radiopharmaceutical and matrix. The matrix may be one of a wide variety of silica-bonded sorbents (*e.g.* bonded alkyl-, amino-, cyano-, or diol-groups), or it may be a cation- or anion-exchange material. SPE is cheap. Plasma samples may be applied directly to individual columns and analyzed in parallel.

The relative advantages and drawbacks of the four analytical chromatographic techniques (radio-HPLC, TLC, OPTLC and SPE) that are currently used are summarised in Table 1.

Table 1. The relative advantages and drawbacks of various techniques applied to plasma metabolite analysis

	HPLC	TLC	OPTLC	SPE
Resolution	high	low	high	low
Sensitivity	high	high	high	high
Rapidity	fast	slow	fast	fast
Pretreatment needed	yes usually	yes	yes	no
Serial analyses possible	yes	yes	yes	yes
Memory effect	rarely	no	no	no
Cost	high	low	significant	low

5. Sources of Errors

Irrespective of the method used for 'plasma tracer analysis', the stability of the radiopharmaceutical during the applied procedure has to be tested. The used procedure has to be validated either by comparing different methods and/or by using an internal standard. The sources of the most frequent errors occurring in such analyses have four different origins:

a. Sample treatment.

Degradation of the radiopharmaceutical can occur during pre-analytical treatment of the biological sample (mechanical disruption, protein elimination). It is then mandatory to check that this treatment does not modify the chemical structure of the radiopharmaceutical. Checks for degradation can be carried out:

— *in vitro*, with a tissue or a plasma sample spiked with a known amount of radiopharmaceutical,

— *in vivo*, by taking the sample only a few seconds after the injection of the radiopharmaceutical.

b. Recovery of unchanged radiopharmaceutical.

Unchanged radiopharmaceutical can be partly adsorbed or bound to the protein or incompletely extracted by the organic solvent. Thus, a recovery factor must be determined after adding a quantity of cold drug to the sample to minimise adsorption losses. Control experiments, in which a known amount of radiopharmaceutical is added, ('reverse isotope dilution analysis') should also be performed to check this factor.

c. Analytical process.

An error may arise because the conditions chosen for chromatography do not allow a complete separation of the unchanged radiopharmaceutical from its metabolites. This type of error is classically detected by comparing the results given by different analytical techniques or systems.

d. Low radioactivity.

If the radioactivity of the sample is too low to be measured with good accuracy statistical counting errors increase and reduce the quality of the results.

6. Pitfalls and Non-Analytical Errors

Many factors contribute to inter-individual variation in radiopharmaceutical metabolism. It is clear that development, genetic constitution, disease and many other factors are important components of this phenomenon (Sitar, 1989). Consequently, whatever the quality of the analytical techniques used, results obtained in various subjects can be conflicting. Among the principal causes of discrepancy, one can find:

a. Polymorphism in metabolism.

Due to intra- or inter-ethnic genetic polymorphism, the metabolism of the radiopharmaceutical can be quite different in people belonging to the extensive or poor metaboliser groups.

b. Drug-drug interactions.

The metabolism of a radiopharmaceutical *in vivo* can be deeply modified by the presence in the blood of various other drugs that can act, for example, as enzyme inhibitors. Well known examples of radiopharmaceutical-drug interaction are in the cases of the radiotracer L-6-[^{18}F]DOPA and the drugs carbidopa, an L-DOPA decarboxylase inhibitor (*e.g.* Melega *et al.*, 1990; McLellan *et al.*, 1991) and nitecapone, a catechol-*O*-methyltransferase inhibitor (Kaakola *et al.*, 1990). Moreover, one must keep in mind the possibility of stereoselective interactions (see *d.*).

c. Physiopathological conditions.

People with hepatic disorders or with a diet particularly rich in carbohydrate can have pharmacokinetic and metabolic profiles that are quite different from those of normals.

d. Stereoselectivity.

It is known that stereoisomers can bind to plasma proteins differently (see Simonyi *et al.*, 1986). Stereoselectivity can also play an important role in the kinetics of radiopharmaceutical metabolism and also in the kinetics of the renal clearance (see Testa, 1986; Walle and Walle, 1986).

7. Review of the Literature

7.1 LABELLED AMINO ACIDS FOR ASSESSING PROTEIN SYNTHESIS RATE

7.1.1. *L-[^{11}C]Methionine.* L-[^{11}C]Methionine is currently used in PET for the evaluation of local amino acid uptake in various physiological and pathological conditions of the human brain. The complex fate of essential amino acids such as L-methionine *in vivo* can be explained by the operation of simultaneous mechanisms to different extents:

— Incorporation into proteins (the main pathway)

— Transformation into biologically important compounds such as enzymes and hormones

— Deamination with loss of ammonia or urea (in man) leading to residues entering the 'common metabolic pool' and being either transformed into carbon dioxide (1–2%) or incorporated into body constituents.

A specific metabolic role of L-methionine is in biological transmethylations enabling the transfer of the *S*-methyl group to suitable acceptors.

Different procedures for the measurement of blood metabolites originating from L-[*S-methyl*-^{11}C]methionine are described in the literature. The method reported by

Lundqvist *et al.* (1985) consists of a fast and sensitive chromatography for the separation of plasma radioactivity into high and low molecular weight fractions. In the low molecular fraction, unchanged L-[*S-methyl*-^{11}C]methionine, as well as derived serine and cysteine, are identified and quantified using liquid chromatographic techniques (on a Lichrosorb™ NH_2 column). All these labelled amino acids, like L-[*S*-methyl-^{11}C]methionine, are approximately 90% utilised in protein synthesis.

The incorporation of L-[*S-methyl*-^{11}C]methionine into proteins and peptides is fast (< 20 min). The degree of incorporation depends on age and nutritional status. Quantitative correlation of L-[*S-methyl*-^{11}C]methionine metabolism with different pathological states therefore requires important corrections to be made as a function of time, based on the amount of labelled proteins which quickly become a large part of the plasma radioactivity.

A simpler method of studying the metabolic fate of L-[*S-methyl*-^{11}C]methionine in human plasma was proposed by Ishiwata *et al.* (1989). This method requires the analysis of four arterial blood samples taken between 5 and 60 min after administration. First, total plasma is counted for radioactivity. Protein-bound and protein-free fractions (unchanged fractions) are isolated and quickly counted. Analysis of the protein-free metabolites is by HPLC, optimally on an Aminex™ A6 column. This method appears adequate for the quantitative measurement of the fast decreasing fraction of labelled methionine in plasma and the protein-free metabolites (10–30%) as well as the labelled proteins. A similar method has been used with other ^{11}C-labelled amino-acids, such as L-[1-^{11}C]tyrosine (Ishiwata *et al.*, 1987; Ishiwata *et al.*, 1988; Paans *et al.*, 1993).

The importance of measuring L-[*S-methyl*-^{11}C]methionine in plasma for quantitative assessment of amino acid metabolism *in vivo* in humans was confirmed by Hatazawa *et al.* (1989). They demonstrated that definite irreversible uptake into lung or brain tumours can be seen when the L-[*S-methyl*-^{11}C]methionine plasma radioactivity is used as the input function.

7.1.2. *L-2-[^{18}F]Fluorotyrosine (2F-TYR).* 2F-TYR is considered to be a true tracer of cerebral protein synthesis (Coenen *et al.*, 1989, Vaalburg *et al.*, 1992). The analysis of the plasma metabolites of 2F-TYR has been thoroughly studied (Kling *et al.*, 1991). Separation of [^{18}F]fluoride and 2F-TYR is achieved simply by using small SAX columns (Adsorbex™ 400 mg, Merck) eluted with phosphate buffer. Precipitation of protein has to be used before the SAX filtration. This technique demonstrated that free 2F-TYR and protein-bound fraction are the only two radioactive pools, since they give an almost quantitative radioactivity balance at all times investigated. While 2F-TYR allows an easy quantitation of PSR in brain, the metabolic behaviour of 2F-TYR is not well-known in malignant tissue and therefore requires a further specific study of amino acid-protein metabolism.

7.2. LABELLED AMINO-ACIDS AS DOPAMINERGIC PRESYNAPTIC TRACERS

7.2.1. *L-6-[^{18}F]Fluoro-DOPA (6-FDOPA).* 6-FDOPA is used to assess presynaptic dopaminergic function *in vivo* with PET in human brain. According to the literature (Boyes *et al.*, 1986; Melega *et al.*, 1990; 1991), 6-FDOPA is metabolised in the periphery to 3-*O*-methyl-6-[^{18}F]fluoro-L-DOPA (3-OMFD) by catechol-*O*-methyl transferase (COMT) and to 6-[^{18}F]fluorodopamine (FDA) by aromatic amino acid decarboxylase. The free amine is then sulphated to give 6-[^{18}F]fluorodopamine sulphate or deaminated by monoamine oxidase to give 6-[^{18}F]fluorodihydroxyphenyl acetic acid (FDOPAC), which is methylated by COMT to give 6-[^{18}F]fluorohomovanillic acid (FHVA).

Plasma metabolite analysis by HPLC has been described (Melega *et al.*, 1990; 1991). After perchloric acid deproteinisation, centrifugation and filtration, plasma samples are injected into a HPLC column (C18, 5 μm, 250 x 4.6 mm) eluted with 80% 0.1M-sodium dihydrogen phosphate, 2.6mM-octanesulphonic acid sodium salt, 0.1mM-EDTA and 20% methanol, at pH 3.5, and at a flow rate of 1 mL/min. Fractions are collected and counted for radioactivity. This method can be considered as the 'gold standard' for the separation and the quantification of all the metabolites but can handle only a limited number of samples during a PET scan.

Alternative and simpler methods have been developed including the use of small alumina column which preferentially retains 6-FDOPA, with the eluate containing the other metabolites (Chan *et al.*, 1992). A more sophisticated method (McLellan *et al.*, 1991) has been described recently and uses a cation and anion exchange column separation followed by an alumina column extraction; the anion exchange column retains FHVA, FDOPAC and the sulphate; the cation exchange and alumina columns retain FDA and FDOPA respectively; the supernatant liquid concentrates the 3-OMFD. These methods allow the analysis of a larger number of samples and the resultant data are comparable with those obtained by HPLC analysis.

7.2.2. *L-4-[^{18}F]Fluoro-m-tyrosine (4-FMT).* 4-FMT acts as a probe for presynaptic dopaminergic function (Barrio *et al.*, 1989a). In the plasma, as in the brain, 4-FMT is decarboxylated. The resultant 4-fluorotyramine is either oxidised by monoamine oxidase to 4-fluoro-3-hydroxyphenylacetic acid (FPAC) or conjugated by phenolsulphotransferase into the 3-*O*-sulfate of 4-fluoro-*m*-alanine (4-FMA). Unlike FDOPA, at two hours post-injection in monkeys, most of the tracer (~ 60%) is still present in plasma while FMA-sulphate is the main metabolite (35%) (Melega *et al.*, 1991b).

These findings were confirmed for the 6-[^{18}F]fluoro isomer (6-FMT) in monkey and human studies. There seemed to be no strong isomer effects and the metabolite ^{18}F-labelled FPAC only accumulated 20 times less in the brain than 6-FMT (Firnau *et al.*, 1991).

All theses metabolites are rather polar; they are not very likely to cross the blood-brain barrier. As the metabolism of 4-FMT is similar to that of 6F-DOPA, the analytical method used for 6F-DOPA (Firnau *et al.*, 1987, Luxen *et al.*, 1992) is therefore suggested as a general reference procedure, consisting of centrifugation of blood samples, precipitation of plasma proteins with perchloric acid and liquid chromatography of the supernatant liquid.

7.3. BENZODIAZEPINE BINDING SITE RADIOLIGANDS

7.3.1. *[*N-methyl-*^{11}C]Flumazenil.* Several benzodiazepine agonists have been labelled with positron-emitters as prospective radioligands for PET studies of central benzodiazepine receptors [*e.g.* flunitrazepam (Comar *et al.*, 1979); for a review see Pike *et al.*, 1993]. A search for more specific and central receptor type-selective benzodiazepine radioligands led to the labelling of the antagonist, flumazenil (Ro 15-1788). [*N-methyl-*^{11}C]Flumazenil is now used routinely for visualizing and quantifying benzodiazepine receptors in pharmacological and clinical PET studies (Mazière *et al.*, 1983; Hantraye *et al.*, 1984; Samson *et al.*, 1985; Persson *et al.*, 1985, 1989; Shinotoh *et al.*, 1986; Savic *et al.*, 1988).

Flumazenil has been labelled with carbon-11 either by *N*-methylation with [^{11}C]iodomethane (Mazière *et al.*, 1984; Ehrin *et al.*, 1984; Suzuki *et al.*, 1985; Halldin *et al.*, 1988) or by esterification with [1-^{11}C]iodoethane (Halldin *et al.*, 1988). The method using [^{11}C]iodomethane is preferred and is the only one used routinely (Pike *et al.*, 1993). Being an ester, flumazenil is expected to be hydrolysed to the free acid (Ro 15-3890) and to the hydroxyethyl ester (Ro 15-4965) in peripheral compartments such as the liver (Halldin *et al.*, 1988; Swahn *et al.*, 1989; Loc'h *et al.*, 1990).

The various chromatographic methods that have been used for the metabolite analysis of [*N-methyl*-^{11}C]flumazenil are the following:

a. TLC.

TLC has been used by several groups (Swahn *et al.*, 1989; Loc'h *et al.*, 1990; Barré *et al.*, 1991; Debruyne *et al.*, 1991). Plasma is mixed with an equal volume of acetonitrile containing reference flumazenil and the two metabolites. After centrifugation the supernatant liquid is evaporated to dryness and the residue dissolved in methanol. The sample is transferred to a silica gel layer which is then developed using a suitable mobile phase. After drying the layer is inspected under ultraviolet light (254 nm). All three compounds are sufficiently resolved to allow measurement of their radioactivity.

Experiments have shown that between 90–95% of the radioactivity in plasma is recovered in the supernatant liquid after protein precipitation (Swahn *et al.*, 1989). The recovery of radioactivity from the TLC plates varies from about 50–80%. One person was studied in four experiments. The amount of [*N-methyl*-^{11}C]flumazenil remaining after 36 min was 59 ± 11%. This gives an estimate of the total variation due to the method and to characteristics of the individual. In baboon studies, about 45% of the radioactivity in plasma represent unchanged compound after 1 h (Loc'h *et al.*, 1990).

The TLC method used for [*N-methyl*-^{11}C]flumazenil has pros and cons. It is simple, inexpensive and convenient because all radioactivity applied to the plates can be accounted for and quantified. One possible source of error is a differential solubility in methanol for the different compounds which could result in an unequal degree of transfer to the TLC plate. Volatile compounds would not of course be detected.

b. Ion Exchange Chromatography (IEC).

IEC uses a basic anion exchanger, Dowex™ 1X2 in the hydroxide form, in disposable Pasteur pipettes (Pauli *et al.*, 1992; Swahn *et al.*, 1992). Plasma is deproteinised as in the TLC experiments but without addition of reference material. The supernatant liquid is applied to the column and forced through the column under pressure. The tip of the column is removed and radioactivities in eluate and column are measured. IEC allows many samples (*ca* 10–15) to be analyzed. However, the accuracy of the method is limited because the more lipophilic metabolite (the hydroxyethyl ester (Ro 15-4965), which usually represents 5% of the total radioactivity, cannot be separated from the unchanged compound.

c. OPTLC.

Compared to the classical TLC method, the advantages of OPTLC are a better resolution and a more rapid migration (Loc'h *et al.*, 1990). These facts make OPTLC generally more favourable than TLC.

d. SPE.

Plasma is diluted tenfold with water-methanol and loaded onto a C18 cartridge. After washing the column with water and 1M-sodium hydroxide solution , the radioactivities on the column and in the eluate are compared. The radioactivity in the eluate corresponds to metabolites. However, the radioactivity retained on the column originates not only from the unchanged compound but also from the lipophilic metabolite (Loc'h *et al.*, 1990).

e. HPLC.

In this method plasma is mixed with an equal volume of acetonitrile containing reference flumazenil, as in the TLC-method (Debruyne *et al.*, 1991, Halldin *et al.*, 1991; Sedvall, 1991; Luthra *et al.*, 1993b). The supernatant liquid (1.0 mL) obtained after centrifugation is counted in the well-counter and subsequently injected into a C18 HPLC column. The total time for separation of unchanged radioligand and the two metabolites is only about 5 min. Experiments show that almost all of the radioactivity in plasma is recovered from the column.

f. SPE plus HPLC.

Cell-free plasma is prepared by centrifuging arterial blood samples containing reference flumazenil and directly injected onto an automated metabolite analysis system (Luthra *et al.*, 1993b). After injection of a plasma sample onto a C18 solid phase extraction (SPE) column, the column is washed with 0.01M-diammonium hydrogen phosphate. The radioactivity retained on the SPE column is then transferred onto a C18 HPLC column using 0.1M-ammonium formate-methanol (60:48 v/v). The ratio of unchanged [*N-methyl*-^{11}C]flumazenil in plasma at a given time is calculated from the integrated radioactivity trace and the activity present in the SPE eluent. Experiments show that > 95% of the loaded radioactivity is recovered from the system. Separation of unchanged [*N-methyl*-^{11}C]flumazenil and its two metabolites is complete within about 15 min.

This technique combines the advantage of HPLC, previously outlined, with the added advantages that it allows the direct use of plasma and permits fast processing of serial samples. Subsequent samples can be loaded and processed on the SPE column while the HPLC analysis of the previous sample is in progress, thus saving time.

In conclusion, all six described analytical methods can and have been used to measure the metabolites of [*N-methyl*-^{11}C]flumazenil in plasma. However, both the IEC and SPE methods cannot resolve [*N-methyl*-^{11}C]flumazenil from its two metabolites. OPTLC and TLC can both be used to measure the metabolism accurately. When combined with SPE for sample processing, HPLC provides a rapid, efficient and reliable technique for routine metabolite analysis.

7.4. DOPAMINE RECEPTOR RADIOLIGANDS

7.4.1. *[*N-methyl-*^{11}C]SCH 23390.* The usefulness of [*N-methyl*-^{11}C]SCH 23390 as a radioligand for the analysis with PET of central dopamine D_1 receptor binding in monkey and in man is well established (Halldin *et al.*, 1986; Farde *et al.*, 1987; for a review see Mazière *et al.*, 1992). SCH 23390 is usually labelled with carbon-11 by alkylation of the desmethyl compound (SCH 24518) with [^{11}C]iodomethane (Halldin *et al.*, 1986; DeJesus *et al.*, 1987; Ravert *et al.*, 1987).

Several metabolic pathways can be suggested for SCH 23390. The most probable one is conjugation by sulphate or glucuronic acid at the phenolic hydroxyl group. Other possible pathways are oxidative processes. Considering the one hour time-span of a PET experiment, oxidative processes are probably too slow to be of quantitative importance.

The various chromatographic methods that have been used for the metabolite analysis of [*N-methyl*-^{11}C]SCH 23390 are the following:

a. TLC.

Plasma is deproteinised by the addition of an equal volume of acetonitrile containing reference SCH 23390, followed by centrifugation (Swahn *et al.*, 1992). The supernatant liquid is evaporated to dryness and the residue in methanol is transferred to the TLC plate. The plate is developed in ethyl acetate-methanol-water and inspected under ultraviolet light (254 nm).

b. IEC.

Two different ion exchangers can be used (Swahn *et al.*, 1992). [*N-methyl*-^{11}C]SCH 23390 is retained on a Dowex™ 50 W X 4 in the pyridine form but is eluted from Dowex™ 1 X 2 in the acetate form, whereas acid compounds such as the sulphate and glucuronide, are retained in the latter ion exchanger. The columns are prepared in disposable Pasteur pipettes. Plasma and an equal volume of acetonitrile are mixed and centrifuged. The supernatant liquid is applied to the column, forced through the column by pressure and collected in a plastic test tube. The column is then washed with 50% acetonitrile which is collected in the same tube as the first eluate. The column and the eluate are counted in a well-counter.

c. HPLC.

Plasma was mixed with an equal volume of acetonitrile containing reference SCH 23390 as in the TLC method (Halldin *et al.*, 1991). The supernatant liquid (1.0 mL), obtained after centrifugation for 1 min, is counted in the well-counter and subsequently injected onto the HPLC column. The mixture is chromatographed through a C18 column and the UV-absorbing and radioactive peaks are integrated using a PC. The total time for separation of unchanged radioligand and the two metabolites is only about 5 min. Experiments show that almost all of the radioactivity in plasma is recovered from the column.

d. SPE and HPLC.

Cell-free plasma is injected directly onto the metabolite analysis system as previously described (*cf.* Section 7.3.1.; Luthra *et al.*, 1993b). The SPE column containing C18 material is eluted with 0.01M-diammonium hydrogen phosphate; the HPLC eluent is methanol-0.1M-diammonium formate-methanol (30:70 v/v). More than 95% of the radioactivity injected is recovered from the system. The metabolism of [*N-methyl*-^{11}C]SCH 23390 (7 human studies) is very rapid. The percent of unchanged [*N-methyl*-^{11}C]SCH 23390 in plasma is found to decrease from 60% at 5 min to 6% at 1 h after injection.

The results from the four methods are consistent and show that [*N-methyl*-^{11}C]SCH 23390 is extensively metabolised, namely 40% after 4 min and 85% after 42 min.

7.4.2. *[*O-methyl-*^{11}C]Raclopride*. Raclopride is a potent and selective antagonist of dopamine D_2 receptors (Köhler *et al.*, 1985; Hall *et al.*, 1988) and has been labelled either by *N*-ethylation with [1-^{11}C]iodoethane (Ehrin *et al.*, 1985) or by *O*-methylation with [^{11}C]iodomethane (Ehrin *et al.*, 1987; Farde *et al.*, 1988). Mainly, the *O-methyl*-labelled raclopride has been used regularly since 1984 for pharmacological and clinical studies (Farde *et al.*, 1986, 1988a,b,c, 1989, 1990; for a review see Mazière *et al.*, 1992).

The different methods used for the study of [*O-methyl*-^{11}C]raclopride metabolism are similar to those described for [*N-methyl*-^{11}C]SCH 23390. The fraction of unchanged [*O-methyl*-^{11}C]raclopride in plasma is 92.5% after 4 min and 75% after 42 min (Swahn *et al.*, 1992, Luthra *et al.*, 1993b).

7.4.3. *Labelled Butyrophenones and Ergolenes.* A variety of butyrophenone neuroleptics has been labelled with various radionuclides for PET studies, of which 3-*N*-[^{11}C]methylspiperone ([^{11}C]MSP), 3-*N*-[^{18}F]methylspiperone ([^{18}F]MSP) and 3-*N*-(ω-[^{18}F]fluoroethyl)spiperone ([^{18}F]FESP) have proved the most useful (for reviews see Stöcklin, 1991; Mazière *et al.*, 1992). From the synthetic ergolenes only [^{76}Br]bromolisuride ([^{76}Br]BLIS) is used for PET (Mazière *et al.*, 1986). Although all of these radioligands are relatively stable in brain (striatal) tissue (Arnett *et al.*, 1985; Coenen *et al.*, 1987; Welch *et al.*, 1988; Barrio *et al.*, 1989b) they are metabolised in the periphery.

The biodegradation of butyrophenones proceeds predominantly via oxidative *N*-dealkylation to give butyrophenone and spirodecanone fractions (Soudijn *et al.*, 1967). Correspondingly, [^{18}F]MSP and [^{11}C]MSP give an almost identical metabolite pattern in baboon plasma (Fowler *et al.*, 1986). Based on rat studies there was some speculation of amide-*N*-dealkylation in [^{18}F]fluoroalkylated spiperones (Welch *et al.*, 1988). However, the observation of identical plasma concentration kinetics for [^{18}F]FESP and 3-*N*-(ω-[^{18}F]fluoropropyl)spiperone, indicates the common cleavage of the butyrophenone moiety (Coenen *et al.*, 1988).

Metabolism of [^{76}Br]BLIS *in vivo* proceeds via debromination, hydroxylation of the benzene ring and hydrolysis of the urea-moiety (Loc'h *et al.*, 1989). Methods of plasma metabolite analysis will now be discussed.

a. OPTLC.

An elaborate analytical OPTLC procedure has been developed for [^{76}Br]BLIS which allows the determine of unchanged radioligand in blood and which distinguishes its bound and free fractions (Mazière *et al.*, 1988; Loc'h *et al.*, 1989). Centrifugation, protein precipitation and SPE are used before final analysis by means of OPTLC on silica gel layers with chloroform-methanol-triethylamine (90:10:0.05 by vol.) as mobile phase. The use of bromine-76 ($t_{1/2}$ = 16 h) allows this complex method to be performed. It is however questionable whether this procedure can be performed on shorter-lived ^{18}F- or ^{11}C-labelled radiopharmaceuticals in a routine setting.

b. HPLC.

A centrifugation method in combination with subsequent HPLC analysis has been used to determine the free plasma fraction of [^{11}C]MSP (Burns *et al.*, 1984). Usually plasma analysis for labelled butyrophenones is performed by HPLC, often after SPE with acetonitrile as for [^{11}C]MSP or [^{18}F]MSP (Arnett *et al.*, 1985; Fowler *et al.*, 1986) or by direct injection of heparinised plasma as for [^{18}F]FESP (Coenen *et al.*, 1988). Many more HPLC conditions have been described for the preparation of labelled butyrophenones which can of course all be used for identifying the above mentioned compounds in plasma samples (Omokawa *et al.*, 1985; Shiue *et al.*, 1985; Chi *et al.*, 1986; Adam *et al.*, 1989; Perlmutter *et al.*, 1989; Hamacher *et al.*, 1991). TLC has also been used to analyze for [^{18}F]FESP (Barrio *et al.*, 1989)

For baboon plasma samples, metabolites with similar elutropic properties appear to make the use of HPLC mandatory (Coenen *et al.*, 1988). However in preliminary tests on human plasma , comparing HPLC data with simple SPE (RP 18 material, methanol-water gradient), almost identical results were obtained (Coenen, unpublished data).

Interestingly [^{76}Br]BLIS and labelled spiperones show a distinct species difference in plasma stability, when going from rodent to baboon to humans (Figure 1). The percentage of unchanged [^{76}Br]BLIS at two hours after injection increases from 3% to 7% to 21%, respectively (Loc'h, unpublished data). For [^{18}F]FESP, the corresponding values at three hours after injection are ~ 9%, ~ 10% and 55% of plasma activity (Coenen *et al.*, 1987, 1988; Wienhard *et al.*, 1989), which correspond directly to those of [^{18}F]MSP (Arnett *et al.*, 1985; Fowler *et al.*, 1986). Given the high level of unchanged radioligand, the irreversible binding of butyrophenones and consequently high striatum-to-blood ratios (15–20 after 2 h p.i.), it is debatable whether plasma analysis is necessary for each individual patient.

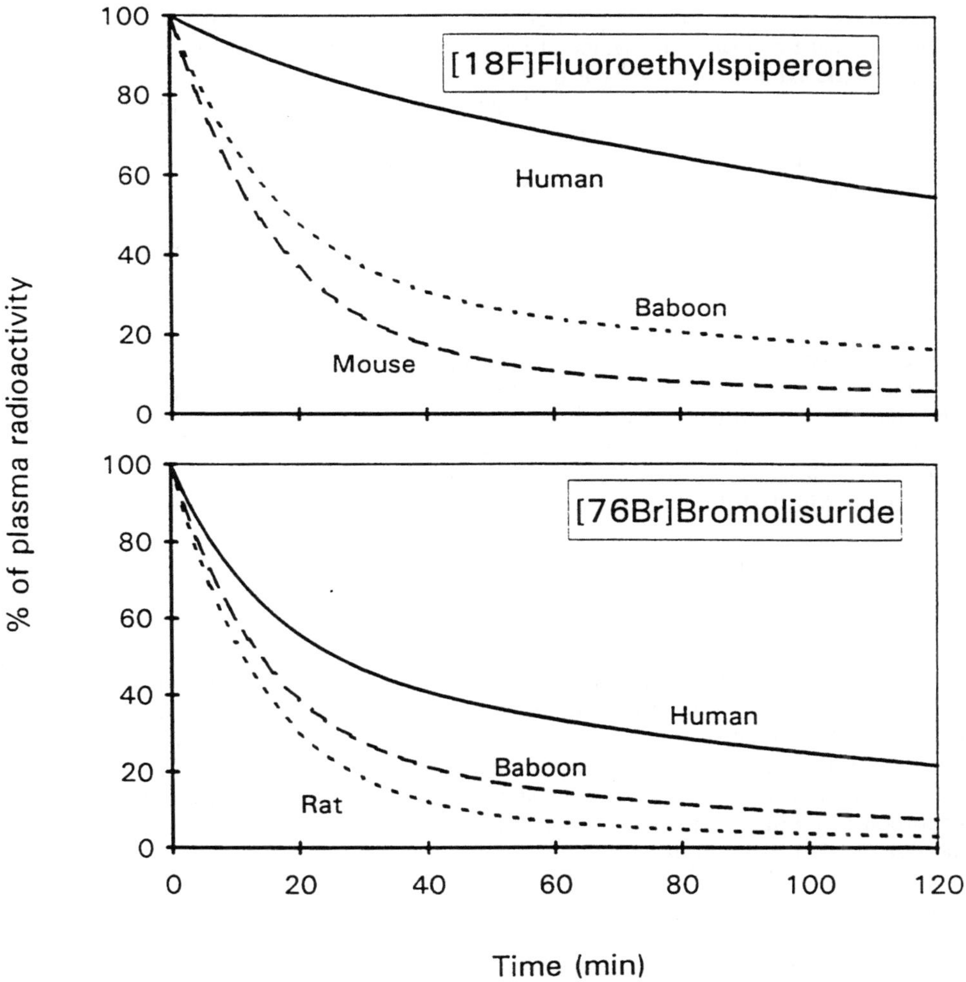

Figure 1. Time dependent concentrations of unchanged [^{18}F]FESP (Coenen *et al.*, 1988; Wienhard *et al.*, 1990) and [^{76}Br]BLIS (Loc'h, Unpublished data) in plasma of different species.

7.5. SEROTONIN RECEPTOR RADIOLIGANDS

7.5.1. *[^{18}F]Setoperone.* Setoperone, a piperidine derivative known for its potent serotonin and moderate dopamine receptor blocking properties, has been labelled with fluorine-18 (Crouzel *et al.*, 1988) and used for the imaging of cortical serotonin receptors *in vivo* (Mazière *et al.*, 1988, Blin *et al.*, 1990). For metabolite analysis, the plasma sample is deproteinised with methanol. The supernatant liquid is evaporated and the residue is dissolved in a minimal amount of acetonitrile and methanol. Analysis of the radioactive compounds is performed by TLC on silica plates using a mixture of dichloromethane-methanol-ethylamine (100:12:0.2 by vol.) as the mobile phase. Using this procedure, the extraction efficiency is over 96%.

The peripheral metabolism of [^{18}F]setoperone has been studied in patients. The percentage of unchanged [^{18}F]setoperone decreased from 82% after 5 min to 24% after 90 min. The main metabolite was identified as reduced [^{18}F]setoperone. This compound was synthesised, labelled with fluorine-18 and studied in humans (Blin *et al.*, 1990). This study has demonstrated that the metabolite, reduced [^{18}F]setoperone, though it crosses the blood-CSF barrier, does not cross the blood-brain barrier and has no affinity for $5HT_2$ receptors.

7.5.2. *[^{18}F]Altanserin.* Among the various ^{11}C- and ^{18}F-labelled radiopharmaceuticals that have already been prepared for mapping $5HT_2$ serotonin receptors with PET (for a review see Crouzel *et al.*, 1992), [^{18}F]altanserin appears to be more selective for $5HT_2$ receptors than other radioligands currently available today (*e.g.* [^{11}C]MSP, [^{18}F]MSP, [^{11}C]ketanserin and labelled alkyl derivatives; [^{11}C]methylbromo-LSD, [^{18}F]setoperone, [^{18}F]ritanserin) (Lemaire *et al.*, 1991; Sadzot *et al.*, 1991, 1992). [^{18}F]Altanserin has been labelled by nucleophilic substitution with [^{18}F]fluoride in the corresponding nitro analogue (Lemaire *et al.*, 1988, 1991).

From a chemical point of view, altanserin is structurally very similar to ketanserin (C=S in place of C=O) and like setoperone, this compound is a 4-fluorobenzoyl-piperidine derivative. Preliminary investigations performed on rats have shown that the major metabolic pathways of altanserin are similar to that of ketanserin (Heykants, Jansens Pharmaceutica, unpublished data). This metabolism involves *N*-dealkylation, aromatic hydroxylation and ketone reduction. The latter leads to ketanserin-ol which was identified as a minor metabolite in rat but as a more important pathway in dogs and particularly in man. Upon these findings, a reverse HPLC method was developed to enable the simultaneous separation of ketanserin and ketanserin-ol in human plasma (Meuldermans *et al.*, 1988). Under these conditions, the proportion of [^{18}F]altanserin-ol was found to be lower than 1% at 90 min after intravenous injection of [^{18}F]altanserin into man.

Determination of unchanged [^{18}F]altanserin in the plasma of rats and humans has been carried out by both HPLC and TLC methods.

a. TLC.

Due to degradation of the radioligand on the silica gel layer during TLC analysis (ethyl acetate-dichloromethane; 60:40 v/v), this technique is not recommended for determining unchanged [^{18}F]altanserin in plasma (Monclus *et al.*, 1992).

b. HPLC.

The plasma sample was diluted with water at pH 4 (0.05 M in acetic acid) and slowly passed through a C18 Sep-Pak™ cartridge that had previously been activated with methanol and water at pH 4. The cartridge was then washed with water containing 0.1% triethylamine. For rat samples the radioactivity was recovered with THF-methanol and injected onto a Lichrosorb™ RP Select-B column (250 x 0.4 cm; Merck). The radioactive compounds were eluted with methanol-THF-water (pH 4) (13:32:55 by vol.) (Lemaire *et al.*, 1991). For human samples, the radioactivity was recovered with methanol only and analyzed with a μ-Bondapak™ C18 column (Waters) eluted with methanol-0.1% *aq.* triethylamine (80:20 v/v) (Sadzot *et al.*, 1991). Before HPLC injection, a small amount of reference altanserin was added to the plasma sample. The various radioactive peaks were collected and measured in a γ-counter. The extraction efficiency of [^{18}F]altanserin was greater than 92% for the two procedures.

In rats the percentage of unchanged radiopharmaceutical was found to be greater than 85% and 96% at 4 hours after radioligand injection, for blood and brain samples respectively. Similar techniques were used by Monclus *et al.* (1992) and comparable results were obtained by Meuldermans *et al.* (1984).

In human, the amount of unchanged [^{18}F]altanserin in plasma decreases from 94% after 5 min to 59% after 90 min. In addition to [^{18}F]altanserin and [^{18}F]altanserin-ol, two other metabolites were also detected but not identified.

7.6. ADRENERGIC RECEPTOR RADIOLIGANDS

Among the radiopharmaceuticals proposed to image noradrenergic neurotransmission three have been studied in terms of metabolic fate in plasma, namely two analogues of noradrenalin, [^{18}F]fluorometaraminol and [^{11}C]*m*-hydroxyephedrine, and a β-receptor antagonist, [*carbonyl*-^{11}C]CGP 12177.

7.6.1. *[*carbonyl*-^{11}C]CGP 12177.* [*carbonyl*-^{11}C]CGP 12177 has been proposed as a radioligand for studying β-adrenergic receptors by PET (Delforge *et al.*, 1991). The *S*-enantiomer of CGP 12177 has about eighty-fold greater affinity than *R*-enantiomer for β-adrenergic receptors *in vitro* (Affolter *et al.*, 1985). Studies with *S*-[^{3}H]CGP 12177 and *R,S*-[^{3}H]CGP 12177 in rats have shown that the *S*-enantiomer gives about a two-fold greater ratio of receptor-bound to non-receptor bound radioligand in heart and in lung compared to the racemate (Law and Burgin, 1989). Hence, the use of the *S*-enantiomer rather than the racemate is preferred for PET studies. *S*-[*carbonyl*-^{11}C]CGP 12177 has been prepared from the *S*-precursor with an enantiomeric excess > 95% (Brady *et al.*, 1991; Hammadi *et al.*, 1991; Aigbirhio *et al.*, 1992). Two methods have been used for the analysis of unchanged radioligand in plasma, TLC/OPTLC and SPE-HPLC.

a. TLC/OPTLC.

Unchanged radioligand in plasma is measured by TLC and OPTLC (Delforge *et al.*, 1991). Dog or rat plasma (0.2 mL) is spiked with unlabelled CGP 12177 and diluted tenfold with methanol; after centrifugation, the precipitate is resuspended and washed in methanol (1 mL). The supernatant methanol is evaporated. The residue is dissolved in methanol (20 μL) and analyzed by TLC or OPTLC on silica gel layers with acetonitrile-water (20:80 v/v) containing 1% triethylamine acetate buffer pH 4. In rats, the percentage of unchanged radioligand is 35% at 10 min after injection. In dogs (beagles), labelled metabolites appear very quickly, the fraction of unmetabolised radioligand ranging from 10 to 15% at 5 min after injection.

b. SPE-HPLC.

Unchanged [*carbonyl*-^{11}C]CGP 12177 is measured by HPLC on a reverse phase column. To improve the sensitivity of radioactivity detection and to eliminate proteins, plasma (3 mL) are loaded onto a Sep-Pak™ cartridge (Jones *et al.*, 1991) or a pre-column containing silica C18 material (Luthra *et al.*, 1993a).

The Sep-Pak™ cartridge is washed with water (5 mL) and eluted with methanol (5 mL). After rotary evaporation to 0.3 mL, the sample is analyzed by reverse phase HPLC using a linear gradient (20 to 50% methanol in aqueous sodium octanesulphonate, pH 6) (Jones *et al.*, 1991).

The C18 pre-column is washed with 0.01M-diammonium hydrogen phosphate at 5 mL/min for 2 min, to eliminate plasma protein (Luthra *et al.*, 1993a). The sample-enrichment column is then back-flushed with the eluent for 2 min to load the sample onto the HPLC column (μ-Bondapak™ C18). [*carbonyl*-^{11}C]CGP 12177 is eluted from the HPLC column with 0.01M-diammonium hydrogen phosphate-methanol (45:55 v/v) at a flow rate of 3 mL/min. The percentage of unchanged radioligand is calculated from the integrated radioactivity trace and the radioactivity present in the SPE eluate.

Significant metabolism of the radioligand was not observed in either dog (greyhounds) (Jones *et al.*, 1991) or man (Luthra *et al.*, 1993a) over 80 min. In rat, the metabolism of racemic and *S*-[*carbonyl*-^{11}C]CGP 12177 are identical. In rat, unchanged *S*-[*carbonyl*-^{11}C]CGP 12177 ranges from 92% at 5 min to 74% at 80 min after injection.

Since a discrepancy had appeared between the results obtained using the two analytical methods, an EEC task group has systematically analyzed the various parameters of the analyses. [*carbonyl*-^{11}C]CGP 12177 was efficiently (> 93%) extracted from plasma whatever the method used (methanol or SPE). In rat plasma samples, two radioactive metabolites were detected using HPLC, the UV-absorbing and radioactivity peaks being well-resolved from each other and from the parent compound. Using TLC the same peaks are not resolved. The results obtained using OPTLC are in broad agreement with those from HPLC but the lower resolution of the OPTLC method can lead to problems of interpretation.

From the work of this EEC task group it appears that the SPE-HPLC method gives more reliable results and should be recommended to measure unchanged radioligand in plasma. Using this SPE-HPLC technique the EEC task group did not find any significant metabolism of *S*-[*carbonyl*-^{11}C]CGP 12177 in man at 15 min post injection. In rats, the percentage of unchanged radioligand was about 75% at 20 min after injection, indicating slow metabolism.

7.6.2. *[^{18}F]Fluorometaraminol.* The measurement of unchanged [^{18}F]fluorometaraminol has been studied by HPLC using reverse phase ion pair chromatography and the radioactivity has been monitored with a flow through radiation detector (Rosenspire *et al.*, 1989). The comparison of unchanged radiopharmaceutical in plasma, heart and liver of different animal species shows a rapid metabolism of this radiotracer in plasma; 40–95% of radiolabelled metabolites are present at one hour after injection. However, HPLC analysis of heart extracted from dog or guinea pig shows virtually no metabolite at that time.

7.6.3. *[*N-methyl-*^{11}C]m-Hydroxyephedrine.* [*N-methyl*-^{11}C]*m*-Hydroxyephedrine has been developed for mapping the sympathetic nerves of the heart (Rosenspire *et al.*, 1990a). Metabolic analysis of plasma, heart and liver samples has been performed after deproteinisation with sulphosalicylic or perchloric acid. The deproteinised samples were analyzed on a C8 reverse HPLC phase column or by SPE on a C18 Sep-Pak™ cartridge. These measurements show that 30 min after injection 20% of the plasma radioactivity is still unchanged radiotracer; at the same time 95% of the radioactivity in the heart is also unchanged radiotracer.

7.7. ACETYLCHOLINE RECEPTOR RADIOLIGANDS

7.7.1. *[N-methyl-^{11}C]Scopolamine.* [*N-methyl*-^{11}C]Scopolamine has been developed for muscarinic cholinergic receptor imaging *in vivo* in human brain (Frey *et al.*, 1992).

Unchanged [*N-methyl*-^{11}C]scopolamine in plasma has been determined by SPE and elution in acetone; a double measurement of [*N-methyl*-^{11}C]scopolamine and of [^{3}H]scopolamine tracer was used to determine recovery yields. Within 5 min after injection in humans, radiolabelled metabolites are significant and account for over 85% of plasma activity by 90 min after injection.

7.7.2. *[N-methyl-^{11}C]MQNB.* Myocardial muscarinic receptors have been measured *in vivo* with [*N-methyl*-^{11}C]methylquinuclinidyl benzilate [*N-methyl*-^{11}C]MQNB, an almost non-metabolized receptor antagonist (Delforge *et al.*, 1990).

The possible presence of labelled metabolites in plasma was checked in dog blood samples. After precipitation of plasma protein in methanol, the concentrated supernatant liquid was analyzed by TLC. The results have shown that unchanged [*N-methyl*-^{11}C]MQNB represents more than 97, 96 and 90% of the total plasma radioactivity at 2, 10 and 30 min after injection, respectively.

7.8. FLOW TRACER

7.8.1. *[^{13}N]Ammonia.* [^{13}N]Ammonia is a widely used tracer for PET myocardial blood flow studies (Hutchins *et al.*, 1990). After extraction by myocardial tissue, [^{13}N]ammonia is metabolically trapped as ^{13}N-labelled glutamine by the action of glutamine synthetase.

Two tracer kinetic models have been validated for the quantification of regional myocardial blood flow in dogs (Nienaber *et al.*, 1991; Bol *et al.*, 1993). For one of these, the [^{13}N]ammonia arterial input function was corrected for metabolites (Bol *et al.*, 1993). The different ^{13}N-labelled metabolites (urea, neutral amino acids, acidic amino acids) were separated from the [^{13}N]ammonia using ion-exchange resins (Rosenspire *et al.*, 1990b).

A simplified has been described (Bol *et al.*, 1993) for the determination of the unmetabolised [^{13}N]ammonia in plasma. Plasma is deproteinised by 0.42M-perchloric acid and the resulting solution is centrifuged. The supernatant liquid is neutralized with sodium bicarbonate and the solution applied to a small column (5 x 70 mm) filled with Dowex™ AG-50 W-8 (Na^{+} form)previously equilibrated with a solution of 30mM-sodium dihydrogen phosphate (pH 7.1). The column is washed with of 30mM-sodium dihydrogen phosphate (pH = 7.1; 1 mL) and dried with air. Eluate, which contains the ^{13}N-labelled metabolites, and the ion exchange resin which retains the [^{13}N]ammonia, are counted for radioactivity. The activity of the resin is divided by the total activity (resin plus eluate) to give the percentage of unmetabolised [^{13}N]ammonia. In sequential samples collected during the 5 min following [^{13}N]ammonia. administration to humans, comparable percentages of unmetabolised [^{13}N]ammonia in arterial plasma (93% and 43% respectively 1 and 5 min post injection) have been found by various groups (Rosenspire *et al.*, 1990b; Luxen, unpublished data).

8. References

Adam M.J., Grierson J.R. and Jivan S. (1989) An improved HPLC system for the analysis and purification of organic amine radiopharmaceuticals. *Appl. Radiat. Isot.*, 40, 91–92.

Affolter H., Hertel C., Jaeggi K., Portenier M. and Staehelin M. (1985) (-)-*S*-[^{3}H]CGP 12177 and its use to determine the rate constants of unlabeled β-adrenergic antagonists. *Proc. Natl. Acad. Sci. USA.*, 82, 925–929.

Aigbirhio F., Pike V.W., Francotte E., Waters S.L., Banfield B., Jaeggi K.A. and Drake A. (1992) S-[1-(2,3-Diaminophenoxy)]-3'-(*N*-t-butylamino)propan-2'-ol — simplified asymmetric synthesis with chiral HPLC and CD analysis. *Tetrahedron: Asymmetry*, 4, 539–554.

Arnett C.D., Fowler J.S., Wolf A.P., Shiue C-Y. and McPherson D.W. (1985) [^{18}F]*N*-Methylspiroperidol: the radioligand of choice for PETT studies of the dopamine receptor in human brain. *Life Sci.*, 36, 1359–1366.

Barré L., Debruyne D., Abadie P., Moulin M. and Baron J.C. (1991) A comparison of methods for the separation of [^{11}C]Ro 15-1788 (flumazenil) from its metabolites in the blood of rabbits, baboons and humans. *Appl. Radiat. Isot.*, 42, 435-439.

Barrio J.R., Perlmutter M.M., Luxen A., Melega W.P., Grafton S.T., Huang S.C., Hoffman J.M., Van Moffaert G., Mazziotta J.C. and Phelps M.E. (1989a) 4-[F-18] Fluoro-L-m-tyrosine, a novel in vivo probe of presynaptic dopaminergic function. *J. Nucl. Med.*, 30, 752. (Abstract).

Barrio J.R., Satyamurthy N., Huang.S.C., Keen R.E., Nissenson C.H.K., Hoffman J.M., Ackermann R.F., Bahn M.M., Mazziotta J.C. and Phelps M.E. (1989b) 3-(2'-[^{18}F]Fluoroethyl)-spiperone: *in vivo* biochemical and kinetic characterization in rodents, non human primates, and humans. *J. Cerebr. Blood Flow Metab.*, 9, 830–839.

Blin J., Sette G., Fiorelli M., Bietry O., Elghozi J.L., Crouzel C. and Baron J.C. (1990) A method for the in vivo investigation of the serotonergic 5-HT_2 receptors in the human cerebral cortex using positron emission tomography and ^{18}F-labelled setoperone. *J. Neurochem.*, 54, 1744–1754.

Bol A., Melin .J, Vanoverschelde J., Vogelaers D., Michel C., Luxen A., Heyndrickx G., Labar D., Cogneau M,. Cauwe F., Robert A. and Wijns W. (1993) Direct comparison of N-13 ammonia and O-15 water estimates of perfusion with quantitation of regional myocardial blood flow by microspheres. *Circulation*, 87, 512–525.

Boyes B.E., Cumming, P., Martin W.R.W. and McGeer E.G. (1986) Determination of plasma [^{18}F]-6-fluorodopa during positron emission tomography: elimination and metabolism in carbidopa treated subjects. *Life Sci.*, 39, 2243–2252.

Brady F., Luthra S.K., Tochon-Danguy H-J., Steel C.J., Waters S.L., Kensett M.J., Landais P., Shah F., Jaeggi K.A., Drake A., Clark J.C. and Pike V.W. (1991) Asymmetric synthesis of a precursor for the automated radiosynthesis of *S*-(3'-*t*-butylamino-2'-hydroxypropoxy)-benzimidazol-2-[^{11}C]one (*S*-[^{11}C]CGP 12177) as a preferred radioligand for β-adrenergic receptors. *Appl. Radiat. Isot.*, 42, 621–628.

Breimer D.D. (1983) Interindividual variations in drug disposition. Clinical implications and methods of investigation. *Clin. Pharmacokin.*, 8, 371–377.

Burns H.D., Dannals R.F., Långström B., Ravert H.T., Zemyan S.E., Duelfer T., Wong D.F., Frost J.J., Kuhar M.J. and Wagner H.N. (1984) (3-*N*-[^{11}C]methyl)Spiperone, a ligand binding to dopamine receptors: radiochemical synthesis and biodistribution studies in mice. *J. Nucl. Med.*, 25, 1222–1227.

Chamberlain J. (1987) *Analysis of Drugs in Biological Fluids.* CRC Press. Boca Raton.

Chan G.L-Y., Hewitt K.A., Pate B.D., Schofield P., Adam M.J. and Ruth T.J. (1992) Routine determination of [^{18}F]-L-6-fluorodopa and its metabolites in blood plasma is essential for accurate positron emission tomography studies. *Life Sci.*, 50, 309–318.

Chatain J.C. (1986) L'O.P.L.C. une nouvelle technique de séparation et de quantification, *Chimie Magazine*, p. 105.

Chi D.Y., Kilbourn M.R., Katzenellenbogen J.A., Brodack J.W. and Welch M.J. (1986) Synthesis of no-carrier-added *N*-([^{18}F]fluoroalkyl)spiperone derivatives. *Appl. Radiat. Isot.*, 37, 1173–1180.

Coenen H.H., Laufer P., Stöcklin G., Wienhard K., Pawlik G., Böcher-Schwarz H.G. and Heiss K. (1987) 3-*N*-2-[^{18}F]-fluoroethyl-spiperone: a novel ligand for cerebral dopamine receptor studies with PET. *Life Sci.*, 40, 80–81.

Coenen H.H., Wienhard K., Stöcklin G., Laufer P., Heboldt I., Pawlik G. and Heiss W.D. (1988) PET measurement of D_2 and S_2 receptor binding of 3-*N*-([2'-^{18}F]-fluoroethyl)spiperone in baboon brain. *Eur. J. Nucl. Med.*, 14, 80–87.

Coenen H.H., Kling P. and Stöcklin G. (1989) Cerebral metabolism of L-[2-^{18}F]fluorotyrosine, a new PET tracer of protein synthesis. *J. Nucl. Med.*, 30, 1367–1372.

Comar D., Mazière M., Godot J.M., Berger G., Soussaline F., Menini C., Arfel G. and Naquet R. (1979) Visualization of ^{11}C-flunitrazepam displacement in the brain of the live baboon. *Nature*, 280, 329–331.

Cooper D., Schleyer H., Levin S.S., Eisenhardt R.H., Novack B.G. and Rosenthal O. (1979) A reevaluation of the role of cytochrome P-450 as the terminal oxidase in hepatic microsomal mixed function oxidase catalyzed reactions. *Drug Metab. Rev.*, 10, 153–185.

Crouzel C., Venet M., Irie T., Sanz G. and Boullais C. (1988) Labelling of a serotoninergic ligand with ^{18}F: [^{18}F]setoperone. *J. Label. Compd. Radiopharm.*, 25, 403–414.

Crouzel C., Guillaume M., Barré L., Lemaire C. and Pike V.W. (1992) Ligands and tracers for PET studies of the 5-HT system — current status. *Nucl. Med. Biol.*, 19, 857–870.

Debruyne D., Abadie P., Barré L., Albessard F., Moulin M., Zarifian E. and Baron J.C. (1991) Plasma pharmacokinetics and metabolism of the benzodiazepine antagonist [^{11}C]Ro 15 1788 (flumazenil) in baboon and human during positron emission tomography studies. *Eur. J. Drug. Metab. Pharmacokinetics*, 16, 141–152.

DeJesus O.T., van Moffart G.J.C. and Friedman A.M. (1987) Synthesis of [^{11}C]SCH 23390 for dopamine D_1 receptor studies. *Appl. Radiat. Isot.*, 38, 345–348.

Delforge J., Janier M., Syrota A., Crouzel C., Vallois J.M., Cayla J., Lançon J.P. and Mazoyer B. (1990) Noninvasive quantification of muscarinic receptors in vivo with positron emission tomography in the dog heart. *Circulation*, 82, 1494–1504.

Delforge J., Syrota A., Lançon J-P., Nakajima K., Loc'h C., Janier M., Vallois J-M., Cayla J. and Crouzel C. (1991) Cardiac beta-adrenergic receptor density measured in vivo using PET, CGP 12177 and a new graphical method. *J. Nucl. Med.*, 32, 739–748.

Ehrin E., Johnström P., Stone-Elander S., Nilsson J.L.G., Persson A., Farde L., Sedvall G., Litton J.E., Eriksson L., Widen L. and Greitz T. (1984) Preparation and preliminary positron emission tomography studies of ^{11}C-Ro 15-1788, a selective benzodiazepine receptor antagonist. *Acta Pharm. Sued.*, 21, 183–188.

Ehrin E., Farde L., De Paulis T., Eriksson L., Greitz T., Johnström P., Litton J-E., Nilsson J.L.G., Sedvall G., Stone-Elander S. and Ögren S-O. (1985) Preparation of ^{11}C-labelled raclopride, a new potent dopamine receptor antagonist: preliminary PET studies of cerebral dopamine receptors in the monkey. *Int. J. Appl. Radiat. Isot.*, 36, 269–273.

Ehrin E., Gawell L., Högberg T., De Paulis T. and Ström P. (1987) Synthesis of [methoxy-^{3}H]-and [methoxy-^{11}C]-labelled raclopride, specific dopamine-D_2 receptor ligands. *J. Label. Compd. Radiopharm.*, 24, 931–940.

Farde L., Hall H., Ehrin E. and Sedvall G. (1986) Quantitative analysis of dopamine D_2 receptor binding in the living human brain. *Science,* 231, 258–261.

Farde L., Halldin C., Stone-Elander S and Sedvall G. (1987) Analysis of human dopamine receptor subtypes using ^{11}C-SCH 23390 and ^{11}C-raclopride. *Psychopharmacol.*, 92, 278–284.

Farde L., Pauli S., Hall H., Eriksson L., Halldin C., Högberg T., Nilsson L., Sjögren I. and Stone-Elander S. (1988a) Stereoselective binding of ^{11}C-raclopride in living human brain — a search for extrastriatal central D_2-dopamine receptors by PET. *Psychopharmacol.,* 94, 471–478.

Farde L., Wiesel F-A., Halldin C. and Sedvall G. (1988b) Central D_2-dopamine receptor occupancy in schizophrenic patients treated with antipsychotic drugs. *Arch. Gen. Psychiatry,* 45, 71–76.

Farde L., Wiesel F.A., Jansson P., Uppfedt G., Wahlen A. and Sedvall G. (1988c) An open label trial of raclopride in acute schizophrenia. Conformation of D2-dopamine receptor occupancy by PET. *Psychopharmacol.*, 94, 1–7.

Farde L., Eriksson L., Blomqvist G. and Halldin C. (1989) Kinetic analysis of ^{11}C-raclopride binding to D2-dopamine receptors studied by PET — a comparison to the equilibrium analysis. *J. Cerebr. Blood Flow Metab.*, 9, 696–708.

Farde L., Wiesel F.A., Stone-Elander S., Halldin C., Nordström A-L., Hall H. and Sedvall G. (1990) D_2-Dopamine receptors in neuroleptic-naive schizophrenic patients. A positron emission tomography study with [^{11}C]raclopride. *Arch. Gen. Psychiatry*, 47, 213–219.

Firnau G., Sood S., Chirakal R., Nahmias C. and Garnett E.S. (1987) Cerebral metabolism of 6-[^{18}F]fluoro-L-3,4-dihydroxyphenylalanine in the primate. *J. Neurochem.*, 48, 1077–1082.

Firnau G., Chirakal R., Nahmias C., and Garnett E.S. (1991) Tracers for the investigation of cerebral presynaptic dopaminergic function with positron emission tomography. In *Frontiers in Nuclear Medicine: In vivo Imaging of Neurotransmitter Function in Brain, Heart and Tumors.* Kuhl D. (Ed.). Amer. Coll. Nucl. Phys. Washington DC. pp. 67–92.

Fowler J.S., Arnett C.D., Wolf A.P., Shiue D-Y., MacGregor R.R., Halldin C., Långström B. and Wagner H.N. Jr (1986) A direct comparison of the brain uptake and plasma clearance of *N*-[^{11}C]methylspiroperidol and [^{18}F]*N*-methylspiroperidol in baboon using PET. *Nucl. Med. Biol.*, 13, 281–284.

Frey K., Koeppe R., Mulholand G., Jewett D., Hichwa R.D., Ehrenkaufer R., Carey J., Wieland D., Kuhl D. and Agranoff B. (1992) In vivo muscarinic cholinergic receptor imaging in human brain with ^{11}C-scopolamine and positron emission tomography. *J. Cerebr. Blood Flow Metab.*, 12, 147–154.

Gisch D.J., Hunter B.T. and Feibush B. (1988) Shielded hydrophobic phase: a new concept for direct injection analysis of biological fluids by high-performance liquid chromatography. *J. Chromatogr.*, 433, 264.

Hall H., Köhler C., Gawell L., Farde L. and Sedvall G. (1988) Raclopride, a new selective ligand for the dopamine-D2 receptors. *Prog. Neuro-Psychopharmacol. & Biol. Psychiat.*, 12, 559–568.

Halldin C., Stone-Elander S., Farde L., Ehrin E., Fasth K.J., Långström B. and Sedvall G. (1986) Preparation of ^{11}C-labelled SCH 23390 for the in vivo study of dopamine D-1 receptors using positron emission tomography. *Appl. Radiat. Isot.*, 37, 1039–1043.

Halldin C., Stone-Elander S., Thorell J.O., Persson A. and Sedvall G. (1988) ^{11}C-Labelling of Ro 15-1788 in two different positions, and also ^{11}C-labelling of its main metabolite Ro 15-3890, for PET studies of benzodiazepine receptors. *Appl. Radiat. Isot.*, 39, 993–997.

Halldin C., Swahn C.G., Farde L., Litton J.E. and Sedvall G. (1991) Determination of [^{11}C]SCH 23390 and its radioactive metabolites in plasma by HPLC. *Eur. J. Nucl. Med.*, 18, 526. (Abstract).

Hamacher K., Nebeling B., Coenen H.H. and Stöcklin G. (1991) No-carrier-added [^{18}F]fluorination ot *N*-Methyl-nitrospiperone via aminopolyether supported direct nucleophilic substitution. *J. Label. Compd. Radiopharm.*, 30, 353. (Abstract).

Hammadi A. and Crouzel C. (1991) Asymmetric synthesis of (2S)- and (2R)-4-(3-t-butylamino-2-hydroxypropoxy)-benzimidazol-2-[^{11}C]one ((S)- and (R-)-[^{11}C]-CGP 12177 from optically active precursors. *J. Label. Compd. Radiopharm.*, 29, 681–690.

Hantraye P., Kaijima M., Prenant C., Guibert B., Sastre J., Crouzel M., Naquet R., Comar D, and Mazière M. (1984) Central type benzodiazepine binding sites: a positron emission tomography study in the baboons brain. *Neurosci. Lett.*, 48, 115–117.

Hatazawa J., Ishiwata K. Masatoshi I., Kameyama M., Kubota K., Ido T., Matsuzawa T., Yoshimoto T., Watanuki S. and Seo S. (1989) Quantitative evaluation of L-methyl-^{11}C methionine uptake in tumor using positron emission tomography. *J. Nucl. Med.*, 30, 1809–1813.

Hutchins G., Schwaiger M., Rosenspire K.C., Krivokapich J., Schelbert H. and Kuhl D.E. (1990) Noninvasive quantification of regional blood flow in the human heart using N-13 ammonia and dynamic positron emission tomographic imaging. *J. Am. Coll. Cardiol.*, 15, 1032–1042.

Ishiwata K., Vaalburg W., Paans A.M.J., Elsinga Ph.H., Vissering H. and Woldring M.G. (1986) A comparison of L-(^{11}C)tyrosine, L-(1-^{11}C)methionine and L-(S-^{11}C)methionine for measuring protein synthesis in tumors with PET. *Proc. 24th Int. Meeting Soc. Nucl. Med.* - Europe Goslar (FRG). Emrich D. and Schmidt H.A.E. (Eds). FK Schattauer Verlag. Stuttgart and New York. pp. 37–42.

Ishiwata K., Vaalburg W., Elsinga Ph.H., Paans A.M.J. and Woldring M.G. (1988) Metabolism studies with L-1-^{11}C-tyrosine for the investigation of a kinetic model to measure protein synthesis rates with PET. *J. Nucl. Med.*, 29, 524–529.

Ishiwata K., Hatazawa J., Kubota K., Kameyana K., Itoh M., Matsuzawa T., Takahashi T., Iwata R. and ldo T (1989) Metabolic fate of L-$^{11}CH_3$-methionine. *Eur. J. Nucl. Med.*, 15, 665–669.

Jenner P. and Testa B. (Eds) (1980) Concepts in drug metabolism. In Part A. *Drugs and the Pharmaceutical Sciences.* Vol. 10., Dekker. New York.

Jones H., Rhodes C., Becket J., Clark J.C., Boobis A.R. and Taylor G.W. (1991) Rapid analysis for metabolites of [^{11}C]-S-(tert.-butylamino-2-hydroxypropoxy)-benzimidazol-2 in the dog. *J. Chromatogr.*, 570, 361–370.

Kaakkola S., Gordin A., Järvinen M., Wikberg T., Schultz E., Nissinen E., Pentikaïnen P.J. and Rita H. (1990) Effect of a novel catechol-O-methyltransferase inhibitor, nitecapone, on the metabolism of L-DOPA in healthy volunteers. *Clin. Neuropharmacol.*, 13, 436–447.

Kling P., Coenen H.H. and Stöcklin G. (1991) Routine plasma analysis for 2-^{18}F fluorotyrosine by SAX-cartridges. *J. Label. Compd. Radiopharm.*, 30, 264–265. (Abstract).

Köhler C., Hall L., Ögren S.O. and Gawell L. (1985) Specific *in vitro* and *in vivo* binding of ^{3}H-raclopride. A potent substituted benzamide drug with high affinity for dopamine D-2 receptors in the rat brain. *Biochem. Pharmacol.*, 34, 2251–2259.

La Dù B.N., Mandel H.G. and Way E.L. (Eds) (1971) *Fundamentals of Drug Metabolism and Drug Disposition.* Williams and Wilkins. Baltimore.

Law M.P. and Burgin J. (1989) Evaluation of CGP 12177 for characterization of beta-adrenergic receptors by PET: in vivo studies in rat. *J. Nucl. Med.*, 30, 766. (Abstract).

Lemaire C., Cantineau R., Christiaens L. and Guillaume M. (1988) N.C.A. Radiofluorination of altanserine a potential serotonin receptor-binding radiopharmaceutical for positron emission tomography. *J. Label. Compd. Radiopharm.*, 26, 336-337. (Abstract).

Lemaire C., Cantineau R., Guillaume M., Plenevaux A. and Christiaens L. (1991) [^{18}F]Altanserin: a radioligand for the study of serotonin receptors with PET: radiolabelling and *in vivo* biological behavior in rats. *J. Nucl. Med.,* 32, 2266–2272.

Loc'h C., Mazière B., Stulzaft O., Ottaviani M. and Syrota A. (1989) Radioligand cerebral regional metabolism and in vivo determination of binding parameters. *J. Nucl. Med.*, 30, 898. (Abstract).

Loc'h C., Hantraye P., Khalili-Varasteh M., Mazière B., Delforge J., Brouillet E., Syrota A. and Mazière B. (1990) C-11 Flumazenil metabolism : analysis of unchanged ligand in baboon plasma. *J. Nucl. Med.*, 31, 897. (Abstract).

Lu A.Y.H. and West S.B. (1980) Multiplicity of mammalian microsomal cytochromes P-450. *Pharmacological Rev.*, 31, 277–295.

Lundqvist H, Stalnacke C.G., Långström B. and Jones B. (1985) Labeled metabolites in plasma after intravenous administration of [$^{11}CH_3$]-L-methionine. In *The Metabolism of the Human Brain Studied with Positron Emission Tomography.* Greitz T., Ingvar D.H. and Widén L. (Eds). Raven Press. New York. pp. 233–240.

Luthra S.K., Osman S., Steel C.J., Law M.P., Rhodes C.G., Vaja V., Ahier R., Brady F., Waters S.L., De Silva R,. Hughes J.M. and Camici P.G. (1993a) Comparison of *S*-[^{11}C]CGP 12177 metabolism in rat, dog and man using solid phase extraction and HPLC. *J. Label. Compd. Radiopharm.,* 32, 504–505. (Abstract).

Luthra S.K., Osman S., Turton D.R., Vaja V., Dowsett K. and Brady F. (1993b) An automated system based on solid phase extraction and HPLC for the routine determination in plasma of unchanged [^{11}C]-L-deprenyl: [^{11}C]diprenorphine:

[11C]flumazenil: [11C]raclopride: and [11C]Sherring 23390. *J. Label. Compd. Radiopharm.*, 32, 518–520. (Abstract).

Luxen A., Guillaume M., Melega W.P., Pike V.W., Solin O. and Wagner R. (1992) Production of 6-[18F]fluoro-L-DOPA and its metabolism *in vivo* — a critical review. *Nucl. Med. Biol.*, 19, 149–158.

Mazière B., Loc'h C., Stulzaft O., Hantraye P., Ottaviani M., Comar D. and Mazière M. (1986) 76Br-bromolisuride: a new tool for quantative *in vivo* imaging of D_2 dopamine receptors. *Eur. J. Pharmcol.*, 127, 239–247.

Mazière B., Crouzel C., Venet M., Stulzaft O., Sanz G., Ottaviani M., Sejourné C., Pascal O. and Bisserbe J.C. (1988) Synthesis, affinity and specificity of 18F-setoperone, a potential ligand for *in-vivo* imaging of cortical serotonin receptors. *Nucl. Med. Biol.*, 15, 463–468.

Mazière B., Loc'h C., Hantraye P., Stulzaft O., Martinot J.L., Syrota A. and Mazière M. (1990) PET imaging of D2 receptors in the living baboon and human brain in normal and pathological conditions using [76Br]bromolisuride. In *Neuropsychopharmacology.* Bunney W.E., Hippius A., Laakmann G. and Schmaub B.M. (Eds). Springer Verlag. pp. 409–417.

Mazière B, Coenen H.H., Halldin C., Någren K. and Pike V.W. (1992) PET radioligands for dopamine receptors and re-uptake sites: chemistry and biochemistry. *Nucl. Med. Biol.*, 19, 497–512.

Mazière M., Prenant C., Sastre J. Crouzel M., Comar D., Hantraye P., Kaijima M., Guibert B. and Naquet R. (1983) 11C-Ro 15-1788 et 11C-flunitrazepam, deux coordinats pour l'ètude par tomographie par positons des sites de liaison des benzodiazepines. *Compt. Rendus. Acad. Sci. (III) (Paris)*, 296, 871–876.

Mazière M., Hantraye P. Prenant C., Sastre J. and Comar D. (1984) Synthesis of ethyl 8-fluoro-5,6-dihydro-5-[11C]methyl-6-oxo-4H-imidazo[1,5a][1,4]benzodiazepine-3-carboxylate (RO 15-1788-11C): a specific radioligand for the *in vivo* study of central benzodiazepine receptors by positron emission tomography. *Int. J. Appl. Radiat. Isot.*, 35, 973–976.

McLellan C.A., Doudet D.J., Brücke T., Aigner T.G. and Cohen R.M. (1991) New rapid analysis method demonstrates differences in 6-[18F]fluoro-L-dopa plasma input curves with and without carbidopa and in hemi-MPTP lesioned monkeys. *Appl. Radiat. Isot.*, 42, 847–854.

Melega W.P., Perlmutter M.M., Luxen A., Nissenson C.H.K., Grafton S.T., Huang S-C., Phelps M.E. and Barrio J.R. (1989). 4-[18F]Fluoro-L-*m*-tyrosine: an L-3,4-dihydroxyphenylalanine analog for probing presynaptic dopaminergic function with positron emission tomography. *J. Neurochem.*, 53, 311–314.

Melega W.P., Hoffman J.M., Luxen A., Nissenson C.H.K., Phelps M.E. and Barrio J.R. (1990) The effects of carbidopa on the metabolism of 6-[18F]fluoro-L-dopa in rats, monkeys and humans. *Life Sci.*, 47, 149-157.

Melega W.P., Grafton S.T., Huang S.C., Satyamurthy N., Phelps M.E. and Barrio J.R. (1991) L-6[18F]fluoro-dopa metabolism in monkeys and humans: biochemical parameters for the formulation of tracer kinetic models with positron emission tomography. *J. Cerebr. Blood Flow Metab.*, 11, 890–897.

Meuldermans W., Hendrickx J., Lauwers W., Swysen E., Hurkmans R., Knaeps F., Woestenborghs R., and Heykants J. (1984) Excretion and biotransformation of ketanserin after oral and intravenous administration in rats and dogs. *Drug. Metab. Disp.*, 12, 772–781.

Meuldermans W., Michiels M., Woestenborghs R., Awouters F., Leysen J.E., Schuurkes J. and Van Nueten J.M. (1988) Pharmacokinetic evaluation of the in vitro and in vivo pharmacological profile of the major metabolites of ketanserin in the rat. *Arzneim Forsch./Drug Res.*, 38, 785–788.

Monclus M., Biver F., Goldman S. and Luxen A. (1993) [^{18}F]Altanserine: a short synthesis of the nitro precursor and preliminary metabolic studies in rat. *J. Label Compd. Radiopharm.*, 32, 523–524.

Newman J.M. (1986) Overpressure layer chromatography (OPLC): a planar HPLC technique. *Chromatography Forum*, pp. 63–66.

Nienaber C.A., Ratib O., Gambhir S.S., Krivokapich J., Huang S–C., Phelps M.E. and Schelbert H.R. (1991) A quantitative index of regional blood flow in canine myocardium derived noninvasively with N-13 ammonia and dynamic positron emission tomography. *J. Am. Coll. Cardiol.*, 17, 260–269.

Omokawa H., Tanaka A., Ito M., Nishihara Y., Inoue O. and Yamazaki T. (1985) Synthesis of *N*-methyl and *N*-^{11}C-methyl spiperone by phase transfer catalysis in anhydrous solvent. *Radioisotopes*, 34, 480–485.

Paans A.M.J., Elsinga Ph.H. and Vaalburg W. (1993) Carbon-11 labeled tyrosine as a probe for modelling protein synthesis rate. In *Developments in Nuclear Medicine*. Kluwer Academic Publishers. pp. 161–174.

Pauli S., Lijequist S., Farde L., Swahn C.G., Halldin C. and Litton J.E. (1992) PET analysis of alcohol interaction with the brain disposition of (^{11}C)flumazenil. *Psychopharmacol.*, 107, 180–185.

Perlmutter J.S., Kilbourn M.R., Welch M.J. and Raichle M.E. (1989) Non-steady-state measurement of *in vivo* receptor binding with positron emission tomography: "Dose-response" analysis. *J. Neurosci.*, 9, 2344–2352.

Persson A., Ehrin E., Eriksson L., Farde L., Hedström C.G., Litton J.E., Mindus P. and Sedvall G. (1985) Imaging of ^{11}C-labelled Ro 15-1788 binding to benzodiazepine receptors in the human brain by positron emission tomography. *J. Psychiat. Res.*, 19, 609–622.

Persson A., Pauli S. Swahn C.G., Halldin C. and Sedvall G. (1989) Cerebral uptake of ^{11}C-Ro 15-1788 and its acid metabolite ^{11}C-RO 15-3890; PET study in healthy volunteers. *Human Psychopharmacol.*, 4, 215–220.

Pike V.W., Halldin C., Crouzel C., Barré L., Nutt D.J., Osman S., Shah F., Turton D.R. and Waters S.L. (1993) Radioligands for PET studies of central benzodiazepine receptors and PK (peripheral benzodiazepine) binding sites — current status *Nucl. Med. Biol.* In press.

Ravert H.T., Wilson A.A., Dannals R.F., Wong D.F. and Wagner H.H. (1987) Radiosynthesis of a selective dopamine D_1 receptor antagonist: R(+)-7-chloro-8-hydroxy-3-[^{11}C]methyl-1-phenyl-2,3,4,5-tetrahydro-^{1}H-3-benzazepine ([^{11}C]SCH 23390). *Appl. Radiat. Isot.*, 38, 305–306.

Rosenpire K.C, Gildersleeve D.L., Massin C.C, Mislankar S.G. and Wieland D.M. (1989) Metabolite fate of the heart agent [^{18}F]6-fluorometaraminol. *Nucl. Med. Biol.*, 16, 735–739.

Rosenpire K.C, Haka M., Van Dort M.E, Jewett D.M, Gildersleeve D.L, Schwaiger M. and Wieland D.M. (1990a) Synthesis and preliminary evaluation of carbon-11-metahydroxyephedrine: a false transmitter agent for heart neuronal imaging. *J. Nucl. Med.*, 31, 1328-1334.

Rosenspire K.C. Schwaiger M., Mangner T.J., Hutchins G.D., Sutorik A. and Kuhl D.E. (1990b) Metabolic fate of [^{13}N]ammonia in human and canine blood. *J. Nucl. Med.*, 31, 163–167.

Sadzot B., Lemaire C., Cantineau R., Hermanne J.P., Plenevaux A., Maquet P., Salmon E., Degueldre C., Guillaume M. and Franck G. (1991)Serotonin-S2 receptor imaging with [^{18}F]-altanserine and PET. Results in young normal controls. *J. Nucl. Med.*, 32, 980. (Abstract).

Sadzot B., Lemaire C., Maquet P., Plenevaux A., Salmon E., Degueldre C., Hermanne J.P., Guillaume M., Cantineau R., Franck G. and Comar D. (1993) Serotonin $5HT_2$ receptor imaging in the human brain using positron emission tomography and a new radioligand, [^{18}F]altanserin. Results in young normal controls. *J. Cerebr. Blood Flow Metab.* Submitted.

Samson Y., Hantraye P., Baron J.C., Soussaline F., Comar D. and Mazière M. (1985) Kinetics and displacement of ^{11}C Ro 15-1788, a benzodiazepine antagonist, studied in human brain *in vivo* by positron emission tomography. *Eur. J. Pharmacol.*, 110, 247–251.

Savic I., Roland P., Sedvall G., Persson A., Pauli S. and Widen L. (1988) In vivo demonstration of reduced benzodiazepine receptor binding in human epileptic foci. *Lancet,* 16, 863–866.

Schenkman J.B., Sligar S.G. and Cinti D.L. (1981) Substrate interaction with cytochrome P-450. *Pharmac. Ther.*, 12, 43–71.

Sedvall G., Farde L., Stone-Elander S. and Halldin C. (1986) Dopamine D_1 receptor binding in the living human brain. In *Neurobiology of Central D1-Dopamine Receptors.* Breese G.R. and Creese I. (Eds). Plenum Press, New York. pp. 119–124.

Sedvall G. (1991) PET scanning as a tool in clinical psychopharmacology. *Triangle,* 30, 11–20.

Shinotoh H., Yamasaki T., Inoue O., Itoh T., Suzuki K., Hashimoto K., Tateno Y. and Ikehira H. (1986) Visualization of specific binding sites of benzodiazepine in human brain. *J. Nucl. Med.*, 27, 1593–1599.

Shiue C-Y., Fowler J.S. Wolf A.P., Watanabe M. and Arnett C.D. (1985) Synthesis and specific activity determinations of no-carrier-added fluorine-18 labeled. *J. Nucl. Med.*, 26, 181–186.

Siler Master B.S. and Okita R.T. (1980) The history, properties, and function of NADPH-cytochrome P-450 reductase. *Pharmac. Ther.*, 9, 227–244.

Simonyi M., Fitos I. and VisyY. (1986) Chirality of bioactive agents in protein binding, storage and transport processes. *TiPS*, 112–116.

Sitar D.S. (1989) Human drug metabolism in vivo. *Pharmac. Ther.*, 43, 363–375.

Soudijn W., Van Wijngaarden I. and Allewijn F. (1967) Distribution excretion and metabolism of neuroleptics of the butyrophenone type. I Excretion and metabolism of haloperidol and nine related butyrophenone-derivatives in the Wistar rat. *Eur. J. Pharmacol.*, 1,1, 47–57.

Stöcklin G. (1991) Radioligands for PET studies of D2-receptors: butyrophenone and ergot derivatives. In *PET Studies of the Brain Dopaminergic Systems. Imaging with PET.* Baron J.C., Comar D., Farde L., Martinot J.L. and Mazoyer B. (Eds.) Kluwer Academic Publishers. pp. 5–22.

Strobel H.W., Digman J.D. and Gum J.R. (1980) NADPH cytochrome P-450 reductase and its role in the mixed function oxidase reaction. *Pharmac. Ther.*, 8, 525–537.

Suzuki K., Inoue O., Hashimoto K., Yamasaki T., Kuchiki M. and Tamate K. (1985) Computer-controlled large scale production of high specific activity [^{11}C]RO 15-1788 for PET studies of benzodiazepine receptors. *Int. J. Appl. Radiat. Isot.*, 36, 971–976.

Swahn C.G., Persson A., Pauli S. and Sedvall G. (1989) Metabolism of the benzodiazepine antagonist ^{11}C-Ro 15-1788 after intravenous administration in man. *Human Psychopharmacol.*, 4, 297–301.

Swahn C.G., Farde L., Halldin C. and Sedvall G. (1992) Ligand metabolites in plasma during PET-studies with ^{11}C-labelled dopamine antagonists, raclopride, SCH 23390 and *N*-methylspiroperidol. *Human Psychopharmacol.*, 7, 97-103.

Taylor and Francis, Eds. (1984) Xenobiotica: the fate of foreign compounds in biological systems. Special issue Cytochrome P-450. London and Philadelphia. p. 14.

Testa B. (1986) Chiral aspects of drug metabolism. *TiPs*, 60–64.

Testa B. and Jenner P. (Eds) (1976) Drug metabolism: chemical and biochemical aspects. In *Drugs and the Pharmaceutical Sciences.* Vol. 4. Dekker. New York.

Theobald A., (Ed.) (1989) *Radiopharmaceuticals using Radioactive Compounds in Pharmaceutics and Medicine.* Ellis Horwood Limited. Chichester.

Vaalburg W., Coenen H., Crouzel C., Elsinga Ph.H., Långström B., Lemaire C. and Meyer G.J. (1992) Amino acids for the measurement of protein synthesis *in vivo* by PET. *Nucl. Med. Biol.*, 19, 227–237.

Van Rijk P.P., Ed. (1986) *Nuclear Techniques in Diagnostic Medicine.* Martinus Nijhoff Publishers. Dordrecht.

Walle T. and Walle U.K. (1986) Pharmacokinetic parameters obtained with racemates. *TiPS,* 155–158.

Welch M.J., Katzenellenbogen J.A., Mathias C.J., Brodack J.W., Carlson K.E., Chi D.Y., Dence C.S., Kilbourn M.R. Perlmutter J.S., Raichle M.E. and Ter-Pogossian M.M. (1988) *N*-(3-[^{18}F]fluoropropyl)Spiperone: the preferred ^{18}F labeled spiperone analogue for positron emission tomographic studies of the dopamine receptor. *Nucl. Med. Biol.,* 15, 83–97.

Westerlund D. (1987) Direct injection of plasma into column liquid chromatographic systems. *Chromatographia*, 24, 155–164.

Wieland D.M., Tobes M.C. and Mangner T.J. (1986) *Analytical and Chromatographic Techniques in Radiopharmaceutical Chemistry.* Spinger-Verlag. New York.

Wienhard K., Coenen H.H., Pawlik G., Rudolf J., Laufer P., Jovakar S., Stöcklin G. and Heiss W-D. (1990) PET studies of dopamine receptor distribution using [^{18}F]fluoroethylspiperone: findings in disorders related to the dopaminergic system. *J. Neural. Transm.*, 81, 195–213.

Williams R.T. (1960) Detoxication mechanism and the design of drugs. In *Symposium on Biological Approaches to Cancer Chemotherapy.* Academic Press. London.

Wilson K. (1984) Sex-related differences in drug disposition in man. *Clin. Pharmacokin.*, 9, 189–202.

Developments in Nuclear Medicine

1. P.H. Cox (ed.): *Cholescintigraphy*. 1981 ISBN 90-247-2524-0
2. P.H. Cox (ed.): *Progress in Radiopharmacology*. Selected Topics. Proceedings of the 3rd European Symposium (Noordwijkerhout, The Netherlands, April 1982). 1982 ISBN 90-247-2768-5
3. M.H. Jonckheer and F. Deconinck (eds.): *X-Ray Fluorescent Scanning of the Thyroid*. 1983 ISBN 0-89838-561-X
4. K. Kristensen and E. Nørbygaard (eds.): *Safety and Efficacy of Radiopharmaceuticals*. 1984 ISBN 0-89838-609-8
5. A. Bossuyt and F. Deconinck: *Amplitude/Phase Patterns in Dynamic Scintigraphic Imaging*. With a Foreword by A. Bertrand Brill. 1984 ISBN 0-89838-641-1
6. M.R. Hardeman and Y. Najean (eds.): *Blood Cells in Nuclear Medicine, Part I*. Cell Kinetics and Bio-distribution. 1984 ISBN 0-89838-653-5
7. G.F. Fueger (ed.): *Blood Cells in Nuclear Medicine, Part II*. Migratory Blood Cells. 1984 ISBN 0-89838-654-3
8. H.J. Biersack and P.H. Cox (eds.): *Radioisotope Studies in Cardiology*. 1985 ISBN 0-89838-733-7
9. P.H. Cox, G. Limouris and M.G. Woldring (eds.): *Progress in Radiopharmacology 1985*. 1985 ISBN 0-89838-745-0
10. P.H. Cox, S.J. Mather, C.B. Sampson and C.R. Lazarus (eds.): *Progress in Radiopharmacy*. 1986 ISBN 0-89838-823-6
11. H. Deckart and P.H. Cox (eds.): *Principles of Radiopharmacology*. 1987 ISBN 0-89838-774-4
12. W.-D. Heiss, G. Pawlik, K. Herholz and K. Wienhard (eds.): *Clinical Efficacy of Positron Emission Tomography*. 1987 ISBN 0-89838-898-8
13. G.B. Gerber, H. Métivier and H. Smith (eds.): *Age-related Factors in Radionuclide Metabolism and Dosimetry*. 1987 ISBN 0-89838-953-4
14. K. Kristensen and E. Nørbygaard (eds.): *Safety and Efficacy of Radiopharmaceuticals 1987*. 1987 ISBN 0-89838-986-0
15. C. Beckers, A. Goffinet and A. Bol (eds.): *Positron Emission Tomography in Clinical Research and Clinical Diagnosis*. Tracer Modelling and Radioreceptors. 1989 ISBN 0-7923-0254-0
16. M. De Schrijver: *Scintigraphy of Inflammation with Nanometer-sized Colloidal Tracers*. 1989 ISBN 0-7923-0272-9
17. Ch. Kessler, M.R. Hardeman, H. Henningsen and J.-N. Petrovici (eds.): *Clinical Application of Radiolabelled Platelets*. 1990 ISBN 0-7923-0729-1
18. H.J. Biersack and P.H. Cox (eds.): *Nuclear Medicine in Gastroenterology*. 1991 ISBN 0-7923-1074-8
19. R.P. Baum, P.H. Cox, G. Hör and G.L. Buraggi (eds.): *Clinical Use of Antibodies*. Tumours, infection, infarction, rejection and in the diagnosis of AIDS. 1991 ISBN 0-7923-1424-7

Developments in Nuclear Medicine

20. J.C. Baron, D. Comar, L. Farde, J.L. Martinot and B. Mazoyer (eds.): *Brain Dopaminergic Systems: Imaging with Positron Tomography.* 1991
ISBN 0-7923-1476-X
21. M.K. Dewanjee: *Radioiodination.* Theory, Practice, and Biomedical Application. 1991 ISBN 0-7923-1491-3
22. P.A. Schubiger and G. Westera (eds.): *Progress in Radiopharmacy.* 1992
ISBN 0-7923-1525-1
23. B.M. Mazoyer, W.D. Heiss and D. Comar (eds.): *PET Studies on Amino Acid Metabolism and Protein Synthesis.* 1993 ISBN 0-7923-2076-X
24. G. Stöcklin and V.W. Pike (eds.): *Radiopharmaceuticals for Positron Emission Tomography.* Methodological Aspects. 1993 ISBN 0-7923-2340-8

Kluwer Academic Publishers - Dordrecht / Boston / London

MIX
Papier aus verantwortungsvollen Quellen
Paper from responsible sources
FSC® C105338

If you have any concerns about our products,
you can contact us on
ProductSafety@springernature.com

In case Publisher is established outside the EU,
the EU authorized representative is:
Springer Nature Customer Service Center GmbH
Europaplatz 3, 69115 Heidelberg, Germany

Printed by Libri Plureos GmbH
in Hamburg, Germany